Hepatitis C Virus: from Laboratory to Clinic

Hepatitis C infects 170 million people worldwide and has been labeled the 'silent epidemic' since it is asymptomatic for years after infection. This multidisciplinary overview covers basic concepts related to the discovery of the virus, development of serological and nucleic acid tests to detect infection, the structure of the virus genome, generation of virus gene products, and proposed replication scheme. It then goes on to introduce the epidemiology, transmission, pathogenesis of infection, the development of hepatocellular carcinoma associated with chronic virus infection, and current strategies for treatment. The book then discusses advances in cell culture systems, animal models of infection, and emerging treatments and vaccine development. Through its coverage of basic science, clinical consequences, and methods of research, this integrated and accessible account will be of immense value to biomedical scientists and clinicians alike, and a useful introduction for all those studying the virus and its effects.

- Combines basic science, clinical aspects and laboratory approaches to investigation
- Extensively cross-referenced for easy access to concepts
- An accessible introduction to a complex field.

Mark A. Feitelson is currently Professor in the Department of Pathology, Anatomy and Cell Biology, Thomas Jefferson University, Philadelphia. He has a secondary appointment in the Department of Microbiology and Immunology and is a member of the Kimmel Cancer Center at Thomas Jefferson University. In addition, he is Head of the Molecular Diagnostics Laboratory in Microbiology for Thomas Jefferson University Hospital. Prior to his transfer to Jefferson Medical College, Dr Feitelson trained with the Nobel laureate Dr Baruch S. Blumberg at the Fox Chase Cancer Center. Dr Feitelson has been working on the biology and pathogenesis of hepatitis B for more than 20 years and has recently started a similar research program in hepatitis C.

Hepatitis C Virus

From Laboratory to Clinic

Mark A. Feitelson

Department of Pathology, Anatomy and Cell Biology,
Department of Microbiology and Immunology,
and Kimmel Cancer Center, Thomas Jefferson University,
Philadelphia, PA, USA

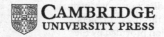

CAMBRIDGE
UNIVERSITY PRESS

University Printing House, Cambridge CB2 8BS, United Kingdom

One Liberty Plaza, 20th Floor, New York, NY 10006, USA

477 Williamstown Road, Port Melbourne, VIC 3207, Australia

314-321, 3rd Floor, Plot 3, Splendor Forum, Jasola District Centre, New Delhi - 110025, India

103 Penang Road, #05-06/07, Visioncrest Commercial, Singapore 238467

Cambridge University Press is part of the University of Cambridge.

It furthers the University's mission by disseminating knowledge in the pursuit of education, learning and research at the highest international levels of excellence.

www.cambridge.org
Information on this title: www.cambridge.org/9780521799591

First published 2002

A catalogue record for this publication is available from the British Library

Library of Congress Cataloging in Publication data
Feitelson, Mark.
Hepatitis C virus: from laboratory to clinic / Mark A. Feitelson.
     p.   cm.
Includes bibliographical references and index.
ISBN 0 521 79959 7 (pbk.)
1. Hepatitis C.   2. Hepatitis C virus.   I. Title.
RC848.H425 F45 2002
616.3′623 – dc21   2001035623

ISBN 978-0-521-79959-1 Paperback

....

Every effort has been made in preparing this book to provide accurate and
up-to-date information which is in accord with accepted standards and practice
at the time of publication. Although case histories are drawn from actual cases,
every effort has been made to disguise the identities of the individuals involved.
Nevertheless, the authors, editors and publishers can make no warranties that the
information contained herein is totally free from error, not least because clinical
standards are constantly changing through research and regulation. The authors,
editors and publishers therefore disclaim all liability for direct or consequential
damages resulting from the use of material contained in this book. Readers
are strongly advised to pay careful attention to information provided by the
manufacturer of any drugs or equipment that they plan to use.

This book is dedicated in the loving memory of my parents,

Ann and Seymour

Contents

Preface

Since the discovery of hepatitis C virus (HCV) in 1989, there has been an explosion of research and information on the virus. This is evidenced by the more than 20 000 papers on HCV (as of December, 2000), as well as the numerous reviews in journals and edited books. The purpose of this book is to present an overview of the different disciplines that have contributed to an understanding of the virus, its diseases, current and proposed treatments, and much more. Importantly, this book attempts to integrate the various disciplines to provide an overall picture of what has been accomplished in the field, and what major questions still remain.

This book is organized so that the reader will first understand how and why it was so difficult to identify HCV and then how the development of antibody and HCV RNA detection tests have nearly eliminated HCV-associated post-transfusion hepatitis. The book then explores the physical characteristics of the virus, the structure of the genome, polyprotein synthesis, and the proposed replication cycle of HCV. With a broad understanding of the virus, and the ability to screen for both viral antibodies and RNA in blood, considerable work has now been done to elucidate the epidemiology and transmission of HCV. For example, population-based viral antibody surveys have revealed the seroprevalence and burden of infection in different geographic regions of the world, which has been central to the identification of risk factors for transmission and the development of preventative measures to reduce risk. Further characterization of the virus genome from various sources has resulted in the discovery of virus genotypes, subtypes and quasispecies, which may contribute importantly to the outcome of infection. The genetic hererogeneity of HCV, and its implications to the natural history and pathogenesis of infection, is discussed in successive sections of the book.

The high rate of acute infections that become chronic, combined with a high frequency of liver diseases among chronically infected people, has placed considerable emphasis upon trying to understand natural history and pathogenesis. This book has likewise placed an emphasis upon these areas, since they are so important for understanding the outcome of natural infection and for therapeutic intervention. For example, it will be very important to know whether HCV triggers direct cytopathic effects, or whether the bulk of chronic liver disease is immune mediated, since the answer to these questions will profoundly influence the types of therapy that are going to be developed in the future. The strong epidemiological association between chronic HCV infection and the development of hepatocellular carcinoma, which is one of the most frequent tumor types worldwide, calls for additional research into the mechanism(s) of hepatocarcinogenesis, which will also be essential for the development of therapeutics for people who develop this cancer. It is now recognized that HCV appears to infect lymphoid cells in addition to hepatocytes. This extrahepatic infection may contribute importantly to both the immune-mediated pathogenesis of chronic liver disease and the development of autoaggressive and autoimmune syndromes. In order to understand these host–virus relationships in more detail, this book presents a section on recent advances that includes attempts to propagate HCV in tissue culture cells, develop HCV animal models to study pathogenesis, and develop protective and/or therapeutic vaccines. A section on experimental approaches provides suggestions as to how some of these challenges will be met. For those who are interested in entering the field of HCV research, a discussion of several protocols and techniques that are uniquely used in the field are presented in the hope that they will provide guidelines for future work. Use of these approaches will promote advances in the field, which will be key to the future management of HCV infection.

The book closes with a series of questions that need to be addressed in the field, and some suggested approaches to solve them. The hope here is to stimulate both thinking and action, and to provide starting points for both. In this regard, it is anticipated that the fairly comprehensive treatment of HCV in this work will be readily accessible and understandable to both the inquisitive undergraduate student and the graduate student or postdoctoral fellow contemplating a project or career in the field of HCV. In addition, it is hoped that this book will be used by people who wish to broaden their education and gain an overall perspective in the field prior to a more detailed reading of the original publications. This includes people who are already working within a narrow area within the field of HCV research. The multi- and interdisciplinary presentation of information should also be useful for clinicians who wish to learn more about the basic biology of the virus and by basic scientists who wish to learn more about the clinical aspects of disease or therapeutic prospects for control. Finally, it is hoped that the contents of this book will provide the tools to help interested individuals with a basic background in biology to ask meaningful questions, and to obtain relevant answers to some of the outstanding problems that face the field today.

This work is supported by NIH grants CA48656, CA66971 and CA79512.

Mark Feitelson, Ph.D.
Philadelphia, PA

Foreword

Infection with the RNA-containing hepatitis C virus, which was isolated little more than 10 years ago, causes damage to the liver resulting in cirrhosis, liver failure and cancer of the liver. In the majority of individuals, hepatitis C infection progresses slowly over many years and approximately 85% of those who contract the disease remain chronically infected, with the virus replicating throughout their lifetime. Lifelong measures are, therefore, required to limit the spread of infection to others. The importance of the disease is clear from the fact that 170 million people are estimated to be chronically infected worldwide. In the USA, where liver failure from chronic hepatitis C infection is one of the most common reasons for liver transplants, some 4 million people are infected by the virus. Hepatitis C is probably also the most common cause of primary liver cancer in the developed world.

There is no doubt that important advances have been made in recent years. As detailed in this book, the development and deployment of assays that specifically detect anti-HCV antibodies and HCV RNA in infected patients have reduced the risk of acquiring HCV from contaminated blood to almost zero. However, there is currently no cure for liver disease caused by hepatitis C, and interferon therapy is of limited efficacy and has significant side-effects. Recently, it has been commented that not only is current therapy for HCV infection woefully inadequate but also some studies estimate that annual deaths from hepatitis C could triple over the first two decades of the twenty-first century unless new, more effective interventions are developed. To this end, genome analysis, virology, immunology, cell and tissue biology, pathogenesis, animal studies, and clinical investigations are being pursued in numerous multidisciplinary scientific and clinical investigations of acute and chronic infections caused by the virus. In the final section of this book, it is pointed out that perhaps one of the biggest challenges to stem the spread of hepatitis C in the future is the development of a safe and effective protective vaccine, and lacking that, a therapeutic vaccine.

The book is designed to appeal to a wide range of readers. Its contents include the pathogenesis of the disease, animal models, molecular approaches, the propagation of the virus in culture systems, screening assays, and the development of effective and safe antiviral agents, therapeutic regimens, and vaccines. In addition, the book covers essential experimental protocols and techniques employed in studies on the virus. At one level, the book aims to convey the essential information needed for a well-informed entry into the subject. It will, therefore, be of value to anyone wishing to obtain an insight into hepatitis C, including postgraduate research students in the medical sciences, clinical investigators registered for a research degree, medical students pursuing research projects, researchers in universities or industry, and university teachers and clinical practitioners looking for an introduction to, or an integrated, "update". On another level, since thousands of papers are published each year on HCV, the book will provide an essential overview and well-documented distillation of work in the field for scientists and clinicians who are investigating specific aspects of the virus and/or its clinical manifestations.

There are many unsolved questions in research on hepatitis C, such as why the virus causes disease immediately in some people but takes years or decades to progress in others; why African-Americans respond so poorly to the current standard of care, and how the disease can persist virtually unnoticed in the body for decades. Understanding such issues will aid in the development of new ways to halt the virus before it causes disease or is passed on to others by people who are unaware that they are infected. Since better treatment and prevention strategies will come from carefully designed, innovative and interdisciplinary research, another important feature of this book is the section on outstanding scientific and clinical questions.

Jack A. Lucy

Emeritus Professor, Royal Free and
University College Medical School,
University of London

Abbreviations

AAV	adeno-associated virus
ALT	alanine aminotransferase
Anti-HBc	antibodies to hepatitis B core antigen
AP-1	activation protein 1
AUG	translation initiation start codon
bDNA	branched chain signal amplification
CLD	chronic liver disease
core	nucleocapsid of hepatitis C virus
CTL	cytotoxic T lymphocytes
E1	envelope glycoprotein 1 of hepatitis C virus
E2	envelope glycoprotein 2 of hepatitis C virus
elF2, elF3	eucaryotic initiation factors 2 and 3 (for translation)
ELISA	enzyme-linked immunosorbant assay
EM	electron microscopy
EMC	essential mixed cryoglobulinemia
ER	endoplasmic reticulum
FasL	Fas ligand
GBV	GB virus
GM-CSF	granulocyte-macrophage colony-stimulating factor
HAV	hepatitis A virus
HBcAg	hepatitis B core antigen
HBsAg	hepatitis B surface antigen
HBV	hepatitis B virus
HBxAg	hepatitis B X antigen
HCC	hepatocellular carcinoma
HCV	hepatitis C virus
HIV	human immunodeficiency virus
HVR	hypervariable region
IFN	interferon
IκB	inhibitor of nuclear factor kappa B

IL	interleukin
IRES	internal ribosome entry site
ISDR	interferon sensitivity-determining region
JNK	Jun amino-terminal kinase
LDL	low density lipoprotein
LOH	loss of heterozygosity
MHC	major histocompatibility complex
NANBH	non-A, non-B hepatitis
NF-κB	nuclear factor kappa B
NK cells	natural killer cells
NKT cells	natural killer T cells
NS3	nonstructural protein 3
NS5B	nonstructural protein 5B
NTP	nucleoside trisphosphate
ORF	open reading frame
PBMC	peripheral blood mononuclear cells
PKR	double-stranded RNA-induced protein kinase
PTB	polypyrimidine-tract-binding protein
PTH	post-transfusion hepatitis
RAG-2	recombinant activating gene 2
Rb	retinoblastoma tumor suppressor gene
RdRp	RNA-dependent RNA polymerase
RIBA	recombinant immunoblot assay
RT	reverse transcriptase
RT/PCR	reverse transcriptase/polymerase chain reaction
SCID	severe combined immunodeficient
SH3	Src homology domain 3
SV40	simian virus 40
TCR	T cell receptor
TGF	transforming growth factor
Th1, Th2	T helper cells types 1 and 2
TNF	tumor necrosis factor
UTR	untranslated region

Part I

Basic principles

Background

An active female business executive, aged 39 years and a mother of three young children, visited her family doctor for an annual check-up. She had never been seriously ill. A few days after her visit, she received a phone call from the doctor's office, informing her that her liver enzymes were slightly elevated. Since this result may reflect an underlying problem in the liver, she was asked to come back in for more tests. She tested positive for antibodies against a recently discovered hepatitis virus that establishes a chronic, asymptomatic infection in most people, which is often accompanied by an underlying liver disease that is serious and often progresses toward cirrhosis. Cirrhosis, or end-stage liver disease, is accompanied by considerable morbidity and mortality. She left the doctor's office with the knowledge that within 10–15 years the virus infection could destroy her liver. She was treated with antiviral therapy, which was expensive, had considerable side effects, and was not effective beyond the period of treatment. She was then informed that her best chances for survival may eventually be a liver transplant. This is the clinical face that is often seen in chronic hepatitis C virus (HCV) infection. This book will present the basic features of the virus and associated diseases as well as discuss present and future treatment options, in the hope that it will stimulate further research and provide a brighter future for those infected with HCV.

1.1 The enigma of non-A, non-B hepatitis

The search for HCV is a great detective story that had to await the definition of hepatitis as an infectious disease entity. In addition, its discovery came about only after several other agents responsible for post-transfusion hepatitis (PTH) were identified and yet a considerable amount of PTH still existed without a known cause. During the 1940s, for example, it was realized that hepatitis could be transmitted by blood transfusion (Beeson, 1943) and that at least two forms of hepatitis existed (MacCallum, 1947). They were termed "infectious" or type A hepatitis and "serum" or type B hepatitis. Further characterization of the responsible agents showed that hepatitis A virus (HAV) (Feinstone, Kapilian & Purcell, 1973) was transmitted by ingestion of contaminated food and drink, while hepatitis B virus (HBV) (Blumberg, Alter & Visnich, 1965) was a major source of PTH. Moreover, HAV was associated with a single bout of acute hepatitis, while HBV was associated with both acute and chronic liver disease (CLD). There was great hope that the development of specific serological tests for HAV and HBV would eliminate most, if not all, PTH, since the rates of PTH in the United States, for example, had exceeded 20% during the 1960s (Alter et al., 1972). However, once screening of blood became widespread, it became apparent that up to 10% of individuals who received blood transfusions in the United States during the late 1970s still developed hepatitis (Feinstone et al., 1975; Knodell, Conrad & Dienstag, 1975; Seeff et al., 1975; Maugh, 1980). As a result, the term non-A, non-B hepatitis (NANBH) was created to account for the presumed existence of one or more infectious agents responsible for inflammatory liver disease that lacked serological markers of HAV and HBV (Prince et al., 1974; Alter et al., 1975; Feinstone et al., 1975). Hence, until the discovery of HCV (Choo et al., 1989), the diagnosis of NANBH was one of exclusion. In addition to the lack of HAV and HBV serology, the diagnosis of NANBH was also based upon differences in clinical presentation (Ch. 8) and epidemiological characteristics (Ch. 3) of NANBH compared with HAV and HBV (Krugman & Gocke, 1978) (Table 1.1).

It soon became apparent that a diagnosis of exclusion included a large number of possibilities that could account for NANBH. First of all, it was not known whether the etiology of endemic, sporadic, post-transfusion, or epidemic NANBH was linked to one or multiple agents (Alter, 1988). In 1984, two groups published provocative evidence that a NANBH agent might be a retrovirus (Prince et al., 1984; Seto et al., 1984). This was based on the findings that sera from patients with NANBH were consistently positive for reverse transcriptase (RT) activity, that retrovirus-like particles could be isolated from chimpanzee liver cell cultures innoculated with a putative NANBH agent, and that experimental inoculation of candidate sera into chimpanzees resulted in the development of NANBH. Retrovirus-like particles were also observed in the cytoplasm of hepatocytes from patients with acute or chronic NANB PTH (Iwarson et al., 1985). However, RT activity was low, had no direct relationship to the severity of liver disease, and was observed in patients receiving transfusions who did not develop PTH. Independent observations also failed to detect RT activity in sera obtained from multiple, pedigreed, NANB PTH cases, or in sera obtained from chimpanzees inoculated with a NANB agent (Itoh et al., 1986; Kahn and Hollinger, 1986).

There was also evidence presented that a NANB agent might be related to HBV. For example, there were antigen and corresponding antibody specificities in NANB sera that crossreacted with the nucleocapsid (core; anti-HBC) and "e"

Table 1.1. Comparison of infections with hepatitis A or B virus and non-A non-B hepatitis

Characteristic	Hepatitis A	Hepatitis B	Non-A, Non-B hepatitis
Presentation			
Average incubation period (days (range))	~25 (15–50)	70 (50–180)	40–60 (15–180)
Onset	Acute	Usually chronic	Usually chronic
Age affected	Children and young adults	All ages	All ages
Symptoms			
Arthralgias	Uncommon	Common	Uncommon
Nausea and vomiting	Common	Common	Common
Fever	Common	Uncommon	Uncommon
Jaundice	Uncommon	Common	Uncommon
Laboratory values			
Alanine/ aspartate aminotransferase elevation	Transient	Prolonged	Prolonged
Duration of alanine aminotransferase elevation	1–3 weeks	1–8 or more months	1–8 or more months
Anti-hepatitis A antibodies	Positive	Negative	Negative
Hepatitis B surface antigen (HBsAg)	Negative	Positive	Negative
Disease association			
Acute hepatitis	Yes	Yes	Yes
Chronic hepatitis	No	Yes	Yes
Cirrhosis hepatocellular carcinomia	No	Yes	Yes
Transmission			
Percutaneous	Rare	Common	Common
Oral	Common	Rare	?
Virus in feces	Positive	Negative	Negative
Sexual	Rare	Common	Rare
Perinatal	None	Common	Rare

Modified from Krugman and Gocke (1978) with permission from W. B. Saunders, and from Seeff (1992) with permission from Williams & Wilkins.

antigens of HBV (Shirachi et al., 1978; Vitvitski, Trepo & Hantz, 1980; Trepo et al., 1983). These sera were also positive for virus-associated DNA polymerase activity (Hantz, Vitvitski & Trepo, 1980), which is also characteristic of HBV. In addition, monoclonal antibodies raised against HBV surface antigen (HBsAg) detected reactive material in both serum and liver samples from patients with NANBH who were HBsAg negative by conventional assays (Wands et al., 1982). When such sera were inoculated into HBV-susceptible or HBV-immune chimpanzees, several animals developed antigen reactivity in serum for this atypical antibody and also developed NANBH (Wands et al., 1986). Although interesting, the contribution of such HBV-like NANB agent(s) to PTH remains to be demonstrated.

Independent studies have demonstrated virus-like particles with morphology and density characteristics of picornaviruses, such as HAV, in the blood and liver samples from patients (Yoshizawa et al., 1980) and chimpanzees (Bradley et al., 1979) with documented NANBH. However, whether such particles are responsible for blood-borne or water-borne NANBH remains to be seen. Since the discovery of HCV (Choo et al., 1989), other blood-borne viruses, such as hepatitis G virus (Simons et al., 1995a,b; Linnen et al., 1996) and transfusion-transmitted virus (Nishizawa et al., 1997), have been discovered, but their relationship to PTH also remains to be firmly established. Greater success was met with the identification of the hepatitis E virus as a major agent responsible for epidemic, water-borne NANBH, which is a major problem in southern Asia and northern Africa (Wong et al., 1980). There is also evidence that several herpes viruses, such as Epstein–Barr and human cytomegalovirus, are also associated with NANBH in some settings (Prince, 1983). Although the detection of anti-HCV has greatly reduced the incidence of PTH during the 1990s, the documentation of non-A, non-B, non-C hepatitis (Alter and Bradley, 1995) has stimulated the search for new viral candidates, which are now regularly described at hepatitis symposia throughout the world.

1.2 The chimpanzee as a model of non-A non-B infection

The transmission and propagation of NANB agent(s) in chimpanzees during the 1970s (Alter et al., 1978; Hollinger et al., 1978; Tabor et al., 1978, 1979; Tsiquaye & Zuckerman, 1979) represented a major breakthrough in the eventual identification and characterization of HCV. These studies demonstrated that NANBH was really caused by one or more infectious agents, that the agent(s) could be transmitted from chronically infected people, and that chronic infection and mild hepatitis could be shown to develop in an animal model. The agent(s) were then shown to be serially transmitted in chimpanzees using serum from animals obtained at the time of acute or chronic hepatitis (Tabor et al., 1979). Additional studies in which outbreaks of NANBH from contaminated factor VIII (Bradley et al., 1979) or factor IX (Wyke et al., 1979) concentrates, used to treat hemophiliacs, also induced NANBH in chimpanzees, firmly establishing the chimpanzee as a reliable animal model of NANB infection. Hepatocytes isolated and cultured from infected chimpanzees during the acute phase of NANBH infection continued to replicate virus for several weeks, as indicated by the ability of tissue culture supernatants to infect susceptible animals (Jacob et al., 1990). These chimpanzees developed elevated alanine aminotransferase (ALT) levels in serum (reflecting the release of an intracellular enzyme into the blood from damaged hepatocytes), inflammatory liver disease, and the appearance of cyto-plasmic tubule structures commonly observed in the livers of those with NANBH (Jacob et al., 1990). Further characterization showed that these tubular structures derived from the proliferation of membranes associated with the smooth endo-plasmic reticulum (ER) (Shimizu et al., 1979). These ultrastructural changes, however, were not specific to the agent(s) responsible for NANBH, since they were also observed in different cell types infected with a variety of RNA viruses, including strawberry latent ringspot virus (a picornavirus) (Roberts & Harrison, 1970), St Louis encephalitis virus (a flavivirus) (Harrison, Murphy & Gardner, 1982), human immunodeficiency virus (HIV) (Sidhu et al., 1983), hepatitis delta virus (Canese et al., 1984), and poliovirus (Dales et al., 1965). These findings were consistent with the hypothesis that a NANB agent may have a RNA genome. Further work supported the existence of at least two agents associated with NANBH (Shimizu et al., 1979) and showed that one of these agents was sensitive to pretreatment with chloroform (Bradley et al., 1983; Feinstone et al., 1983), suggesting the presence of an envelope. Infection with the chloroform-sensitive virus was also associated with the development of cytoplasmic tubular structures. To determine the appropriate size of the NANB agent(s), infectious samples were passed through membranes with different pore sizes, and the eluants used for chimpanzee challenge studies. Using this approach, the size of this putative NANB agent was estimated to be 30–60 nm, with a 37 nm inner core (Bradley et al., 1985; He et al., 1987; Jacob et al., 1990), which was consistent with it being a toga- or flavivirus. The buoyant density of the infectious agent, 1.08–1.11 g/ml, in sucrose gradients was also consistent with a togavirus (Bradley et al., 1991; Miyamoto et al., 1992). Although a chloroform-resistant NANB agent was also reported (Bradley et al., 1983), the enveloped NANB agent had many of the characteristics that were later shown to be associated with HCV.

The presence of one or more NANB agents is further suggested by the finding of multiple episodes of NANBH in patients with biopsy-proven hepatitis (Mosley et al., 1977) and in hemophiliacs given multiple doses of factor VIII (Hruby and Schauf, 1978). At least two agents were also suggested by the existence of PTH of both short- and long-term incubation (Craske & Spooner, 1978; Norkrans et al., 1980). The appearance and transmission of tubular structures in the livers of chimpanzees that were serially infected with some but not other sources of infectious material also suggested the existence of at least two NANB agents (Shimizu et al., 1979). In addition, immunity appeared to develop against agent(s) from a single source, but cross-protection against putative NANB agents in different inocula was not consistently observed (Tsiquaye & Zuckerman, 1979; Bradley et al., 1980; Feinstone et al., 1981; Yoshizawa et al., 1981), since in some challenges, chimpanzees would experience a new bout of hepatitis. Following the discovery of HCV, it became evident that these results reflected the genetic heterogeneity of the virus (Chs. 3 and 14). Independent observations also showed two separate episodes of NANBH in chimpanzees inoculated with chloroform-resistant followed by chloroform-sensitive strains (Bradley et al., 1983). Consequently, it was not clear how many NANBH agents were present.

The difficulty in identifying agents associated with NANBH was further highlighted by the failure to isolate any infectious virus particle from human or chimpanzee sera. In addition, many laboratories reported "unique" antigen–antibody systems that appeared to be associated with NANBH (Kabiri, Tabor & Gerety, 1979; Shirachi et al., 1978; Spertini & Frei, 1982; Prince, 1983; Jacob et al., 1990). In one promising approach, lymphocytes obtained from chimpanzees with NANBH were transformed by Epstein–Barr virus, and tissue culture supernatants were used to stain for NANB antigens in infected liver (Shimizu et al., 1985). Although two antibodies stained infected but not uninfected liver, their cross-reactivity with delta antigen encoded by hepatitis delta virus (Shimizu et al., 1986) suggested that either the NANB agent was delta-like or that the reactions were nonspecific. This work, and others cited above, have not been independently confirmed in the literature, nor did any of them correctly identify a NANBH agent in samples of pedigreed human sera from infected patients, from normal individuals, or from chimpanzees known to be infected with a NANBH virus. Attempts to find antigens encoded by a NANB agent in the liver and serum were also disappointing, implying that their levels of expression may be too low for detection. Likewise, electron microscopic (EM) examination of serum and liver samples revealed a variety of virus-like particles (Bradley et al., 1979; Yoshizawa et al., 1980), but the relationship between any of these particles and the agents responsible for NANBH remained elusive. The reason for all of these difficulties, it turns out, was the very low titer of virus particles in most infectious sera from patients or experimentally infected chimpanzees, which was below the levels of detectability of most methodologies used at the time to detect markers of the NANB agent(s). This was supported by the fact that most sera had titers less than 1×10^3 chimpanzee infectious doses (Bradley et al., 1979). Consequently, it was realized that much more sensitive assays would have to be developed if reproducible detection of the NANB agent(s) was going to succeed. This early work in chimpanzees did show that a major agent for NANBH consisted of a chloroform-sensitive agent that was less than 80 nm in diameter and was associated with acute and chronic NANBH. Infections could also be shown to result in characteristic ultrastructural changes in the liver. Together, these results suggest that a major etiological agent of NANBH was a small, enveloped, RNA virus that probably replicated in the cytoplasm of infected hepatocytes.

1.3 Surrogate markers

The difficulties in establishing reproducible markers of HCV infection during the 1970s and 1980s (Section 1.1 and 1.2) prompted studies aimed at the evaluation of surrogate markers in the hope that such an effort would further reduce the incidence of NANB PTH. Exclusion of donor blood with ALT levels (ALT levels throughout refer to serum levels) greater than two standard deviations above the logarithmic mean prevented about 30% of NANB PTH (Alter et al., 1981; Aach et al., 1991). In attempts to reduce the incidence of NANB PTH further, antibodies against HBV core antigen (anti-HBc), which had been used to detect low levels of HBV in a PTH setting (Hoofnagle et al., 1973, 1978), were evaluated. For example, a large transfusion-related study of 1151 patients showed that 18.7% of those transfused with a single unit of anti-HBc-positive blood developed NANBH, while this was observed in only 7.2% of individuals receiving a single transfusion of anti-HBc-negative blood (Stevens et al., 1984). Similar results were obtained in independent studies (Koziol et al., 1986; Sugg, Schenzle & Hess, 1988), although still other studies showed no benefit of anti-HBc screening (Hanson & Polesky, 1987; Hoyos et al., 1989). Among the studies with positive results, anti-HBc screening prevented another 20–30% of NANB PTH. While the significance of isolated anti-HBc detection in PTH remains to be fully elucidated, it is clear that some anti-HBc-positive blood is infectious (Debure et al., 1988), and that isolated anti-HBc may reflect either very low levels of HBV or an HBV-like NANB agent that triggers a cross-reactive anti-HBc response (Lai et al., 1990a). While the combined use of ALT and anti-HBc as surrogate markers significantly reduced NANB PTH, the utility of these tests was limited by problems with standardization of "normal" ALT values and the nonspecificity of anti-HBc testing (Kroes, Quint & Heijtink, 1991). Use of these tests resulted in the rejection of a significant proportion of the donor blood supply (Kline et al., 1987). Even so, surrogate markers provided a temporary solution to the problem of partially eliminating NANB PTH.

With the discovery of HCV, and the establishment of first-generation serological tests, a number of studies were conducted to examine whether it was still worthwhile to continue surrogate marker testing. An early study in the Netherlands showed that surrogate and first-generation anti-HCV tests were roughly comparable (van der Poel et al., 1990b), implying that specific anti-HCV testing may not be needed in countries that already did surrogate testing (van der Poel et al., 1990a). However, the finding that many anti-HCV-positive blood donors had normal ALT (Alter et al., 1989a; Katayama et al., 1990; van der Poel, 1999) suggested that surrogate testing missed many HCV-infected individuals. In addition, surrogate testing using ALT excluded 2–4% of donated blood units whereas only 0.2–0.4% of donated blood was excluded by anti-HCV testing, making it obvious that the specific antibody assay was a better test (Zuck, Sherwood & Bove, 1987; van der Poel et al., 1990b; Watanabe et al., 1990). Independent studies showed no difference in the incidence of NANB PTH in transfusion recipients receiving blood that had been screened for ALT and anti-HBc compared with those receiving unscreened blood (Esteban et al., 1990; Blajchman, Bull & Feinman, 1995). Further work showed that three cases of HCV "window" period donations (i.e., before the appearance of anti-HCV) out of a million transfused units could have been prevented by continuing ALT testing and demonstrated that continued ALT testing in the light of anti-HCV screening was of little value (Busch et al., 1995). Although it was possible that continued screening for anti-HBc would eliminate HBsAg-negative HBV mutants (Carman et al., 1990; Feitelson et al., 1995), it would also exclude 1–4% of donors in western countries (Sugg et al., 1988; Hetland et al., 1990; Koziol et al., 1986) and the great majority of donors in HBV endemic countries, such as Taiwan (Lin-Chu et al., 1990). A number of studies also showed no correlation between anti-HBc and anti-HCV positivity (Hetland et al., 1990; Lin-Chu et al., 1990; van der Poel et al., 1990a). Consequently, once anti-HCV testing was validated, surrogate testing was largely dropped as screening against NANB PTH.

1.4 The discovery of hepatitis C virus

The finding that most infectious sera had very low titers of virus (Section 1.2) meant that large volumes of high-titered serum or plasma samples would have to be created if attempts at cloning the virus genome were going to succeed. Accordingly, HCV was passaged from chimpanzee to chimpanzee so that the virus might "adapt" to its new host and grow to higher levels, as was done with HAV. Other chimpanzees were immunosuppressed in the hope that this would result in higher levels of virus (Bradley et al., 1984a,b). Eventually large pools of high-titered sera ($> 1 \times 10^5$ chimpanzee infectious doses/ml) were collected and used as starting material for the attempted cloning and further characterization of a major agent responsible for NANB PTH (reviewed in Bradley, 2000).

In 1989, a group led by investigators at Chiron Corporation described a molecular clone obtained from a chimpanzee infected with the tubule-forming agent associated with NANBH that had been well characterized in animal transmission studies (Choo et al., 1989). Accordingly, plasma with a high concentration of the NANB agent(s) was centrifuged to pellet the putative virus(es) and the pellets extracted for total nucleic acid, since it was not known whether the genome of the agent(s) consisted of DNA or RNA. The extracted material was denatured, subjected to complementary DNA (cDNA) synthesis with random primers, and the products cloned into a lambda gt11 expression vector. In this vector, protein fragments encoded by the putative NANB agent were expressed as a fusion protein with β-galactosidase. The library of cloned inserts, which was then screened with a serum from a patient with NANBH, detected an epitope made by a 155 base pair (bp) clone (designated 5-1-1) that did not hybridize to human DNA or chimpanzee DNA from animals with NANBH. These results implied that the NANB agent(s) did not have a DNA genome. Further characterization showed that the 5-1-1-encoded epitope was recognized by sera collected from many patients with NANBH. This probe, as well as a larger overlapping clone (353 bp long), hybridized with RNA from the liver and sera of infected chimpanzees, but not with that from uninfected animals, suggesting that the NANB agent(s) had an RNA genome. Further characterization showed that the RNA detected was single stranded, was about 9.6 kilobases (kb) in length, had plus strand polarity, and had a genome organization similar to that of flaviviruses (Houghton et al., 1991; Weiner et al., 1991). This agent was referred to as HCV (Choo et al., 1989; Kuo et al., 1989), and its discovery was the culmination of many painstaking years of chimpanzee transmission studies (Section 1.2). The difficulty in identifying HCV earlier was a consequence of its usually low titers in the blood, the fact that HCV is genetically heterogeneous (Section 3.2), and its natural history, which often has a lengthy asymptomatic phase during the early years of chronic infection (Ch. 4). The low titer made it difficult to detect the genome and virus-encoded proteins by conventional methods. The sequence heterogeneity of HCV-encoded proteins made it difficult to detect them reproducibly in different infections. Finally, the asymptomatic course of early chronic infections provided few pathological landmarks to follow in the development of chronic hepatitis (Ch. 5).

1.5 The detection of viral antibodies

Following the discovery of clone 5-1-1, it was used to probe for other overlapping clones in the lambda gt11 expression library. Reconstruction of the clone 5-1-1 sequences within overlapping clones resulted in a larger recombinant, referred to as C 100, which was located mostly within the nonstructural (NS) protein 4 (NS4) region of HCV (Fig. 1.1). C 100 was then fused with the gene for human super-

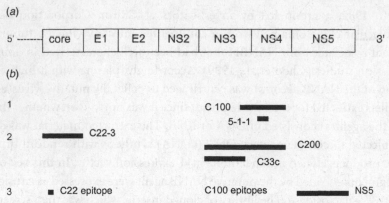

Fig. 1.1   Summary of hepatitis C virus (HCV) antigen specificities used to detect anti-HCV in the first-
(1), second- (2) and third- (3) generation assays. (*a*) Schematic of the regions within the
HCV genome. (*b*) Position of the recombinant proteins or epitopes (synthetic peptides) in
each of the different assays. (Modified from van der Poel, Cuypers & Reesink (1994) with
permission from Elsevier Science Ltd.)

oxide dismutase, expressed in recombinant yeast, and the product (C 100-3) used
to construct the first generation of commercial assays capable of detecting anti-
HCV in the sera of blood donors and in patients with NANBH. These assays
consisted of a standard enzyme-linked immunosorbant assay (ELISA) (developed
by Ortho Diagnostic Systems) and an indirect ELISA based upon the coating of
C 100-3 on polystyrene beads (Abbott Labs). First-generation confirmatory tests
were also developed. These included a recombinant immunoblot assay (RIBA;
Ebeling, Naukkarinen & Leikola, 1990), which is an ELISA type assay carried out
with the above antigens spotted onto nitrocellulose strips instead of coated in
micotiter wells. Alternatively, an HCV neutralization ELISA was developed in
which soluble C 100-3 was used to block the binding of antibodies in human sera
to the identical antigen coated on polystyrene beads (Dawson et al., 1991).
Application of these first-generation assays detected anti-HCV in more than 80%
of individuals with NANBH (Alter, 1990) and in the great majorty of those who
developed NANB PTH (Alter et al., 1989a; Aach et al., 1991). In addition, anti-
HCV was detected in the majority of blood donors who transmitted NANB PTH
(Alter et al., 1989a) and in most hemophiliacs at high risk for the development of
NANB PTH (Maisonneuve et al., 1991). These studies led to the widespread use of
these assays for screening blood, which resulted in a greater than 80% reduction in
the incidence of PTH (Donahue et al., 1992). However, it soon became apparent
that the first-generation assays were positive for anti-HCV in a high proportion of
patients with autoimmune hepatitis (Esteban et al., 1989; Lenzi et al., 1990)
(Ch. 7). Closer examination of this phenomenon revealed a correlation between

anti-HCV positivity and hypergammaglobulinemia (McFarlane et al., 1990), suggesting that the use of these tests in patients with autoimmune hepatitis probably resulted in a high frequency of false positives (McFarlane et al., 1990; Onji et al., 1991). False-positive results, coupled with low sensitivity and specificity, were also major problems when screening individuals from low-risk populations, such as blood donors from countries with a low rate of infection (Alter et al., 1989a; Esteban et al., 1990). In addition, not all patients infected with HCV developed antibodies against C 100-3, nor did this antibody specificity always persist during chronic infection. In most cases, anti-C 100-3 first became detectable weeks or months after acute infection, suggesting a significant "window" period in NANB infection before a definitive diagnosis could be made (Ch. 3).

In response to these limitations, several second-generation assays for anti-HCV were developed. The assay formats were similar or identical to those of the first-generation assays, with the exception that they also detected antibodies against the HCV nucleocapsid or core protein and NS3 (Fig. 1.1). Antibodies to these additional antigens were commonly found in serum samples from humans and chimpanzees with HCV or NANBH infections and provided the rationale for their inclusion in the second-generation tests. In one formulation, Ortho Diagnostics, in collaboration with Chiron, added the C 22-3 (recombinant core) and C 33c (recombinant NS3) to the C 100-3 (NS4) protein of the first-generation assay. C 33c and C 100-3 were expressed as a fusion protein (C 200) in the second-generation assay. Independently, Abbott laboratories constructed a bead-based assay using C 22-3, C 33c, and C 100-3. These companies also developed supplemental assays that included these additional antigens but otherwise retained the same format as the first-generation assays. In the supplemental assays, a positive result consisted of detectable reactivity with at least two of the recombinant antigens, while an indeterminate reaction consisted of specific reactivity to only one virus antigen, and a negative result consisted of no reactivity (Busch et al., 1993). These second-generation tests proved to be more sensitive, detected antibodies earlier after acute infection, and were capable of detecting anti-HCV more consistently than the first-generation tests (Chien et al., 1992; van der Poel et al., 1991a, 1992). More extensive second-generation testing showed that it detected anti-HCV in up to 95% of patients with NANB PTH (Chien et al., 1992) and in a larger percentage of patients with hemophilia (Maisonneuve et al., 1992) or on long-term hemodialysis (Chauveau et al., 1992). Based upon these and similar results, second-generation anti-HCV testing further reduced the risk for the transmission of NANB PTH to an estimated less than 1 per 100 000 transfusions (Schreiber et al., 1996a).

Additional work has most recently resulted in the development of more refined, third-generation primary and confirmatory tests for the detection of anti-HCV.

The third-generation tests are more sensitive than the second-generation tests by virtue of improved reactivity to NS3 (by inclusion of C 100 epitopes) (Fig. 1.1); this allows detection of anti-HCV earlier after acute infection than previous tests and also detection of isolated anti-NS3 in some chronic infections (Vernelen et al., 1994). NS5 was also added, although there is no solid evidence that its presence significantly alters the overall sensitivity or specificity of anti-HCV detection, and there is some evidence that it may lead to false-positive results (Vernelen et al., 1994). By comparison, the inclusion of epitopes from C 22 (core) and C 200 (NS3 plus NS4) (Fig. 1.1) has reduced the incidence of false-positive reactions, which was a problem in the first- and/or second-generation assays (Uyttendaele et al., 1994). Hence, anti-HCV testing has been critical in the reduction of NANB PTH, although there is still some nonspecificity associated with these assays, as well as circumstances (such as immunosuppression) where the results are not reliable.

The development of an anti-HCV test has permitted the identification of NANB PTH as being associated with HCV infection. The test has become increasingly important in assessing seroprevalence in different populations, monitoring the natural history of infection, as well as in initiating and following therapeutic trials. If a serum sample tests positive for anti-HCV, then supplemental testing is advised. This can take the form of the RIBA or other immunoblot assays currently available for such purposes (Ichimura et al., 1994), although in many cases, HCV infection is confirmed by testing for HCV RNA in serum using reverse transcriptase/polymerase chain reaction (RT/PCR) or some other type of amplification methodology (Fig. 1.2; Section 1.6 and Ch. 19). If the supplemental testing is negative and ALT is normal, it is likely that the anti-HCV test results may reflect a false positive. In cases where ALT is elevated, other causes should be explored. In the event that the confirmatory test is positive, ALT levels should be periodically monitored over the following 6–8 months. A persistently normal ALT may indicate either an asymptomatic chronic infection or recovery from acute infection. The latter is suspected when initially elevated ALT values return to normal and confirmatory tests become negative. Among patients with persistently elevated ALT, it is likely that there is underlying liver disease, and a liver biopsy should be performed (Davis, 1992). The information obtained from ALT testing and liver biopsy, combined with the results of HCV serology and supplementary testing, is very important in deciding whether to monitor the patient or initiate antiviral therapy. An algorithm for HCV testing has been developed for these purposes (Fig. 1.2). For those patients who undergo therapy, continued monitoring for anti-HCV, HCV RNA, and ALT levels in blood will be very important in assessing the outcome of therapy. Such information will also be central toward making decisions on whether to continue or discontinue therapy, especially as current

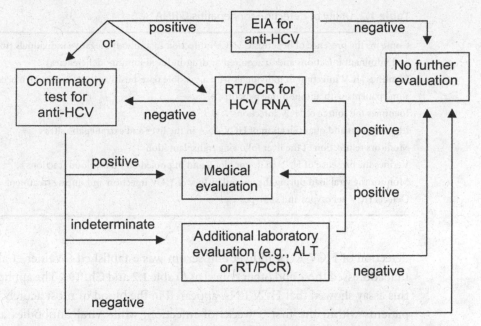

Fig. 1.2.   Algorithm for testing asymptomatic individuals for infection with hepatitis C virus (HCV). The algorithm is used to determine whether people identified as having one or more risk factors are infected with HCV. Initially, a blood sample is tested for anti-HCV; if positive, the result is confirmed independently by recombinant immunoblot assay (RIBA) or enzyme immunoassay (EIA) for antibody and/or by reverse transcriptase–polymerase chain reaction (RT–PCR) for HCV RNA. Patients with confirmed positive test results are then counseled and followed by periodic additional testing. If and when symptoms develop, then treatment options could be considered. If a RIBA test for antibody is indeterminate (not clearly positive or negative), then RT–PCR will be carried out to assess HCV infection. In addition, alanine aminotransferase (ALT) will be determined to assess whether there is underlying liver disease. If either of these tests are positive, the patient will be followed and retested periodically. The development of greatly elevated ALT (> 10-fold above background) or symptoms during follow up would result in counseling and possible treatment. (Modified from Davis (1992) with permission from Williams & Wilkins.)

treatments for HCV (interferon (IFN) and ribavirin (tribavirin)) are expensive and have considerable side effects (Ch. 10).

1.6 Testing for hepatitis C RNA

Anti-HCV may not be present during the first few weeks or months of acute infection nor does it discriminate between ongoing or resolved infection; this suggested that other approaches needed to be explored in the hope of addressing these limitations. Shortly after the discovery of HCV, an RT/PCR method for the

Table 1.2. Utility of detection for hepatitis C RNA

Confirms the presence of hepatitis C (HCV) infection in antibody-negative individuals (in acute and fulminant infections and in acquired or drug-induced immunodeficiencies)

Identifies HCV infection in individuals with a possible false-positive anti-HCV, which occurs in some patients with autoimmune hepatitis

Identifies the source of HCV infection

Identification and quantification of HCV RNA in the liver and extrahepatic sites

Monitors reinfection of the liver following transplantation

Verifies the presence of HCV in donor blood and in pooled blood or blood fractions

Monitor the viral load during the natural history of HCV infection and during treatment

Detects HCV genotypes and subtypes

---

detection of HCV RNA in liver and serum was established (Weiner et al., 1990) that addressed these and other concerns (Table 1.2 and Ch. 19). The application of this assay showed that HCV RNA appeared in the blood of most acutely infected patients within the first 3 weeks of infection, while viral antibodies appeared roughly 8–10 weeks later (Farci et al., 1991; Schreiber et al., 1996b). Since a bout of NANBH occurs roughly 6 weeks after virus exposure, the early detection of HCV RNA provides a definitive diagnosis (Puoti et al., 1992; Schreiber et al., 1996b) that is important in considering treatment options, especially since chronic infections are so prevalent following acute exposure to virus. This is also important when a positive diagnosis of HCV results from needlestick injuries (Ch. 3). The early detection of HCV RNA has also helped to reduce further the incidence of PTH by identifying HCV-contaminated donor blood that is anti-HCV negative. HCV RNA detection in blood donations is also a good measure of infectivity (Saldanha & Minor, 1996b). The last underscores the significance of a positive HCV RNA. It also suggests that if nucleic acid bearing defective interfering particles exist in HCV infection, they make up a minor population of such particles, since the relationship between HCV RNA and infectivity would break down if these particles constituted a major proportion of circulating virus (Section 3.2). HCV RNA also discriminates between past and ongoing infection. Ongoing infection is characterized by the sustained detection of HCV RNA in blood, while past infection is characterized by clearance of HCV RNA that is consistently found over many years.

There are other situations in which HCV RNA detection provides information about infection that is not obtainable by any other means (Table 1.2). As mentioned above, false-positive anti-HCV is an important problem among patients with several types of autoimmune disease, and in these cases, the presence of HCV RNA clarifies whether or not such patients are actually infected. In the context of transplantation, HCV-positive donor organs have been shown to infect the liver in > 90% of recipients, and nearly half of the transplant recipients go on to develop CLD (Pereira et al., 1992; Wreghitt et al., 1994). Graft reinfection usually occurs in > 85% of patients receiving liver transplants within a few days of transplant (Feray et al., 1994; Gretch et al., 1995a), and the virus titers produced in the new liver are often higher than those observed pretransplant (Fukumoto et al., 1996). These observations are consistent with the idea that there is more replication space (i.e., more susceptible hepatocytes) in the transplant compared with the pretransplant liver. In addition, the immunosuppression of patients following transplantation would also permit more rapid viral spread and higher levels of sustained virus replication within the newly transplanted organ.

HCV RNA determination (Ch. 19) has also been useful in identifying the source of infection. For example, a case study has documented heterosexual transmission of HCV (Rice et al., 1993), although negative reports seem to indicate that sexual transmission is uncommon (Gordon et al., 1992; Bresters et al., 1993). Interestingly, maternal–infant transmission of HCV has been shown to occur in 3–5% of babies born to HCV RNA-positive mothers, with the likelihood of transmission greatest among mothers with the highest viral load (Lin et al., 1994a; Aizaki et al., 1996). Since anti-HCV may be passively transferred from mother to child during breast-feeding, the ability to screen for HCV RNA in babies' blood readily distinguishes between passive antibody transfer and active infection (Boudot-Thoraval et al., 1993). In another context, the ability to detect HCV RNA (Ch. 19) has helped in tracking down the source of nosocomial infections in various hospital settings (Schvarcz et al., 1995; Esteban et al., 1996; Munro et al., 1996). The last has had important implications in preventing the spread of infections from infected health care workers (e.g., surgeons and blood bank technicians) and from contaminated equipment (e.g., renal dialysis units) (Ch. 3).

Quantitative HCV RNA determination is very important for deciding whether to treat patients with antiviral drugs, in following the course of treatment, and in deciding whether to continue or terminate treatment (Ch. 10). For example, the finding that responders to IFN treatment had signficantly lower levels of pretreatment HCV RNA compared with patients who relapsed or were unresponsive (Hagiwara et al., 1993; Rumi et al., 1996) highlights the value of quantitative HCV RNA determination in making clinical decisions. As described in Ch. 9, there is also evidence that the sequence of the virus, which is different in individual patients, may influence whether a patient is an appropriate candidate for therapy and, if so, which type of therapy.

2

The virus

2.1 Physical characteristics of the virus

Prior to the discovery of HCV, chimpanzee studies showed that a NANB agent passed through a filter that excluded agents greater than 80 nm in size, suggesting that the responsible pathogen was probably a virus (Bradley et al., 1985; He et al., 1987). In addition, the sensitivity of the pathogen to chloroform indicated that the NANB agent was probably enveloped (Bradley et al., 1983; Feinstone et al., 1983). Molecular cloning and sequencing of the HCV genome further supported these findings (Choo et al., 1989). When virus particles were characterized by banding on sucrose density gradients, infectious sera contained HCV with densities less than 1.06 g/ml while noninfectious sera contained particles banded at approximately 1.12–1.17 g/ml (Miyamoto et al., 1992; Hijikata et al., 1993c). Although both peaks contained detectable HCV RNA, it was subsequently shown that the lighter peak was associated with low density lipoproteins (LDLs) (Miyamoto et al., 1992; Thomssen, Bonk & Thiel, 1993), while the fractions with higher density were associated with immunoglobulins (Hijikata et al., 1993c; Choo et al., 1995). This was verified in experiments showing that the lighter peak was immunoprecipitated with anti-apolipoprotein sera, while the heavier peak was immunoprecipitated with anti-immunoglobulin (Yoshikura et al., 1996). Some of the material in the heavier fractions may also contain nucleocapsids (Kaito et al., 1994; Kanto et al., 1994), which may arise directly from the lysis of hepatocytes supporting virus replication during a bout of liver disease. It has been postulated that LDLs may partially protect HCV from antibody-mediated neutralization and may stimulate uptake of HCV through the LDL receptor (Section 2.5). In addition, the complexing of putative virus particles with immunoglobulins may partially block virus attachment to susceptible cells, thereby favoring the development and/or persistence of chronic infections. Although provocative, there are no direct experimental data supporting the role of LDL or antibody in infectivity or infection. Moreover, the finding of virus at a density of 1.12 g/ml in tissue culture supernatant from a human T cell line (MPB-Ma) that supports virus replication (Nakajima et al., 1996), and where there is presumably no anti-HCV, suggests that antibody may not contribute to the higher density peak observed here. Other studies have reported density values for HCV that varied from 1.03 to 1.20 g/ml (Bradley et al., 1991; Carrick et al., 1992; Miyamoto et al., 1992; Kanto et al., 1994), implying considerable heterogeneity in the types and amounts of host components associated with the virus particles (see related question 1 in Ch. 24).

Given the low concentrations of HCV in most serum samples and the low levels of HCV recovered from current tissue culture systems, it took some time before the virus could be visualized by EM. However, once virus-positive material was concentrated, EM images showed virus-like particles at 60–75 nm in diameter surrounded by a fringe of projections extending 8–15 nm from the surface of the particle (Li et al., 1995). NP-40 treatment of virus preparations resulted in the appearance of 45–55 nm diameter icosahedral nucleocapsids (Kaito et al., 1994; Li et al., 1995; Prince et al., 1996), which had a density of approximately 1.35 g/ml and was immunoprecipitable with antibodies against the core of HCV (Shindo et al., 1994). Similar sized nucleocapsid-like particles, 45 nm in diameter, were observed in HeLa G cells transiently transfected with a plasmid expressing full-length HCV (Mizuno et al., 1995). These results suggest that HCV is an enveloped virus with a nucleocapsid that appears to encapsulate the genome of the virus.

2.2 Genome structure and organization

The genome of HCV is single-stranded, positive sense RNA approximately 9.6 kb long (Choo et al., 1991b). HCV has a genetic organization similar to that of flaviviruses and pestiviruses (Miller & Purcell, 1990) and has been classified as a separate genus (*Hepacivirus*) within the family Flaviviridae (Francki et al., 1991) (Table 2.1). This classification is based upon limited sequence homology and similar hydrophilicity profiles among some of the proteins in the two groups. There is also striking nucleic acid sequence homology and similar secondary structural features between the untranslated region (UTR) at the extreme 5' end of the HCV genome and the analogous region in pestiviruses, but not with flaviviruses (Miller & Purcell, 1990; Han et al., 1991; Brown et al., 1992; Bukh et al., 1992). Flaviviruses include a number of agents that are transmitted by various arthropod vectors. Infection often results in the development of hemorrhagic fever (e.g., by yellow fever virus) or encephalitis (e.g., by Japanese encephalitis virus). Pestiviruses of animals include bovine viral diarrhea virus (BVDV) and classical swine fever virus. The genomic organization of HCV is also closely related to that of the hepatitis G virus isolates GBV-A, GBV-B and GBV-C (Simons et al., 1995a,b; Linnen et al., 1996) with GBV-B being the most closely related to HCV among all comparisons made to date. The overall amino acid identity between HCV and GBV-B is roughly 30%, with up to 50% homology in the HCV-encoded protease (NS3) and RNA-dependent RNA polymerase (RdRp; NS5B) (Miller &

Table 2.1. Characteristics of hepatitis C compared with flaviviruses

Characteristic	Hepatitis C	Flaviviruses
Spherical enveloped virus	Yes	Yes
Genome size (kb)	9.6	11
Genome polarity	Positive	Positive
Genome nucleic acid single-stranded RNA	Yes	Yes
Polyprotein production from single open reading frame (ORF)	Yes	Yes
Internal ribosome entry site	Yes	No
Co- and post-translational cleavage of polyprotein	Yes	Yes
Structural proteins on 5' end of genome	Yes	Yes
Nonstructural proteins on 3' end of genome	Yes	Yes
5' and 3' untranslated regions (UTR) flanking ORF	Yes	Yes

Purcell, 1990; Muerhoff et al., 1995). Despite these similarities, there is no clear association between the hepatitis G viruses and liver disease, suggesting that these viruses may have a different pathogenesis than HCV or be nonpathogenic. Further, there is no known association between HCV and either hemorrhagic fevers or encephalitis, indicating that the pathogenic spectrum of HCV is quite different from that of other members of Flaviviridae.

The RNA of HCV encodes the viral proteins from a single, large open reading frame (ORF) (Fig. 2.1) (Chambers et al., 1990). The translation of this ORF results in the production of a polyprotein 3010–3033 amino acid residues long, depending upon the isolate (Yamada et al., 1994b). The genetic organization of the virus is such that the amino-terminal end of this polyprotein encodes the structural proteins of HCV while the remainder encodes a family of NS proteins that are involved in virus maturation and replication. From amino- to carboxy-terminus, the polyprotein encodes C–E1–E2–p7–NS2–NS3–NS4A–NS4B–NS5A–NS5B (Fig. 2.1). The core or nucleocapsid polypeptide (C protein) of HCV is at the extreme amino-terminus of the polyprotein, followed by two envelope glycoproteins (E1 and E2), which are cleaved by one or more host proteases. p7 is a small polypeptide of unknown function that results from the inefficient cleavage of E2 (Lin et al., 1994a; Mizushima et al., 1994). The adjacent sequences encode the NS2/3 protease, which undergoes autocatalytic cleavage to yield mature NS2 and NS3 (Section 2.4). NS3, which is also a protease, is responsible for the cleavage of the remaining nonstructural polypeptides: NS4A, NS4B, NS5A, and NS5B. These contribute importantly to the formation of the replication complex of HCV (Fig. 2.1; Section 2.4). The genome of HCV also has 5' and 3' UTRs that flank the ORF at each end of the genome. As outlined in Section 2.3, the 5' UTR plays a

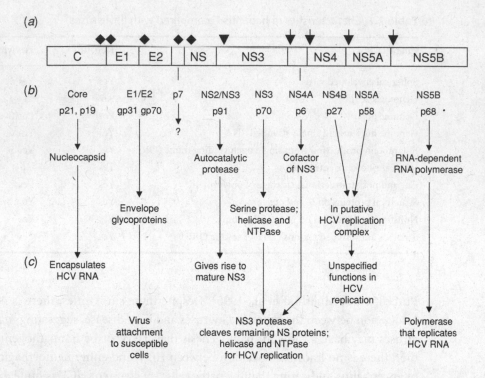

Fig. 2.1.   Hepatitis C (HCV) polyprotein (*a*), the names and sizes (in kDa) of the individual mature gene products (*b*), and the known or putative function of each (*c*). (*a*) Core–E1, E1–E2, E2–p7, and p7–NS2 junctions are cleaved by a cellular signal peptidase (♦) to yield the structural proteins of the virus. The NS2/NS3 protein then undergoes autocatalytic cleavage (▼), which releases the mature NS3 serine protease. The latter cleaves the remainder of the nonstructural (NS) polypeptides (↓), which then assemble into membrane-associated replication complexes, where NS5B then replicates the RNA strands of the virus. p, protein; gp, glycoprotein. (Modified from Major & Feinstone (1997) with permission from W. B. Saunders.)

major role in the initiation of translation, while the 3' UTR is thought to contribute importantly to virus replication.

2.3 The 5' untranslated region

Translation initiation in eucaryotic cells usually follows the "first AUG rule," where a ribosome scans a mRNA molecule until it reaches the first translation initiation codon (AUG), where translation begins (Kozak, 1989). In addition, most eucaryotic mRNAs contain a 5' terminal ^{m7}GpppG cap structure, which promotes the formation of translation initiation complexes. This process is also favored by short scanning distances at the 5' end of the mRNA and by the lack of stable secondary and tertiary structure in this region.

In contrast, primary sequence analysis of RNAs isolated from picornaviruses (e.g., poliovirus), HCV, and the closely related GBV agents paints a different picture. The 5' UTR in these viruses is up to 10% the length of the viral genome. Translation initiation maps to an internal AUG codon (not the first), the mRNAs lack a cap structure, and the 5' UTR is characterized by complex and stable secondary structures in each case. These features suggest a novel mechanism in which translation initiation is directed by the existence of an internal ribosome entry site (IRES) (Jang et al., 1988; Ehrenfeld & Semler, 1995).

The 5' UTR of HCV is 341 nucleotides long (Han et al., 1991), although other studies have reported slightly different lengths (Fig. 2.2) (Takamizawa et al., 1991; Trowbridge & Gowans, 1998). It is not clear whether this microheterogeneity is real, whether it reflects different methods of cloning, or whether the differences are biologically significant (see related question 2 in Ch. 24). However, the primary sequence of the 5' UTR is one of the most conserved regions in the viral genome, with up to 85% nucleotide sequence identity among HCV isolates, suggesting that this region is functionally important. Thermodynamic modeling of the 5' UTR shows considerable secondary structure that is conserved among different HCV isolates as well as in the 5' UTRs of pestiviruses and GBV-B (Brown et al., 1992; Wang et al., 1995; Honda, Brown & Lemon, 1996a). The existence of these stable secondary structural features has been partially confirmed by analyses of nuclease sensitivity of synthetic RNAs (Brown et al., 1992; Honda et al., 1996a). In HCV, these features include several proposed stem–loop structures and a pseudoknot, which are separated into four regions of secondary structure (reviewed in Rijnbrand & Lemon, 2000) (Fig. 2.2). From the 5' end of the UTR, these regions are referred to as I, II, III, and IV, with region IV containing the translation initiation codon. Based upon mutational analyses, the IRES spans regions II, III, and IV, from approximately residue 40 to 344 of the 5' UTR, although the sequences delimiting the IRES are slightly different among independent studies (Brown et al., 1992; Wang et al., 1995; Honda et al., 1996a,b; Kamoshita et al., 1997). These sequences were shown to function as an IRES in vitro, in cell lysates, and when transfected into eucaryotic cells (Wang, Sarnow & Siddiqui, 1993; Iizuka et al., 1994; Rijnbrand et al., 1995). Several of these fragments directed translation from uncapped mRNAs (Reynolds et al., 1996; Rijnbrand et al., 1996). Although the 5' UTR contains multiple AUG codons, translation occurred at the third or fourth AUG codon at nucleotides 342–344 within the proposed stem–loop structure of domain IV. Point mutations upstream of the latter AUG codon had little effect upon translation initiation, suggesting that the ribosomes bind very close to this initiator AUG, with little or

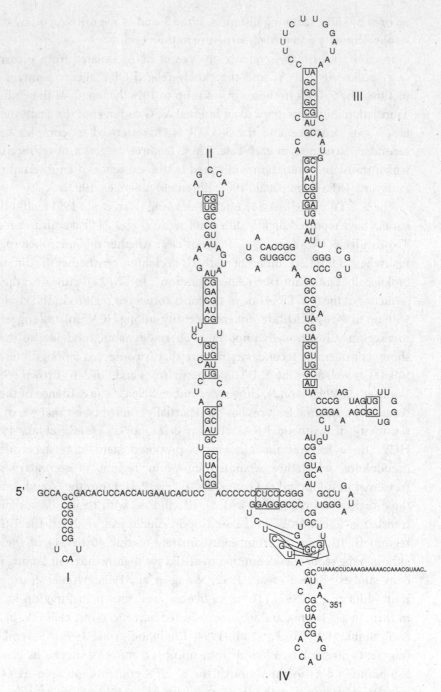

Fig. 2.2.   Secondary structure of the 5' untranslated region (UTR) showing the four domains of the internal ribosome entry site (IRES) (I, II, III, and IV). Base pairings validated by genetic analyses or by natural sequence covariation are indicated by boxes. (Modified from Rijnbrand & Lemon (2000) with permission from Springer-Verlag.)

no scanning prior to the beginning of translation (Reynolds et al., 1996; Rijnbrand et al., 1996). However, mutations that disrupted base pairing and the seconday structure within the IRES disrupted IRES activity (Wang, Sarnow & Siddiqui, 1994; Honda et al., 1996a,b), suggesting that the secondary structure of the 5' UTR is important in regulating the efficiency of translation. Other work has confirmed that IRES activity requires most of the 5' UTR (Fukushi et al., 1994; Reynolds et al., 1995; Rijnbrand et al., 1995), since when secondary structure is destroyed by mutation, IRES activity is similarly affected. Beyond the 5' end of the IRES, most studies have shown that stem–loop 1 has either no impact or a mildly negative influence upon IRES function (Honda et al., 1996b; Kamoshita et al., 1997). On the 3' end, although the IRES extends to the translation initiation codon, there is some evidence that the 5' end of the core-encoding region may stimulate IRES activity (Reynolds et al., 1995; Lu & Wimmer, 1996). However, this has not been universally observed, and it has been proposed that the RNA structure just downstream from the translation initiation site may significantly affect the efficiency of translation (Wang et al., 1993; Rijnbrand et al., 1995; Honda et al., 1996a). In this context, the fact that 5' UTR RNA transcripts terminating just prior to domain IV are still capable of binding to 40S ribosomal subunits (Pestova et al., 1998) suggests that these downstream sequences are not essential for IRES activity, although they may modulate translation efficiency. Hence, while the complex secondary structure of the 5' UTR is important in defining the site of translation initiation of the HCV polyprotein, adjacent sequences in the coding region may further influence the efficiency of translation.

The consequences of the conserved secondary structural features of the HCV IRES are that they likely result in the positioning of the 40S ribosomal subunit at the translation initiation codon without the need for scanning. This scenario is compatible with the finding that the loop in domain III of the IRES is complementary to an unpaired loop segment of 18S rRNA (Brown et al., 1992; Deng & Brock, 1993), although there is no experimental evidence that firmly supports HCV 5' UTR/rRNA base pairing. In addition, the finding that translation is not initiated if the AUG codon is moved either upstream or downstream from the initiation site (Reynolds et al., 1996; Rijnbrand et al., 1996) is also compatible with precise positioning and no scanning. Given that purified 40S subunits bind to 5' UTR RNA lacking the stem–loop domain IV structure and the initiation codon, the initial contacts probably occur at domains II and III and do not require an initiation codon (Honda et al., 1996b). The binding of the 40S ribosomal subunit to viral RNA may also be modified by its interaction with other host components in addition to selected structural features of the 5' UTR. For example, the interaction of eucaryotic initiation factor 3 (eIF3) with domain III may promote the correct alignment of the 40S subunit with the viral RNA (Pestova et al., 1998).

The role of other 5' UTR binding proteins, such as the polypyrimidine tract-binding protein (PTB) (Ali & Siddiqui, 1995), the La autoantigen (Ali & Siddiqui, 1997), and poly(C)-binding protein (Spangberg & Schwartz, 1999) in polyprotein translation initiation is not clear, even though they are known to contribute importantly to picornaviral translation (Ehrenfeld & Semler, 1995). Interestingly, PTB also binds to the 3' UTR of HCV, and it has been suggested that the 3' UTR enhancement of HCV translation (Ito, Tahara & Lai, 1998) may be promoted by dimerization of PTB molecules binding to the 5' UTR and 3' UTR regions (Rijnbrand & Lemon, 2000). However, in vitro reconstruction of translation initiation complexes seems to require the presence of viral RNA, the 40S and 60S ribosomal subunits, GTP, eIF2 and eIF3 (Pestova et al., 1998). Another protein, referred to as heterogeneous nuclear ribonucleoprotein, binds specifically near the translation initiation codon of HCV and reportedly increases translational activity of reporter constructs containing the HCV IRES and 5' core region sequences (Hahm et al., 1998). However, the contribution of this protein or other IRES-binding proteins, to the initiation of HCV translation (Yen et al., 1995; Fukushi et al., 1997; Buratti et al., 1998; Pestova et al., 1998) remains to be elucidated in a tissue culture system supporting HCV replication.

2.4 Polyprotein processing and virus maturation

Polyprotein processing in HCV is accomplished by a cellular protease that cleaves the structural components, and by two virus-encoded proteases that are responsible for cleavage of the nonstructural polypeptides of the virus (Fig. 2.1). It is likely that the cellular enzyme responsible for the cleavage of core, E1, E2, p7 and the amino-terminus of NS2 consists of at least one cellular enzyme with signal peptidase activity. The evidence for this activity is indirect, since the responsible cellular enzyme has not been purified and further characterized. However, the sequences just upstream from the amino-termini of E1, E2, p7 and NS2 consist of hydrophobic, putative signal peptides that are not in the mature protein products (Hijikata et al., 1991; Lin et al., 1994a; Mizushima et al., 1994). In addition, cleavage appears to be membrane dependent and takes place at the lumen of the ER (Hijikata et al., 1991; Lin et al., 1994a; Mizushima et al., 1994; Hussy et al., 1996). Further, cleavage is inhibited when charged amino acids are placed within the signal sequence (Mizushima et al., 1994). An additional membrane-dependent cleavage has been observed at the core–E1 junction but upstream from the signal peptidase site. It is not known whether this cleavage is carried out by the same signal peptidase, or whether another enzyme is involved. However, this additional cleavage results in the generation of two core polypeptides with different carboxy-termini (Santolini, Migliaccio & La Monica, 1994; Hussy et al., 1996), although their termini have not been precisely mapped. It is not known whether the two forms of the mature core polypeptide play distinct roles in virus maturation or replication. Hence, there is one, and perhaps more than one, host protease that cleaves the structural polypeptides of HCV. In all likelihood, the cleavage of the structural polypeptides is important for the encapsidation of viral RNA during HCV replication (Section 2.5).

Processing of the HCV polyprotein at the NS2–NS3 junction appears to occur autocatalytically by a zinc-stimulated activity within the NS2–NS3 polypeptide sequences (Grakoui et al., 1993a; Hijikata et al., 1993a). Once mature NS3 appears, it acts as a second virus-encoded protease to cleave the remaining nonstructural polypeptides at the junctions NS3–NS4A, NS4A–NS4B, NS4B–NS5A, and NS5A–NS5B (Bartenschlager et al., 1993; Eckart et al., 1993; Grakoui et al., 1993b). Evidence for the existence of these two virus-encoded proteases comes from studies in which different mutations were shown to inactivate one or the other activities independently (Bartenschlager et al., 1993; Eckart et al., 1993; Grakoui et al., 1993a). On the one hand, mutations affecting His-952 and Cys-993 of NS2 (numbered from the translation initiation codon of HCV), for example, completely abolished NS2–NS3 cleavage (Grakoui et al., 1993b; Hijikata et al., 1993a) but did not effect the NS3 protease activity. On the other hand, sequence alignment of NS3 with the trypsin family of proteases, and with trypsin-like proteases encoded by flaviviruses and pestiviruses, suggested that His-1083, Asp-1107, and Ser-1165 may constitute the active site of a serine protease (Bazan & Fletterick, 1989; Gorbalenya et al., 1989; Chambers et al., 1990; Miller & Purcell, 1990). The finding that mutations affecting Ser-1165 completely inactivated NS3 protease activity (Bartenschlager et al., 1993; Eckart et al., 1993; Grakoui et al., 1993b; Hijikata et al., 1993a), but had no effect upon NS2–NS3 cleavage, also strongly suggested the existence of two separate virus-encoded protease activities.

The stimulation of NS2–NS3 cleavage by zinc, and its inhibition by ethylenediaminetetraacetic acid (EDTA) (which removes zinc by binding), suggested that the NS2/NS3 protease may be a metalloprotease (Hijikata et al., 1993a). However, the NS2/NS3 protease lacks the typical active site characteristic of metalloproteases (Jiang & Bond, 1992). The more recent suggestion, that NS2/NS3 is a cysteine protease (Gorbalenya & Snijder, 1996), has been supported by studies in which mutation affecting His-952, Cys-993, and Glu-972, which are in the putative active site of cysteine proteases, result in either a decrease or complete loss of NS2/NS3 protease activity (Grakoui et al., 1993a,b). The recent expression of NS2–NS3 in vitro and in various eucaryotic cells (Grakoui et al., 1993a,b; Hijikata et al., 1993a, Hirowatari et al., 1993; Reed, Grakoui & Rice, 1995) has provided an opportunity to characterize the NS2–NS3 cleavage reaction further. Interestingly, the findings that NS2–NS3 cleavage is rapid and that it occurs in *cis* (on the expressed NS2/NS3 polypeptide) but very poorly in *trans* (where NS2 and NS3 polypeptides are added to an appropriate substrate) suggest that the cleavage is autocatalytic. This cleavage reaction appears to be dependent upon the overall conformation of the NS2/NS3 molecule, since it could tolerate many point mutations outside of the active site, although it is sensitive to mutations that disrupt overall polypeptide conformation (Hirowatari et al., 1993; Reed et al., 1995). Hence, cleavage of the HCV structural proteins is followed by a rapid, autocatalytic cleavage of the NS2–NS3 sequences, which releases NS3. As explained below, NS3 plays a number of roles in virus maturation and virus replication.

The NS3 serine protease domain was originally localized to the amino-terminal third of the molecule, based upon conserved sequences with other viral and cellular serine proteases (Bazan & Fletterick, 1989; Miller & Purcell, 1990) and later confirmed by mutagenesis studies (Bartenschlager et al., 1994; Tanji et al., 1994a; Failla, Tomei & DeFrancesco, 1995; Han et al., 1995). Further work has shown that cleavage at the NS3–NS4A site occurred in *cis*, while processing at the other nonstructural protein sites, resulting in the appearance of NS4A, NS4B, NS5A, and NS5B, occurred in *trans* (Bartenschlager et al., 1993; Grakoui et al., 1993b, Lin et al., 1994b). The kinetics of cleavage have shown that the NS3–NS4A site is processed rapidly and prior to the action of NS3 on other sites (Bartenschlager et al., 1994; Lin et al., 1994b; Failla et al., 1995). Another rapid cleavage then occurs at the NS5A–NS5B site, resulting in the appearance of the virus RdRp, NS5B. The precusor NS4A/NS4B/NS5A is then more slowly processed into the corresponding mature polypeptides (Bartenschalger et al., 1994; Lin et al., 1994b). Significantly, NS4A has been shown to bind (Bartenschlager et al., 1995b; Failla et al., 1995; Lin, Thomson & Rice, 1995) and activate (Bartenschlager et al., 1995b; Lin et al., 1995; Tanji et al., 1995a) NS3; it also promotes the association of NS3 with cellular membranes (Hijikata et al., 1993b; Tanji et al., 1995a), which may contribute to protease activation. Amino-terminal sequencing of the NS3 products showed that polyprotein cleavage occurred at Thr-1657 for NS3–NS4A processing, and at Cys-1711, Cys-1972, and Cys-2420 for NS4A–NS4B, NS4B–NS5A, and NS5A–NS5B cleavage, respectively (Grakoui et al., 1993b, Pizzi et al., 1994). These cleavage sites were also observed using appropriate synthetic peptide substrates, suggesting that processing specificity is related to the primary sequence around the cleavage site and is not conformationally dependent. NS3-mediated cleavage events also showed that NS4A is required for processing of NS3–NS4A, NS4A–NS4B, and NS4B–NS5A. In addition, the processing of NS5A–NS5B by NS3 was greatly enhanced by NS4A. Detailed structural analysis showed that the middle portion of NS4A, which forms a hydrophobic β-strand structure, is sufficient to bind to and fully activate NS3 (Lin et al., 1995; Shimizu et al., 1996;

Tomei et al., 1996). With regard to NS3, the amino-terminal 22 amino acid residues have been found to bind NS4A and are all that is needed for the functional activation of NS3 (Failla et al., 1995; Satoh et al., 1995). The finding that the NS4A peptide that binds to NS3 inhibits NS2–NS3 autocatalytic cleavage (Darke et al., 1999) suggests that the conformation of NS3 in the NS2/NS3 precursor is different than in mature NS3, and that NS2–NS3 cleavage must occur prior to the appearance of NS4A. These observations suggest that NS4A is truly a cofactor of NS3 and that their association is likely to be biologically relevant for HCV serine protease function and the order of polypeptide maturation.

The finding that the 180 residues at the amino-terminus of NS3 and a synthetic peptide spanning the middle region of NS4 (approximately residues 20–34) fully reconstituted serine protease activity (Shoji et al., 1995; Suzuki et al., 1995b; Steinkuhler et al., 1996), has provided the foundation for the successful crystallization and further characterization of the HCV serine protease. Crystallographic analysis of the truncated NS3/NS4A complex has shown that it adopts a chymotrypsin-like fold (Kim et al., 1996; Yan et al., 1998). It also showed that the NS4A peptide is completely buried within the complex and contributes significantly to the formation of the hydrophobic core of this complex (Kim et al., 1996). This suggests that NS4A is an integral structural component of the protease and helps to explain how NS4A activates the NS3 protease. Independent observations, in which the cystallographic structure of the truncated NS3 serine protease was solved in the absence of NS4A, showed a much less structured amino-terminus of NS3 (Love et al., 1996), which provides a basis for the observation that NS4A stabilizes NS3 (Tanji et al., 1995a). Hence, NS4A binding alters the conformation of the amino-terminal 22 amino acid residues of NS3, from an unstructured to a helical conformation, and in doing so activates the NS3 protease. Other subtle conformational changes have also been proposed to occur in NS3 following NS3/NS4A complex formation (Yan et al., 1998). An alternative interpretation of NS4A binding is that it contributes centrally to the formation of the substrate-binding site in NS3 (Kim et al., 1996). However, recent work has shown that binding of NS4A results in increased stability and enzymatic activation of NS3 (Wolk et al., 2000). These changes are associated with conformational rearrangement and altered substrate binding, suggesting that the consequences of NS4A binding are not mutually exclusive.

An intriguing feature of the NS3 protein is the presence of three strictly conserved Cys residues at positions 1123, 1125, and 1171, as well as a single conserved His residue at position 1175 (within the carboxy-terminal portion of NS3), which collectively could serve as a metal-binding domain (DeFrancesco et al., 1996a). When the crystallographic structure of NS3 was published (Kim et al., 1996; Love et al., 1996), these residues were indeed positioned to bind metal, and further work showed that NS3 bound stoichiometric amounts of zinc at this site (DeFrancesco et al., 1996a; Stempniak et al., 1997). Although the binding site for zinc was nowhere near the catalytic site for the NS3 protease in the crystal structure, appropriate NS3 conformation and activity was zinc dependent (De-Francesco et al., 1996a; Stempniak et al., 1997; Urbani et al., 1998). These data suggest that NS3-associated zinc serves a structural role in the stability and function of the molecule. This is in contrast to the role of zinc in the NS2/NS3 protease, where autocatalytic processing of this protease is zinc dependent (Hijikata et al., 1993a; Pieroni et al., 1997). Whether the contribution of zinc to NS2–NS3 cleavage is catalytic, structural, or both, remains to be clarified. In addition, the relationship, if any, between the metal-binding residues in NS2 and NS3 remains an open question. Hence, a number of sequential proteolytic events are required for maturation of the virus polyprotein into both the structural and the nonstructural polypeptides that self-assemble into virus replication complexes and, after secretion, into virus particles.

2.5 Gene expression and replication

The development of the chimpanzee as a model for HCV infection and disease (Section 1.2 and Ch. 13) has provided opportunities to study some aspects of virus gene expression and replication. For example, HCV antigens were detectable only in hepatocytes and endothelial cells; within these cells, the antigens were localized exclusively in the cytoplasm (Krawczynski et al., 1992a). Human studies have reported the presence of HCV antigens using sera or IgG fractions from infected patients (Ballardini et al., 1995a; Nouri-Aria et al., 1995) or monoclonal or polyclonal antibodies raised against individual HCV antigens (Blight et al., 1994; Gonzalez-Peralta et al., 1994b; Nouri-Aria et al., 1995; Sansonno et al., 1995). Most studies showed staining in the cytoplasm of hepatocytes, which is where replication is proposed to occur, but some also demonstrated staining in the infiltrating mononuclear cells (Blight et al., 1994; Nouri-Aria et al., 1995) and in a small fraction of biliary epithelial cells (Nouri-Aria et al., 1995) (see related question 3 in Ch. 24). The percentage of positive hepatocytes and the intensity of staining varied widely from study to study, ranging from less than 5% to up to 100% (Blight & Gowans, 1995). These results likely reflect differences in the antibodies used, in tissue fixation and preparation procedures, and in the time during infection when the tissue samples were obtained. However, the cell types in the liver with detectable HCV antigens are the same cell types that appear to support HCV replication in vitro (Ch. 11).

HCV RNA has been detected in the livers of experimentally infected chimpanzees by in situ hybridization (Negro et al., 1992; Shindo et al., 1992). Signals could be detected in 50–95% of hepatocytes by two days after innoculation of 10 million chimpanzee infectious doses per animal and preceded the appearance of HCV RNA in the blood by a day or two. A number of human studies have detected the presence of plus and/or minus strand HCV RNA, which are both amplified during virus replication, in infected liver (Negro et al., 1998). In situ RT/PCR, which combines the power of in situ hybridization to identifiy infected cells with the sensitivity of RT/PCR, showed HCV RNA in the cytoplasm of hepatocytes from infected patients, occasionally in mononuclear cells, but not in bile duct epithelium or sinusoidal cells (Lau et al., 1994). Plus strand HCV RNA has been consistently detected in liver and plasma, and to a more variable extent in peripheral blood mononuclear cells (PBMC) (Takehara et al., 1993). The ratio of plus to minus strands in the liver has been estimated to be on the order of 10 : 1 to 100 : 1 (Fong et al., 1991b; Sakamoto et al., 1994). Additional work showed that the levels of HCV RNA replicative forms in the liver roughly paralleled the extent and intensity of HCV core antigen expression in the same tissue (Negro et al., 1998). In this context, the levels of detectable core antigen derived from virus particles in the sera of infected patients directly correlated with the levels of HCV RNA in the same serum samples (Dickson et al., 1999). These studies imply that core antigen expression is directly related to the levels of HCV replication. Evidence for HCV replication has also been found in hepatocellular carcinoma (HCC) cells by in situ hybridization and RT/PCR (Gerber et al., 1992; Horiike et al., 1993; Ohishi et al., 1999); the impression from this work is that replication is supported but less efficient in HCC cells compared with that in surrounding nontumor liver (Ch. 6). However, detection of plus and minus strands of HCV RNA in the liver and blood of naturally infected patients (Fong et al., 1991b) and experimentally infected chimpanzees (Shindo et al., 1992) raises the question as to the origin of the RT/PCR products. Other studies have localized the minus strand HCV RNA only to the liver (Takehara et al., 1993; Sakamoto et al., 1994; Niu et al., 1995). This may be true for some patients but may also reflect the difficulty in assuring specific minus strand amplification and detection using RT/PCR, even when precautions are taken (Sangar & Carroll, 1998) (Ch. 21).

In the absence of a cell culture system that supports consistently high levels of HCV replication (Ch. 11), there is indirect evidence that viral replication occurs at the membranes of the ER, and/or possibly at other cellular membranes. The membranes of the ER, for example, appear to be important for the cleavage of core and envelope polypeptides during virus maturation, as well as for the processing of the amino-terminal end of NS2 (Hijikata et al., 1991; Lin et al., 1994a; Mizushima et al., 1994; Hussy et al., 1996) (Section 2.4). The processing of virus envelope and core polypeptides at these membranes may be a very important step in the formation of a virus envelope and in the secretion of virus particles. The fact that NS4A stabilizes NS3 and targets NS3 to the membranes of the ER (Hijikata et al., 1993b; Tanji et al., 1995a; Wolk et al., 2000) suggests that NS4A contributes importantly to both polypeptide processing (virus maturation) and virus replication. This is because NS3 is centrally involved in the cleavage of proteins that make up the replication complex of HCV (Section 2.4) and is also likely to act as a helicase within that complex (see below). Hence, the probable function of membrane targeting is to bring together physically all of the components needed for virus replication and maturation; in doing so, this targeting provides an important aspect of the HCV life cycle.

The rate of virus replication has been estimated from the dynamics of HCV clearance among patients treated with IFN (Ch. 9) and in the reappearance of HCV in patients undergoing plasma exchange. In the case of IFN-treated patients, the half-life of viral clearance was estimated to be 2.7 hours (Neumann et al., 1998), which is similar to that calculated for the rapid decline of HCV following liver transplantation (Fukumoto et al., 1996). Very similar numbers were independently obtained based upon the reappearance of HCV in patients who had undergone plasma exchange (Manzin et al., 1999). Given that the IFN-treated patients had a stable baseline of steady-state virus levels prior to treatment, this means that the virus production and clearance rates were probably similar. In the study of Neumann et al. (1998), the average virus production and clearance rate was about 10^{12} virions/day. Assuming that 1–10% of hepatocytes (out of about 2×10^{11} in the liver) are replicating virus, 5–50 virus particles appear to be produced per hepatocyte per day (Neumann et al., 1998). Combined with the high frequency of HCV genome mutation (1.4×10^{-3} to 1.9×10^{-3} base substitutions per site per year) (Ogata et al., 1991; Okamoto et al., 1992a), which stems from the lack of proofreading capability of the virus-encoded RNA polymerase (Holland, de la Torre & Steinhauer, 1992), it is not surprising that chronic infections are commonly characterized by multiple quasispecies. Quasispecies comprise very closely related sequences of viral RNA in the blood and liver of a single infection (Martell et al., 1992) (Section 3.2 and Ch. 22). The high rate of replication and clearance, combined with a short half-life, may also explain the rapid appearance of these quasispecies that accompanies treatment failure (Enomoto et al., 1994; Le Guen et al., 1997) (Ch. 9) as well as the failure of the immune system to clear virus following acute infection. Together, these characteristics of virus replication promote virus persistence and may provide part of the explanation as to how such a large proportion of acutely infected patients become chronically infected.

The lack of a stable, highly productive tissue culture system for HCV (Ch. 11) has prevented a clear understanding of the virus replication cycle; consequently, much of what is known about HCV replication has been deduced from the replication scheme of flaviviruses. In both cases, the initial step in the virus life cycle involves the attachment and entry of virus particles into susceptible cells. For HCV, it has recently been shown that both virions and E2 bind strongly to the cell surface component CD81 (Pileri et al., 1998). Neutralizing sera from chimpanzees that were immunized with E1/E2 blocked the binding of HCV to CD81 in vitro, suggesting that envelope antibodies may contribute to blocking of virus infection (Pileri et al., 1998). The presence of CD81 on both hepatocytes and B cells correlates with the susceptibility of both cell types to HCV infection and may provide a partial explanation for the high frequency of autoimmune diseases and lymphoproliferative disorders associated with HCV infection (Strassburg, Obermayer-Straub & Manns, 1996; Zignego & Brechot, 1999) (Ch. 7). Further work has recently indicated that other molecules besides CD81 may be important for binding of the virus (Takikawa et al., 2000). The presence of LDLs on HCV particles (Section 2.1), and association of HCV (and other flaviviruses) with the LDL receptor (Thomssen et al., 1992), suggests another candidate receptor that may mediate virus uptake into susceptible cells (Agnello et al., 1999). In the latter study, the binding of HCV to cells correlated with the levels of LDL receptor and was inhibited by pretreatment of cells with anti-LDL receptor. In addition, there was a direct correlation between cell surface LDL receptor and the number of cells positive for HCV RNA by ISH. Further, the binding of HCV to cells lacking the receptor was observed only after it was transfected into the cell line (Monazahian et al., 1999). While these lines of evidence suggest that HCV binds and enters a cell through the LDL receptor, it remain to be seen whether this interaction results in a productive infection.

Once inside the cell, the genomic (plus strand) RNA of HCV acts as a substrate for translation of the HCV polyprotein and for the production of minus strand HCV RNA. The latter then serves as a replication intermediate for the production of additional plus strand, which becomes incorporated into new virus particles. While the details of this process are sketchy, most of the evidence suggests that HCV replication takes place in the cytoplasm in association with cellular membranes, especially those of the ER (Section 2.4). For example, following cleavage, mature core polypeptide has been shown to be associated with the perinuclear and ER membranes (Harada et al., 1991; Santolini et al., 1994). In the context of the virus life cycle, HCV core has been shown to autopolymerize (Matsumoto et al., 1996; Nolandt et al., 1997) (Section 5.4), bind RNA (Santolini et al., 1994; Hwang et al., 1995), and interact with E1 (Lo, Selby & Ou, 1996). These features suggest that core protein promotes virion assembly. HCV core protein has also been found associated with 60S ribosomal subunits (Santolini et al., 1994), which may be involved in uncoating. The association of core protein with lipid droplets and colocalization with apolipoprotein II (Barba et al., 1997) is consistent with the observations that core promotes steatosis in some transgenic mouse lines (Moriya et al., 1997) (Ch. 13) and that HCV particles are associated with LDL in the circulation (Thomssen et al., 1992, 1993) (Section 2.1).

In addition to HCV core, the envelope glycoproteins E1 and E2 are also lipophilic. This property has been localized to the carboxy-terminal domain of each polypeptide. During the virus life cycle, they anchor the lumen exposed glycoproteins to the ER membrane. This membrane association appears to be important for correct envelope polypeptide folding, resulting in the formation of E1/E2 heterodimers, which are also thought to exist in native virus particles (Deleersnyder et al., 1997). Further work has shown that E2 is required for the proper folding of E1 (Michalak et al., 1997). Given these considerations, it is likely that HCV, like other flaviviruses, buds through the ER membrane. These observations not only have ramifications for understanding the life cycle of HCV but also in the formulation of vaccines (Ch. 14).

The role of NS2 in the life cycle of HCV appears to involve autocatalytic cleavage at the NS2–NS3 junction in order to generate mature NS3 (Section 2.4). This cleavage reaction is stimulated by the addition of microsomal membranes to an NS2/NS3 in vitro translation mix, suggesting that the conformation of the NS2/NS3 polypeptide in a hydrophobic environment may be important for cleavage to occur (Grakoui et al., 1993a; Santolini et al., 1995). As indicated in Section 2.4, one of the functions of mature NS3 is to catalyze the cleavage of the remaining nonstructural proteins of the virus. This likely occurs as a membrane-bound complex that compartmentalizes the functions required for virus replication. This suggests that maturation of the nonstructural proteins and replication may be coupled in time and space. The finding that NS3 has RNA helicase and NTPase activities (Jin & Peterson, 1995; Kim et al., 1995; Preugschat et al., 1996) is also consistent with its role in virus replication. It is proposed that the helicase activity is important in denaturing the extensive secondary structure of the viral RNA in preparation for replication and/or that it may promote denaturation of the double-stranded RNA replication intermediate after synthesis of the complementary strand (Tai et al., 1996). It turns out that the energy that drives the helicase activity depends upon NTP hydrolysis, which is also provided by NS3. Both of these activities have been mapped to the carboxy-terminal two-thirds of NS3 (Jin & Peterson, 1995; Kim et al., 1995) but are separable by mutagenesis (Heilek & Peterson, 1997). In this regard, it has been shown that NS3 binds to partially or completely single-stranded RNA or DNA and that such binding results in an increase in NTPase activity (Jin & Peterson, 1995; Gwack et al., 1996; Preugschat et al., 1996). Binding activity of NS3 to synthetic oligonucleotides has been demonstrated by X-ray crystallography (Cho et al., 1998; Kim et al., 1998), which has also provided insights into the mechanism of helicase (unwindase) activity. The fact that poly(U) and poly(dU) sequences stimulate NTPase activity the most, and that a poly(U) stretch exists in the 3' UTR region of HCV, suggests a function for this untranslated viral sequence, although it has not yet been shown that NS3 specifically binds to this region of the viral genome. Although additional functions for NS3 have not been identified, other members of the RNA helicase protein family in nature are also involved in the regulation of transcription, translation, and recombination (Gorbalenya & Koonin, 1993; Fuller-Pace, 1994). Preliminary data have shown that NS3 appears to inhibit signal transduction mediated by protein kinase A (Borowski et al., 1997), although the impact of this inhibition upon transcription, translation, and cellular phenotype remain to be studied.

The NS4 region of HCV RNA encodes two proteins, NS4A and NS4B, which presumably contribute to viral replication, but their functions are far from clear. Nothing is known about the role of NS4B in virus replication, although it is assumed that it is present and functions within the replication complex of the virus. NS4A binds to and stabilizes NS3 serine protease and helicase/NTPase, which is likely to promote polyprotein maturation and viral replication, respectively, as described in Section 2.4. NS4A may also promote the formation of replication complexes by directing NS3 to cellular membranes via its amino-terminal hydrophobic domain (Hijikata et al., 1993b; Kim et al., 1996; Wolk et al., 2000). A consistently productive tissue culture system will be needed to demonstrate a role for the NS4-encoded proteins in the HCV life cycle.

NS4A also appears to stimulate the phosphorylation of NS5A (Kaneko et al., 1994; Tanji et al., 1995b) (Fig. 2.3) by direct binding (Asabe et al., 1997). This phosphorylation is a conserved feature among HCV isolates (Reed, Gorbalenya & Rice, 1998), suggesting that it is functionally important. It appears to be mediated by a cellular serine/threonine kinase in the same family as the cyclin-dependent and mitogen-activated protein kinases (Reed, Xu & Rice, 1997), and not by NS4A, since the introduction of NS5A into cells without other HCV proteins still results in phosphorylation. Independent work has shown that NS5A is phosphorylated in vitro by addition of protein kinase A (Ide et al., 1997). If NS5A alters any of these or related pathways in vivo, it may have profound effects upon the cell cycle and/or signal transduction. As indicated in Ch. 10, this appears to be true for IFN-associated responses mediated through the Jak/Stat pathway (Heim, Moradpour & Blum, 1998). It is also supported by recent preliminary evidence showing that NS5A interacts in vitro with a cellular protein containing Src homology and SH3 (Src homology domain 3) binding domains (Herion et al., 1998). In this context, it has been shown that amino-terminally truncated NS5A, but not full-length NS5A, has *trans*-activating activity (Fig. 2.3) (Pawlotsky & Germanidis, 1999). This *trans*-activating activity could be correlated with the ability of NS5A to mediate IFN resistance (Fukuma et al., 1998; Ch. 10), suggesting that IFN signal

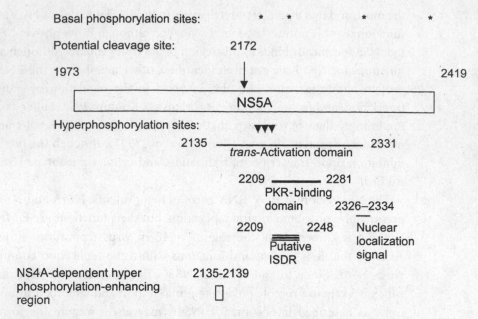

Fig. 2.3.   Selected properties of NS5A (nonstructural protein 5A). The different putative functional domains are discussed in the text. PKR, double-stranded RNA-induced protein kinase; ISDR, interferon sensitivity-determining region. (Modified from Pawlotsky & Germanidis (1999) with permission from Blackwell Science, Inc.)

transduction is affected in vivo. In addition, the finding that NS5A transcriptionally suppresses the cell cycle regulatory gene $p21^{WAF1/CIP1/SDI1}$ while it upregulates proliferating cell nuclear antigen (Ghosh et al., 1999) also suggests that NS5A has *trans*-activating activity in vivo that promotes cell growth and survival. This may not only promote persistent virus replication but also contribute importantly to hepatocarcinogenesis (Ch. 6). Although truncated NS5A has not been detected in natural infections, the amino-terminal domain of NS5A may mask or inhibit the transcriptional activation region; binding to other virus polypeptides or cellular components (Lin et al., 1997) may relieve this inhibitory effect through promoting conformational changes in NS5A (Ide et al., 1996). NS5A also has a putative nuclear localization signal (Fig. 2.3), and it is possible that NS5A capable of *trans*-activation may be transported to the nucleus using this signal (Ide et al., 1996), although it is not known whether this actually occurs. Hence, NS5A may play important but indirect roles in the life cycle of HCV (see related question 4 in Ch. 24).

The NS5B gene product is the RdRp, which is responsible for virus replication. The natural substrate for RdRp is the genome of HCV, which is plus strand RNA; in addition to being a template for replication, plus strand RNA could also be translated into the virus polyprotein (Koonin, 1991; Buck, 1996). Characteriz-ation of RdRp activity in replication complexes has been difficult because of the low levels of virus and variable autolysis that accompanies clinical samples. The absence of a suitable tissue culture system has also been a limitation to these types of analysis. Reconstitution of a functional replication complex is another possible approach to studying the properties of NS5B; although this has not yet been achieved, several laboratories are moving in this direction. Plus strand RNA viruses do not package their polymerase in the mature virions, suggesting that the first step after uncoating is the translation of the viral RNA into the HCV polyprotein (Roizman & Palese, 1996). Once the polyprotein is translated, and mature RdRp is generated, the latter uses the plus strand released from translation for minus strand synthesis. RdRp activity on a plus strand template results in synthesis of minus strand RNA. This process may not be very efficient, since the ratio of plus to minus strand RNA in the infected cell is between 10 : 1 and 100 : 1 (Novak & Kirkegaard, 1991). In order to achieve these ratios during the early stages of infection, both plus and minus strands must be made, while at later stages, mostly plus strand is synthesized. The criteria that determine how much plus and minus strand RNA is made at different times after infection are not known. Although largely incomplete, the current data suggests that HCV core protein binds to the 5' section of the HCV genome (Shimoike et al., 1999), and that this binding, combined with core polypeptide self assembly (Matsumoto et al., 1996), results in the packaging of the HCV genome within core particles. This binding also represses translation at the IRES, suggesting a potential mechanism whereby translation/replication could be switched to packaging. While it is not known whether core particle formation takes the form of a nucleocapsid or an alternatively structured ribonucleoprotein complex, these subviral particles then associate with the envelope polypeptides at the ER membranes. The targeting of E1 and E2 to the ER membranes (Cocquerel et al., 1999; Duvet et al., 1999) provides the environment for budding of mature virus particles to take place, and it is likely that virus is exported at this site by a constitutive secretory pathway.

The putative mechanism of RdRp action has been partially deduced from comparison of NS5B primary sequences and secondary structural motifs with those of other well-characterized polymerases. For example, the predicted second-ary structure of HCV NS5B is similar to that of the corresponding poliovirus polymerase (Hagehorn, van Beers & DeStaercke, 2000). Based upon secondary structure predictions, there are four evolutionary conserved motifs in RdRps from many viruses (Kamer & Argos, 1984; Poch et al., 1989), one of which includes the Gly–Asp–Asp (GDD) motif within the active site (Choo et al., 1991b; Shukla, Hoyne & Ward, 1995). Among 45 HCV isolates (Koonin, 1991), eight conserved motifs were noted, although with the exception of the active site (GDD) motif, the function of the others remain to be established. These NS5B sequences have between 16 and 23 Cys residues. Ten of these were conserved in all isolates, suggesting that disulfide bonding may contribute to the correct three-dimensional folding of NS5B. In addition, NS5B is phosphorylated in eucaryotic cells (Hwang et al., 1997), although none of the putative phosphorylation sites are conserved among NS5B sequences, nor is it known whether phosphorylation is important for NS5B function. Other residues, such as Val-284 and Arg-345 are unique to HCV NS5B compared with RdRp of other viruses (Poch et al., 1989). Mutation of Arg-345 to Lys results in an increase in RdRp activity of more than 50% (Lohmann et al., 1997). Hence, the primary sequence of HCV NS5B isolates has provided clues as to the regions of the protein that may be functionally important.

Building upon this knowledge, expression systems have been generated to characterize NS5B further (Ch. 23). For example, isolation of NS5B under non-denaturing conditions from insect cells expressing recombinant baculovirus (Behrens, Tomei & DeFrancesco, 1996; Lohmann et al., 1997) or from recombinant *Escherichia coli* (Al et al., 1997, 1998; De Staercke et al., 1998; Yamashita et al., 1998) yielded products with RdRp activity, proving that NS5B is the HCV-encoded polymerase. This activity was optimal at pH 7.5 and was Mg^{2+} dependent. Although recombinant NS5B was capable of replicating a number of natural or synthetic templates in vitro (including HCV RNA), other viral and/or host factors probably dictate specificity of template selection and synthesis in the context of virus-infected cells (see related question 5 in Ch. 24). This is indirectly supported by the observation that NS5B does not specifically bind to the 3' UTR of the HCV genome (Lohmann et al., 1997). RdRp activity was strictly primer dependent and was completely inactivated by mutations in the GDD active site (Yamashita et al., 1998). In addition, deletion of up to 40 amino acid residues from the amino-terminus of NS5B resulted in complete loss of RdRp activity (Lohmann et al., 1997), indicating that the integrity of the amino-terminus is important for enzyme activity. Addition of several amino acid residues to the amino-terminus of NS5B also resulted in reduced polymerase activity. While the significance of these observations remains to be understood, the fact that the poliovirus RdRp functions as an oligomer, in which the amino-terminal region of one molecule contributes to the active site of another (Hansen, Long & Schultz, 1997), provides a possible explanation for the HCV results. More recently, kinetic analysis with purified NS5B has shown an incorporation rate of about 200 nucleotides/min using full-length HCV RNA as template. The finding that this elongation rate was independent of NS5B protein concentration suggests that NS5B is a processive enzyme (Lohmann et al., 1998). Preliminary evidence has also demonstrated that recombinant NS5B could be expressed in baby hamster kidney cells and in the human hepatoma cell line Huh-7 (Heller et al., 1998). These findings raise the possibility that additional HCV proteins, and perhaps the virus replication complex, could eventually be reconstructed in liver cells.

Further biochemical characterization of NS5B using synthetic, single-stranded templates resulted in the production of double-stranded RNA products (Behrens et al., 1996). These observations were consistent with the hypothesis that the 3' end of the template RNA acts as a primer for the synthesis of the opposite strand, resulting in the generation of a hairpin structure through a "copy-back" mechanism (Tanaka et al., 1995; Kolykhalov, Feinstone & Rice, 1996). Dimer sized genomic RNAs have been seen in tissue culture cells replicating poliovirus (Young, Tuschall & Flanegan, 1985), suggesting that they may be replication intermediates in the HCV life cycle. A copy-back mechanism of replication has also been suggested from independent data (Lohmann et al., 1997). More recent data have shown that HCV NS5B requires single-stranded RNA "primer" at the end of the 3' UTR for copy-back replication to occur (Zhong et al., 2000). These results suggest that secondary structural flexibility of the 3' UTR may be an important feature permiting HCV replication. Other studies have shown that NS5B is capable of copy-back synthesis, resulting in a hairpin dimer- and a monomer sized product, suggesting de novo RNA synthesis from the input template (Luo et al., 2000). These models will need to be tested in cells consistently replicating HCV.

NS5B has a hydrophobic domain at its carboxy-terminus (Yamashita et al., 1998), and transfection of cells with NS5B expression vectors results in the accumulation of NS5B in the perinuclear region, suggesting that it may be associated with the nuclear membrane and/or the membranes of the Golgi or ER (Hwang et al., 1997). Although it is not known whether NS5B has this cellular distribution in replication complexes, attempts at reconstructing these complexes in cells have revealed an association between NS3, NS4A, and NS5B (Ishido, Fujita & Hotta, 1998). Independent work has shown coexpression and binding of NS5A, NS4A, and NS4B (Lin et al., 1997). It has been found that NS4A stimulates the phosphorylation of NS5A (Asabe et al., 1997), which may affect the nature of protein–protein interactions within replication complexes and, with it, the ability of such complexes to mediate HCV replication.

There are accumulating data that the 5' and 3' UTRs are important for the regulation of replication. In the case of the 5' UTR, it is likely that the ability of viral and/or cellular proteins to bind to the IRES regulates polyprotein translation and, after maturation, replication complex formation (Section 2.3). In this context, the cellular protein PTB has been shown to bind several domains in the 5' UTR (Ali & Siddiqui, 1995). If this binding is the mechanism whereby PTB promotes polyprotein translation, then there may be one or more other host proteins that compete with PTB so that some of the viral RNA templates would be available for replication instead of translation, although this remains to be shown.

Evidence for the role of the 3' UTR in viral replication is stronger, since deletion of 3' UTR sequences destroys infectivity of the corresponding truncated RNA in chimpanzees (Kolykhalov et al., 1997). Like the 5' UTR, the extreme 3' end of the HCV genome has considerable secondary structure, and it is possible that this RNA structure consists of protein-binding motifs for the assembly of ribonucleo-protein complexes for viral replication. Several cellular proteins have been found to be associated with the 3' UTR sequences in vitro (Tsuchihara et al., 1997; Inoue et al., 1998), although their role, if any, in promoting virus replication remains to be demonstrated.

3

Epidemiology and transmission

Epidemiological investigations of HCV actually began with the realization that there was still a high frequency of PTH after exclusion of HAV, HBV (Prince et al., 1974; Alter et al., 1975), and other viral and toxic causes of hepatitis (Reesink & van der Poel, 1989). In the 1970s and early 1980s, the frequency of NANB PTH in different countries ranged from 2–11 per 1000 transfusions in the Netherlands and 3 per 1000 in England to 10–28 per 1000 in the United States and 23 per 1000 in Italy (Reesink & van der Poel, 1989). Among patients receiving transfusions, more than 80% of PTH was designated as NANB PTH, with 10–20% symptomatic in the acute phase. Additional observations showed about half of those with NANB PTH developed chronic hepatitis, and up to 20% of those with chronic hepatitis went on to develop cirrhosis. Cirrhosis was also shown to be an important risk factor for the appearance of HCC (Dienstag, 1983; Reesink & van der Poel, 1989). Among people with NANB PTH, more than 40% had a history of intravenous drug abuse and 5–10% had a history of possible or known occupational exposure to blood (mostly among health care providers). In addition to PTH, NANBH was also reported in up to 40% of those with acute sporadic hepatitis in the United States in which there was no history of blood transfusion (Alter et al., 1982). Hence, considerable progress had been made understanding the epidemiology of PTH and sporadic NANBH hepatitis years before the underlying etiology became known.

With the discovery of HCV, and the development of specific serological tests for its detection, it soon became obvious that HCV was the major cause of blood-borne and sporadic NANBH (Alter et al., 1989a,b; van der Poel et al., 1989; Houghton, 1996). As indicated in Section 1.5, the sensitivity and specificity of the first-generation assays missed approximately 10–20% of serologically positive infections. In addition, the first-generation assays were plagued by a high rate of false positivity. Even with these limitations, an estimated 0.5–1.5% of the world's population was infected with HCV (Purcell, 1994). Anti-HCV was detected in 0.2–0.8% of blood donors from northern European countries (Kuhnl et al., 1989; Contreras et al., 1991), in 0.5–1.7% of donors from southern Europe (Janot, Courouce & Maniez, 1989; Esteban et al., 1990; Par, 1990), and in 1.0–1.5% of donors from Japan (Katayama et al., 1990). Interestingly, anti-HCV was found in

Table 3.1. Risk factors for transmission of hepatitis C virus

Risk for transmission	Factors
High	Multiple transfusions of whole blood (prior to July, 1992) or blood fractions (e.g., immunoglobulins or clotting factors; prior to 1987), especially from paid donors for the treatment of hemophilia and thalassemia
	Intravenous drug abuse (sharing contaminated needles); intranasal cocaine?
Moderate	Long-term hemodialysis (shared machines and/or cross-contamination of supplies in procedures)
	Multiple sexual partners: heterosexual or homosexual relationships; Risk depends upon number of partners
	Medical history of sexually transmitted diseases
	Maternal transmission (to baby at or before birth)
	Transplantation (infected organs into uninfected recipients)
	Vaccination campaigns (in countries where glass syringes are reused by doctors)
Low	Sexual transmission in monogamous relationships (documented but rare)
	Tattooing (contaminated instruments)
	Acupuncture (contaminated instruments)
	HIV infection (coinfected people have accelerated pathogenesis in the liver)
	Other nosocomial infections (e.g., during surgery, use of contaminated gloves, contaminated syringes for intravenous catheter)
	Dental procedures (contaminated gloves or instruments)
	Intrafamilial transmission (sharing toothbrushes, razors, etc.)
Minimal	Needlestick (health care workers)
	Transmission of screened blood or blood products

roughly 0.5% of volunteer blood donors in the United States, but among paid donors, the rate was in excess of 10% (Dawson et al., 1991). The latter reflected high-risk behaviors, the most common of which was intravenous drug abuse (Table 3.1). Independent work from several groups showed that 80–90% of intravenous drug users had detectable anti-HCV within their first year of drug abuse (Esteban et al., 1989; Smyth et al., 1995; van der Poel, 1999). While the exclusion of intravenous drug users significantly reduced the incidence of HCV-associated PTH, considerable transmission of HCV was documented even among those with a distant history of intravenous drug abuse (e.g., during the 1960s), who were asymptomatic and continued to donate blood during the 1970s and

1980s unaware that their past behavior posed a risk for transmission (van der Poel, 1999). Hence, the drug abuse of the 1960s may have contributed significantly to the transmission of the 'silent epidemic' of the 1980s and 1990s (see related question 6 in Ch. 24). When the role of intravenous drug abuse in the transmission of HCV was fully realized, and both sensitive and specific anti-HCV assays became available, many countries reevaluated the seroprevalence of HCV in their blood donors. This work revealed an incidence of less than 0.1% among donors from The Netherlands, Iceland, India, and the United Kingdom (Garson et al., 1992; Love et al., 1995; Arankalle, Tungatkar & Banerjee, 1996; van der Poel et al., 1991b; van der Poel, 1999), while an incidence of greater than 1% of blood donors was observed in Saudi Arabia, China, and Thailand (Abdelaal et al., 1994; Wu et al., 1995; Sawanpanyalert et al., 1996). However, the fact that chronic HCV infection could be asymptomatic for 20 or more years, and that screening blood donors for risk factors from their medical histories often underestimated the true frequency of HCV, suggested that the prevalence of HCV in the general population was likely to be higher than that reported in blood donor studies conducted worldwide (Garcia-Bengoechea et al., 1995) (see related question 7 in Ch. 24). As a consequence, the incidence of HCV transmission in the post-transfusion setting has not been reduced to zero. HCV can be transmitted from acutely infected donors, since samples of donor blood taken during this "window" period are often negative for anti-HCV. In addition, the transmission of HCV in "sporadic" or "community acquired" hepatitis is often not detected, since transmission occurs outside of hospital settings where screening is not readily available.

While current or past intravenous drug use or a history of blood transfusions were significant risk factors for the transmission of HCV, needle stick exposure among health care workers, tattooing, and acupuncture were also identified as sources of HCV infection (Kaldor et al., 1992; Kolho & Krusius, 1992; van der Poel, 1999) (Table 3.1) (see related question 8 in Ch. 24). The preparation of pooled blood fractions, including immunoglobulins (Meisel et al., 1995) (Ch. 4) and clotting factors (Dodd, 1992; Lee, 1996), also transmitted HCV at a high rate. In addition, some studies showed that sexual promiscuity was a significant risk factor for transmission (Kaldor et al., 1992). This was not independently confirmed (Kolho & Krusius, 1992; van der Poel, 1999), suggesting that another major risk factor, such as unreported current or past intravenous drug abuse, may instead be responsible for transmission in these populations (Kaldor et al., 1992). Sexual transmission from infected women to their spouses has been reported, but the frequency is very low (Meisel et al., 1995; Davis & Kowalik, 1996), suggesting that heterosexual transmission in monogamous relationships is uncommon. Male-to-female transmission has also been documented among women under treatment at clinics for sexually transmitted disease (Thomas et al., 1995).

Transmission has been reported from infected mothers to infants, where HCV RNA has been detected in the blood of exposed infants (Kudesia, Ball & Irving, 1995). The frequency of transmission is quite variable, with some studies reporting no evidence of transmission (Ohto et al., 1994; Zanetti et al., 1995; Fischler et al., 1996), while other studies report up to 40% transmission (Matsubara, Sumazaki & Takita, 1995; Resti et al., 1995; Sabatino et al., 1996). However, the number of cases evaluated in each study was small. Breast-feeding by HCV-infected mothers does not seem to be an important source of transmission to their offspring (Zanetti et al., 1995). However, the risk of transmission was significantly increased in HIV-coinfected mothers (Ohto et al., 1994; Zanetti et al., 1995). Hence, there are a variety of risk factors other than blood transfusions and intravenous drug abuse that contribute to HCV transmission (Table 3.1).

Prior to the discovery of HCV, the most common route of transmission was percutaneous, while after the deployment of second- and third-generation anti-HCV detection tests, intravenous drug abuse became the most predominant means of transmission. In fact, intravenous drug abuse accounts for up to 60% of the HCV transmission that currently occurs in the United States (CDC, 1998). Another 10–20% of HCV is transmitted sexually, while roughly 5–10% of HCV is transmitted to health care workers during occupational exposure (CDC, 1998). With regard to occupational exposure, HCV RNA has been detected in cerebrospinal fluid, ascites, semen, saliva, and in tears (Liou et al., 1992; Chen et al., 1995; Fiore et al., 1995; Mendel et al., 1997). Experimentally, HCV has been transmitted to a single chimpanzee by intravenous innoculation of saliva (Abe & Inchauspe, 1991), but it is not known whether any of the other fluids contain infectious virus. As mentioned in Table 3.1, needlestick exposure and contaminated supplies or instruments may also be sources of HCV infection for the health care worker.

3.1 Seroprevalence and burden of infection

As outlined earlier in this chapter, an estimated 0.5–1.5% of the world's population appears to be infected with HCV (Purcell, 1994), with the actual percentage varying among different countries. This translates into an estimated 170 million chronically infected people worldwide who are at high risk for the development of hepatitis, cirrhosis and HCC (Bradley et al., 1983; Choo et al., 1989; Houghton, 1996; Delwaide & Gerard, 2000; Wild & Hall, 2000) (Ch. 6). In the United States, the incidence of acute, symptomatic NANBH fell from an average of approximately 15 in 100 000 transfusions during the 1980s to approximately 3 in 100 000 by 1995 (Alter, 1993a) with the introduction of anti-HCV testing. This corresponded to an estimated 230 000 acute infections per year in the mid-1980s, which fell to approximately 28 000 new infections by 1995 and 36 000 in 1996 (Alter, 1997;

CDC, 1998). However, given that the largest group of infected people are 30–49 years of age (McQuillan et al., 1997), the lengthy asymptomatic phase of chronic HCV infection, and the continued high incidence of intravenous drug abuse, it is expected that the burden of disease will increase in the coming years. Recent serological surveys in the United States have shown an estimated 1.8% of the general population, or nearly 4 million people, are chronically infected with HCV (McQuillan et al., 1997). CLD is the tenth leading cause of death in the United States, resulting in approximately 25 000 or 1% of deaths annually (Dufour, 1994). Among these, 8000–10 000 have been attributed to HCV (CDC, 1998). It is estimated that the health care costs of those with chronic HCV infection is up to a billion dollars per year (CDC, 1998). This does not include the costs for liver transplantation for those with end-stage liver disease (cirrhosis) or HCC associated with HCV. Given that HCV frequently establishes chronic infections with an associated high risk for the development of hepatitis, cirrhosis, and HCC, and that there are few treatment options, this underscores the magnitude of the public health problem and disease burden associated with this virus infection.

3.2 Genotypes and subtypes

Sequence analysis of the full-length HCV genome from many isolates worldwide has shown a consistent genetic organization in the number and position of the UTRs, the structural, and the nonstructural proteins of the virus (Fig. 2.1). However, no two full-length isolates have exactly the same sequence, and comparison of clones from different parts of the world (Kato et al., 1990; Choo et al., 1991b; Chan et al., 1992; Mori et al., 1992; Okamoto et al., 1992b) has resulted in their grouping into broad categories called genotypes. There are six genotypes of HCV (1–6) so far identified, based upon sequence differences in the E1, NS4, core (Bukh, Purcell & Miller, 1993, 1994; Bhattacherjee et al., 1995), and NS5 regions (Enomoto et al., 1990; Chan et al., 1992) (Table 3.2). Clones that make up each genotype have < 70% overall homology with clones that make up a separate genotype (Simmonds et al., 1993). Genetic heterogeneity within each genotype is designated as subtypes (a, b, c, . . .), where clones within each subtype typically have 70–85% homology (Table 3.2). The dominant subtype in a geographic region or in an individual is referred to as 1a, 1b, 2a, etc. Although this standard nomenclature was adopted to distinguish various genotypes and subtypes, not all new isolates of HCV fit into these categories (Tokita et al., 1994, 1995, 1996), suggesting that the genetic complexity of HCV is greater than currently appreciated. Even with these limitations, epidemiological studies have shown that subtypes 1a, 1b, 2a, 2b, and 3a have a worldwide distribution (Bukh, Miller & Purcell, 1995). However, subtypes 1a and 1b are predominant in North and South

Table 3.2. Sequence heterogeneity in hepatitis C virus

Features	Characteristics
Mutation rate	Approximately 1.4×10^{-3} to 1.9×10^{-3} base substitutions/nucleotide per year; this is similar to RNA viruses and contributes importantly to the sequence heterogeneity of HCV
	The high rate of mutation reflects misincorporation of bases during replication and the lack of proofreading by RNA–dependent RNA polymerase (RdRp)
Genotypes	There are at least six major genotypes of HCV (1–6) worldwide; distinct genotypes have < 70% homology overall
	Each genotype has two or more subtypes (a,b,c, etc.); distinct subtypes are 70–85% homologous overall
Quasispecies	Each subtype often has multiple quasispecies that are > 98% homologous within a single patient
	Quasispecies in chronic HCV infections are characterized by sequence heterogeneity in the amino-terminal hypervariable region (HVR1) of E2, which is thought to be a major neutralizing determinant
Microheterogeneity	Sequence microheterogeneity has also been reported within the interferon sensitivity-determining region (ISDR) of NS5A (HVR2), which may contribute to the responsiveness of HCV to interferon treatment
	Sequence heterogeneity in other regions of the HCV genome have been described, but their impact upon the virus life cycle and/or outcome of infection remains to be examined

America as well as Europe (Bukh et al., 1993). Subtype 1b is predominant in most Asian countries (Bukh et al., 1993; Cho et al., 1993; Chen et al., 1994; Hadiwandowo et al., 1994), whereas subtype 1c has been found only in Indonesia (Hotta et al., 1994), and subtype 3b in Japan, Thailand, Nepal, and Indonesia (Doi et al., 1994). Interestingly, genotype 4 is predominant in northern and central Africa (Bukh et al., 1993, 1994; McOmish et al., 1994; Xu et al., 1994), while genotype 5 is predominant in southern Africa (Bukh et al., 1993, 1994). When the sequences for all of the available HCV clones are compared, the differences show that the major genotypes diverged within the past 100–200 years, with many of the subtypes appearing within the past half century. While these calculations are only estimates, it is significant that blood transfusions have really only been widely used in the twentieth century, and that prior to the establishment of HCV screening, this was a major route for transmission and spread, which in turn may have contributed to greater sequence diversity.

The clinical significance of genotype and subtype sequence variation and their varied geographical distribution is not known. However, there is an increasing consensus that genotype 1 is more resistant to IFN treatment than genotypes 2 and 3 (Yoshioka et al., 1992; Martinot-Peignoux et al., 1995) (Ch. 9). These same studies also point out that IFN responsiveness is inversely related to pretreatment virus titer. For these reasons, HCV quantification and genotyping by molecular diagnostic laboratories is becoming more widespread, although the reliability of the various assays for genotyping and subtyping are limited (Chs. 19 and 20). There have also been reports that some HCV genotypes may be more virulent (Pozzato et al., 1994; Feray et al., 1995), with subtype 1b being associated with a higher frequency of elevated transaminases and a higher frequency of cirrhosis compared with other subtypes (Nousbaum et al., 1995; Silini et al., 1995). These observations, however, have not been independently confirmed (Mita et al., 1994; Yamada et al., 1994a; Zeuzem et al., 1996), suggesting that other factors may also contribute to the outcome of chronic infection (Brechot, 1994).

Although most individuals are infected with a single subtype, different virus particles within a single infection have slightly different sequences. This sequence microheterogeneity within a single subtype is referred to as quasispecies (Ogata et al., 1991; Martell et al., 1992). Quasispecies are >98% homologous and are characteristic of HCV infections. Most of the sequence microheterogeneity that defines quasispecies is localized in two hypervariable regions (HVR): the first within the E2 region (HVR1) and the second within the NS5A region (HVR2), although mutations have been documented throughout the HCV genome (Table 3.2 and Ch. 20). This genetic heterogeneity may permit the development of neutralization (in E1 and E2) and cytotoxic T lymphocyte (CTL) escape mutants (in core), the development of drug resistance (in NS5A and NS5B), the development of altered cell tropism (in E1 and E2), and may give rise to mutants with differing replicative fitness and/or pathological potential (Gomez et al., 1999) (see related question 9 in Ch. 24). Overall, the appearance of quasispecies is a mechanism of adaptation used by a number of RNA viruses, including HIV, that promotes the development and persistence of chronic infections in the face of multiple and persistent attempts by the immune system to eliminate the virus.

In the absence of a consistently productive tissue culture system, the actual mutation rate for HCV cannot be accurately calculated. Instead, the stable mutations that accumulate over time during infection, or "fixed mutation rates", have been reported (Ogata et al., 1991; Okamoto et al., 1992b) (Table 3.2). Although the rates for HCV are similar to those for retroviruses (Domingo & Holland, 1994), they are not evenly distributed along the HCV genome. For example, the lowest frequency of mutations has been consistently reported in the 5' UTR. The integrity and secondary/tertiary structures of the 5' UTR and the IRES are important for correct polyprotein initiation and for viral replication (Sections 2.3 and 2.5). The highly conserved 5' UTR among subtypes has also been exploited in the laboratory for the consistent detection of HCV RNA in clinical samples (Garson et al., 1990; Okamoto et al., 1990) (Ch. 18). Similarly, the low prevalence of mutations affecting NS3 is consistent with its protease, helicase, and NTPase activities being central to the life cycle of HCV (Sections 2.4 and 2.5). In contrast, high rates of fixed mutations have been reported in the amino-terminal portion of the E2 region that spans the HVR1 (Okamoto et al., 1992a; Bukh et al., 1995). In the case of E2 (and E1 as well), many of the mutations result in altered amino acid sequence (nonsynonymous or nonconserved mutations), while a similar high rate of mutation within the NS2 region resulted in few changes on the amino acid level (synonymous or conserved mutations). Significantly, acute infections that are characterized by nonsynonymous mutations in E1, but few nonsynonymous mutations in E2, are much more likely to result in viral clearance than acute infections in which the nonsynonymous mutations are low in E1 compared with E2 (Ray et al., 1999). This suggests that the immune responses against E1, and the appearance of E1 mutations, are associated with virus clearance, whereas immune responses against the HVR1 sequences in E2 are not. Variability in the fixed mutation rate has also been seen in other regions of the HCV genome, although the significance of most other mutations to viral replication and the outcome of infection are uncertain. For example, the frequency of the fixed mutations in the genes for envelope and NS2 is more than fivefold higher than that observed within core and NS3. While the envelope mutants of HCV may provide escape from neutralization (Weiner et al., 1992; Farci et al., 1994), the impact of most naturally occurring mutations upon the biology and replication of the virus is unknown. It appears that highly mutated regions may not be essential to the virus life cycle, and their selection may be immune driven. Alternatively, regions that are highly conserved do not tolerate mutations because they encode functions required for binding to cellular proteins and/or for the virus life cycle (Domingo & Holland, 1994). These conserved regions are and will continue to be exploited as targets for antiviral drug development (Chs. 16 and 17). In the end, the genetic variability of HCV permits competition among quasispecies that insures the survival of the virus under a variety of conditions, which may partially explain how such a high proportion of infections become chronic.

Knowledge of the evolution of quasispecies is influenced by a number of factors. These include the viral load in a given patient (Domingo et al., 1996), the region of the genome (Martell et al., 1992; Kurosaki et al., 1995; Cabot et al., 1997), and whether the virus sample was derived from liver, serum, or other tissues (Cabot et al., 1997; Maggi et al., 1997). Other factors are whether the sample came from an acutely or chronically infected patient (Honda et al., 1994; Koizumi et al., 1995) and whether the patient was immunocompetent (Toyoda et al., 1997). The first factor, viral load, is inversely correlated with the amount of replicative space in the liver. Poorly replicating quasispecies will be present in detectable quantities when there is a lot of replicative space (e.g., when there are many uninfected hepatocytes), such as during the early part of acute infection or when a highly replicative quasispecies is eliminated and extra replicative space is created. Detection of quasispecies has been dependent upon the subgenomic region chosen for analysis, since different regions have different fixed mutation rates (Gomez et al., 1999). For this reason, it is difficult to ascribe a particular outcome of natural infection or treatment to the presence of a single or multiple mutations. When such mutations are documented, it is impossible to decide whether they are the cause or the effect of the observed outcome. Interestingly, sequence analysis of HCV in the liver and blood from individual patients revealed qualitative differences (Oshima et al., 1991; Cabot et al., 1997; Maggi et al., 1997). HCV quasispecies from blood have a narrower sequence spectrum relative to liver-derived sequences from the same patient (Cabot et al., 1997). These findings suggest that only a fraction of the liver-derived HCV RNA species are replication competent and are preferentially packaged. Replication-deficient genomes that become packaged may act as defective interfering particles in the next round of infection within the chronically infected liver. Some mutants that are less hardy than wild-type HCV may replicate inside the cell at the expense of the wild-type virus, possibly decreasing the overall titer of virus produced. If HCV exhibits limited cytopathology, as discussed in Section 5.1, then the downregulation of overall virus titer by defective interfering particles that do not replicate well or at all in the absence of wild-type virus may effectively limit HCV-associated cytopathic effects (Kirkwood & Bangham, 1994) (Section 5.1). This hypothesis has been supported by the finding of defective genomes in serum from chronically infected individuals (Martell et al., 1992; Higashi et al., 1993).

The differential distribution of quasispecies in liver compared with serum (Cabot et al., 1997) is also mirrored by differences in the CTL specificities at these same anatomical locations (Koziel & Walker, 1997). Assuming that individual virus mutants demonstrate different levels of virus gene expression and replication, immunological priming in the liver may be against different viral epitopes than priming in the periphery. Since most T cells are primed at extrahepatic sites (e.g., lymph nodes), these primed cells may not have the appropriate specificity to recognize and eliminate intrahepatic HCV efficiently (Rehermann & Chisari, 2000). Given that NS5B has no proofreading function (Holland et al., 1992; Mizokami, Gojobori & Lau, 1994), which contributes to the high mutation rate of HCV (Table 3.2), it is not surprising that this activity could result in the appearance of many replication defective genomes or subgenomic fragments during infection. It is proposed that highly replicating variants of HCV will also express higher levels of intrahepatic virus antigens, which, in turn, will attract more virus-specific CTL. This will result in more severe liver disease, which is accompanied by a higher rate of hepatocellular turnover. Since the majority of virus appears to result from *de novo* infection and turnover of infected cells (Fukumoto et al., 1996), and not by release of virus from chronically infected cells, the changing quasispecies distribution may contribute importantly to the persistance of virus and progression of CLD (Ch. 5). This suggests that the increased number of quasispecies among people who develop chronic infection (Honda et al., 1994) may provide the viral genetic diversity which contributes importantly to repeated bouts of liver disease during chronic infection. In other words, the genetic diversity and associated replicative fitness of various quasispecies will influence the amplitude and specificity of the corresponding immune responses, and in doing so, will influence the severity and progression of CLD. Since diversity of quasispecies increases with time following acute infection, it is not surprising that strong and rapid cell-mediated immune responses against multiple HCV antigens are characteristic of acute, resolving hepatitis. During acute infection, the diversity of quasispecies is often quite limited, and appropriate immune responses would prevent the appearance of escape mutants.

Having said this, some studies have shown a clear relationship between quasispecies diversity and liver disease (Hayashi et al., 1997; Yuki et al., 1997), while others have not (Naito et al., 1995). While the basis for these differences remain to be explained, it is clear that there are different virus variants in the liver compared with serum (Cabot et al., 1997). In addition, liver disease correlates with intrahepatic but not serum levels of virus (Gonzalez-Peralta, Davis & Lau, 1994a). These observations suggest that the relationship between quasispecies diversity and liver disease will be better understood by studying the virus dynamics within the target organ.

3.3 Prevention of infection

Prior to the discovery of HCV, the incidence of NANBH was reduced by up to 50% by the use of surrogate markers for infection (anti-HBc and ALT) (Section 1.3) and by the regular screening of blood samples for HIV (Alter et al., 1990; Donahue et al., 1992). The introduction of effective procedures to inactivate viruses in pooled concentrates of factor VIII and factor IX (Manucci et al., 1990, 1992; Mosley, 1992) also contributed importantly to the dramatic reduction of HCV transmission among hemophiliacs and other patients who needed to have multiple transfusions on a regular basis. Hence, inroads were made into the prevention of HCV infection even prior to the discovery of the virus.

The single most important advance that helped to prevent HCV infection was the implementation of widespread anti-HCV testing of donated blood, and the demonstration that up to 90% of patients with NANB PTH were infected with HCV (Kuo et al., 1989; Esteban et al., 1990; Donahue et al., 1992; Alter et al., 1989a) (Section 1.5). The increased sensitivity and specificity of the second- and third-generation anti-HCV assays has almost totally eliminated PTH associated with HCV (Barrera et al., 1995b; Lee et al., 1995; Schreiber et al., 1996b), although blood donated during the "window" period of acute infection (prior to the appearance of anti-HCV) still transmits HCV in 1 in 100 000 to 1 in 500 000 transfusions (Vrielink et al., 1995; Kitchen, Wallis & Gorman, 1996). HCV RNA has also been a good supplementary test (Ch. 19) to help to exclude infection, especially when a questionnaire or medical history suggests that a prior exposure may have occurred. In the context of blood fractions, special categories of patients have been at particularly high risk for HCV after receiving blood fractions for either prophylactic (e.g., hyperimmune gammaglobulins) or therapeutic (e.g., factor VIII or IX concentrates) purposes. These groups include patients with hemophilia and thalassemia, who often require lifelong transfusions of clotting factors, and patients who are injected with hyperimmune gammaglobulins directly after exposure to some viruses. As the sources of infection were identified, and then eliminated, the risk of these various groups of patients for acquiring infection has diminished greatly. For example, immunoglobulins prepared by alcohol fraction have not been shown to transmit HCV (Rousell et al., 1991). Likewise, pasteurization and detergent treatment of blood clotting fractions have almost totally eliminated the risk of HCV transmission to hemophiliacs (Mauser-Bunschoten et al., 1995). Patients requiring hemodialysis also used to be at high risk for the development of HCV infections through use of the same dialysis machines (Allander et al., 1994; de Lamballerie et al., 1996) (Table 3.1), although the allocation of anti-HCV-positive and anti-HCV-negative patients to different machines has significantly reduced the transmission of HCV (Blumberg, Zehnder & Burckhardt, 1995). The transmission of HCV by health care personnel using the same gloves or using the same instruments on multiple patients also used to be an important source of transmission, but this has now been eliminated given vigorous application of universal precaution practices (Gilli et al., 1995; Okuda et al., 1995). Appropriate disinfection and sterilization of medical and dental instruments used in surgical procedures has also been recommended in preventing the transmission of HCV (Piazza, Borgia & Picciotto, 1995). In the context of organ transplantation, the use of anti-HCV-negative organ and tissue donors has nearly eliminated the transmission of HCV from the transplantation setting (CDC, 1998). Hence, anti-HCV testing has done a remarkable job in the identification of infected sources, which has resulted in the development of meaningful preventative practices in a wide variety of settings.

The identification of intravenous drug abuse as the major cause of acute HCV infections in the United States (Alter, 1990, 1997; Garfein et al., 1998) (Table 3.1) has focused much attention upon the development of preventative measures. These include drug rehabilitation programs, counseling and community service projects that promote the development of low-risk behaviors, and an exchange program that supplies sterile, single-use needles for continued users. Although consistent evidence for the sexual transmission of HCV is lacking, perhaps because of the often low levels of virus present in most infections, individuals with multiple sex partners are at risk for acquiring sexually transmitted diseases, which, in addition to HCV, include HBV, HIV, syphilis, gonorrhea, and chlamydia. Given this reality, such individuals should be advised to (i) limit the number of sexual partners or abstain from having sex, (ii) use condoms consistently, and (iii) be offered HBV and, in some cases, HAV vaccines (CDC, 1998). Among patients on renal dialysis, the finding that HCV incidence correlates with increasing years on dialysis, and not with blood transfusions (Niu et al., 1992; Niu, Coleman & Alter, 1993), implies that transmission may be a result of incorrect practices in the sharing of medication vials and supplies (Favero & Alter, 1996). The assignment of patients to specific dialysis stations, the use of ancillary equipment (trays, clamps, scissors, etc.) that is not shared, and the use of properly sterilized or single-use supplies has gone far to reduce the transmission of HCV in dialysis units. The more rigorous adoption of universal precautions against blood-borne pathogens through educational programs for physicians and support staff has also been important in eliminating the transmission of HCV in hemodialysis and other settings. This additional awareness has reduced other types of nosocomial and occupational exposure to both patients and staff within the hospital as well as in home nursing settings. The practice of universal precautions in the United States outside of the hospital setting has also reduced the incidence of HCV transmission from tattooing, body piercing, and acupuncture, for example, to undetectable levels (Alter et al., 1982, 1989b), although HCV transmission is still associated with these practices in several other parts of the world (Mansell & Locarnini, 1995; Sun et al., 1996). Hence, many steps have been taken that have successfully reduced the risk of HCV transmission.

In this context, the Centers for Disease Control and Prevention in the United States (CDC) has recently compiled a list of recommendations aimed at the prevention and control of HCV. Among the *primary* activities for preventing HCV infection, the CDC recommends the screening and testing of blood and blood fractions, as well as tissue and semen samples, for HCV and the regular inactivation of blood fractions prior to use. These recommendations also include the implementation of counseling aimed at the identification and reduction of behavioral and environmental risk factors and the adoption of infection control measures based upon universal precautions against blood-borne pathogens (CDC, 1998). In addition, the CDC has outlined *secondary* prevention activities aimed at reducing risk for the development of CLD and other chronic diseases in HCV-infected patients. These activities involve the identification of infected patients at risk for disease, as well as the counseling and treatment of such patients, the development of professional and public education, and monitoring both disease trends and prevention methods as a foundation for future improvement of these activities (CDC, 1998). Among the people who should be tested for HCV (Table 3.1), those with current or past intravenous drug use, those receiving clotting factor concentrates prior to 1987, those on long-term renal dialysis, and those with unexplained elevated transaminases clearly qualify. In addition, individuals who received a transfusion of blood or blood fractions, an organ transplant prior to July 1992, or who received a transfusion from a donor who later tested positive for anti-HCV should be tested for HCV. Further, medical personnel exposed to HCV and children born to HCV-positive mothers should also be tested since both groups are at risk for the development of CLD if they test HCV positive (CDC, 1998). Finally, perhaps the most difficult group of all includes individuals who had used intravenous drugs several decades ago and do not consider themselves at risk for HCV infection. The testing algorithm used by physicians encountering this group of patients, most of whom are asymptomatic, is presented in Fig. 1.2.

An important goal of epidemiological studies is to improve the public health surveillance of HCV in order to identify new cases of infection and to determine disease incidence and trends. Surveillance will not only depend upon the continued availability of anti-HCV testing and, where applicable, HCV RNA determination but also upon the identification of acute infections and the sources of such infections by local and regional public health departments. The further development of registries of HCV-infected patients will also be valuable for counseling and medical follow-up at the individual level, and for better assessment of the incidence of infection and natural history of HCV infection at regional and national levels. The conduct of serological surveys on a local and regional basis will be important for monitoring the geographical incidence of infection and disease, for assessing the quality of prevention programs, for identifying risk factors (and their relative importance over time), and for assessing the impact of therapeutics upon the burden, incidence, and distribution of chronic disease (CDC, 1998).

4

Natural history of infection

Prior to the discovery of HCV, a series of studies in patients with acute NANB PTH (which was mostly caused by HCV) (Hopf et al., 1990; Di Bisceglie et al., 1991; Tremolada et al., 1992; Koretz et al., 1993a,b; Mattsson, Sonnerborg & Weiland, 1993) showed that only 4–13% of 406 patients became symptomatic over an 8–14 year follow-up. Histologically defined cirrhosis was identified in 8–24% of patients, and HCC was observed in 0.7–1.3%. While these studies did not provide a longer follow-up, they did help to establish a link between NANB PTH, cirrhosis, and HCC. Independent observations in HCV-infected patients with chronic hepatitis who were followed for 4–11 years (Roberts, Searle & Cooksley, 1993; Takahashi et al., 1993; Yano et al., 1993) revealed cirrhosis in 8–46% and HCC in 11–19%. In these studies, however, the time and duration of infection were not known. Additional longitudinal studies among patients chronically infected with HCV, where the time of transmission through transfusion was known, estimated that chronic hepatitis developed within 10 years of transfusion, cirrhosis by 21 years, and HCC by 29 years (Kiyosawa et al., 1990). Some patients developed HCC only after 40–50 years of infection. These results were independently confirmed (Tong et al., 1995) and highlight both the protracted asymptomatic phase of infection, lasting for 10–20 years, and the seriousness of the sequelae. By comparison, clinical observations have shown that cirrhosis could appear several years after infection. Hence, the clinical spectrum of chronic HCV infection is variable and the course of disease development unpredictable.

An outbreak of HCV infection associated with transmission from contaminated lots of anti-D immunoglobulin (Rho-gam) in the 1970s has provided a rare opportunity to document further the natural history of HCV PTH, since the time of infection was known with certainty. In this case, 417 (0.8%) of 53 178 recipients of immunoglobulin later seroconverted to anti-HCV. After 17 years of follow-up with 232 of these patients, liver biopsy specimens showed that 55% had mild liver disease, 38% had mild-to-moderate disease, and 68% had severe disease (Crowe et al., 1995). Less than 5% of infected patients had evidence of fibrosis or early cirrhosis, suggesting very slow progression of disease in this population. Another outbreak of HCV, again from contaminated lots of immunoglobulin, resulted in the appearance of anti-HCV in 160 out of 2533 treated patients (Dittmann et al.,

1991). Of the anti-HCV-reactive patients, 54% developed chronic hepatitis within a 10-year follow-up, again suggesting that HCV-associated CLD takes many years to develop. Given that chronic infection and disease are often asymptomatic for up to 20 years postinfection, and the majority of chronic infections today are increasingly the result of previous drug abuse, it is likely that the HCV-related morbidity will increase in the coming years as these infections become symptomatic. Hence, despite the elimination of most HCV from the blood supply, it is expected that the frequency of HCV will increase for the foreseeable future. Since the evolution to cirrhosis is central to increased morbidity and mortality (Niederau et al., 1998), a major question remains as to whether most or all chronically infected patients progress on to cirrhosis (Seeff, 1998).

Studies at the National Heart, Lung and Blood Institute from 1968 to 1980 in the United States evaluated the incidence of NANB PTH in patients following transfusion(s) given at the time of cardiac surgery. After an 18 year follow-up, there was a small but significant difference in the mortality of acutely infected patients compared with controls (Seeff et al., 1992). Among the patients with NANB PTH, approximately one-third developed mild symptoms of acute NANBH, another third developed chronic hepatitis, as judged by sustained elevated transaminases, while the remainder also had chronic infection. This last group also had persistent viral RNA in the blood but normal or near normal transaminases. Among those chronically infected, morbidity and mortality was low, with the exception of those diagnosed with cirrhosis. In addition, the frequency of progression, if any, from biopsy-proven chronic hepatitis to cirrhosis was uncertain. Most of the mortality observed was among alcoholics, and further observations showed that mortality was also caused by liver failure among patients with cirrhosis or HCC (Tong et al., 1995). The cirrhosis-related mortality was so high (> 50%) that HCV-associated end-stage liver disease has become the most common indication for liver transplantation in the United States. Other studies, however, have shown that HCV infection could follow a more benign course, with cirrhosis developing in only 10% of patients over 20 years (Crowe et al., 1995). Similar results have been reported elsewhere (Fattovich et al., 1997). Therefore, these longer-term follow-up studies have further established that variability is a key element in the natural history of chronic HCV-associated liver disease.

While the elements that promote disease progression remain to be clearly established, the viral dose, quasispecies, and/or genotype may have an impact upon the severity and progression of CLD. The contribution of viral dose is uncertain, since the frequency of chronic hepatitis in groups with parenterally transmitted virus (i.e., transmitted in a high volume of transfused blood) is similar to frequencies calculated from populations with a low rate of parenteral transmission (Alter et al., 1992). With regard to virus genotype, there are some data to suggest that genotype 1b is associated with more severe liver disease than genotype 1a or 2 (Dusheiko et al., 1994). However, independent observations failed to see any relationship between genotype and disease severity (Romeo et al., 1996b). As mentioned in Section 3.2, the diversity of quasispecies decreased in acutely infected patients who went on to resolve disease, while it remained the same in those who developed mild liver disease. Diversity of quasispecies increased in patients who developed severe chronic hepatitis (Farci et al., 1996a; Hayashi et al., 1997). Hence, quasispecies diversity is likely to contribute significantly to the natural history of infection.

There is some evidence to suggest that the natural history of infection is dependent upon age at infection, since individuals older than 55 years appear to develop more severe liver disease than younger persons with the same duration of infection (Poynard, Bedosa & Opolon, 1997; Garcia-Monzon et al., 1998). In addition, it is now well documented that HBV coinfection increases both the severity of CLD (Fong et al., 1991a) and the risk of developing HCC (Benvegnu et al., 1994). Although there is also convincing evidence that in coinfected individuals HCV suppresses HBV replication (Liaw et al., 1998), the recent detection of "cryptic" HBV infections in HCV-associated HCC (Liang et al., 1993; Paterlini et al., 1993) and the observation that the HBV-encoded X antigen (HBxAg) alone contributes centrally to the development of HCC (Diamantis et al., 1992; Paterlini et al., 1995; Feitelson & Duan, 1997; Tamori et al., 1999) suggest an explanation for the increased risk of HCC in coinfections. In addition to HBV, HIV coinfection of HCV-positive patients appears to exacerbate HCV-associated hepatitis (Thomas et al., 1996) and cirrhosis (Soto et al., 1997) (Table 4.1 and Ch. 14). This is consistent with the finding that CD4$^+$ helper T cell (Th cells) function, which is compromised in HIV infection, is important for the control of HCV (Gerlach et al., 1999) (Section 5.4), resulting in increased HCV gene expression and replication. Independent observations that the levels of HCV RNA correlated well with the severity of liver disease (Alberti et al., 1992; Lau et al., 1993; Prieto et al., 1995) may contribute to the understanding of the HCV/HIV-1 relationship. Finally, there is accumulating evidence that chronic alcoholism greatly exacerbates HCV-associated CLD (Rosman et al., 1993; Koff & Dienstag, 1995), in part, by stimulating HCV replication (Sawada et al., 1993; Oshita et al., 1994). In fact, alcohol exacerbates CLD so much that the National Institutes of Health (NIH) consensus statement strongly discourages alcohol consumption among any chronically infected patients (NIH, 1997). In summary, the outcome of HCV infection depends upon a variety of interacting parameters, with considerable variability in the development of disease and in clinical outcome.

The high morbidity and mortality associated with cirrhosis has prompted investigations aimed at identifying the host and virus factors that are most closely

Table 4.1. Host factors that contribute to the development of cirrhosis in hepatitis C infection

---

Parenteral transmission of hepatitis C virus

Chronic alcoholism (> 50 g/day)

Male gender

Age (> 50 years when infected)

Lack of specific HL-A haplotypes

Diabetes

Hemophilia

Coinfection with hepatitis B virus or human immunodeficiency virus

Immunosuppression

From Minuk (1999)

linked to the development of end-stage liver disease. These include the acquisition of HCV by blood transfusion, the presence of HBsAg, and chronic alcoholism (Minuk, 1999) (Table 4.1). As mentioned above, the mean time for the development of cirrhosis following infection was significantly faster in patients older than 50 years compared with younger patients. The same age-related trend was observed for HCC (Tong et al., 1995). The reasons for the age-related increase in disease intensity may have to do with an age-related increasing propensity to sustain hepatocellular damage, coupled with a decreased ability to repair damage during and after a bout of liver disease. In addition, the regenerative ability of mature hepatocytes decreases with age (Gupta, 2000). Interestingly, men were more likely to be positive for HCV RNA and antibodies, as well as for elevated ALT, than were women, suggesting that women may resolve infection more often than men (Yamakawa et al., 1996). This may be a result of generally stronger female immune responses against the virus and also because estrogens decrease the expression of transforming growth factor (TGF) beta 1 ($TGF\beta_1$), which promotes fibrogenesis (Sporn & Roberts, 1989). Hence, decreased virus load resulting from strong immunity, coupled with decreased fibrogenic potential, may significantly reduce the development of cirrhosis in females relative to males. There is also evidence that some HL-A haplotypes are present in people who are more likely to clear virus (Cramp et al., 1998) whereas patients with hemophilia have, reportedly, more severe liver disease than those without (Bianchi et al., 1987). Among diabetics, the frequency of anti-HCV is almost fivefold that of nondiabetics (Simo et al., 1996), and disease is reportedly more severe; however, the underlying mechanisms for these associations remain to be elucidated. Significantly, HCV-infected patients with cirrhosis are likely to be moderate or heavy alcohol drinkers, while patients without cirrhosis, on average, consume little or no alcohol (Serfaty et al., 1997; Wiley et al., 1998), underscoring alcohol as an important cofactor in the development of cirrhosis. These observations are consistent with the findings that the immunosuppressive properties of alcohol often result in increased virus load (Corrao & Arico, 1998; Ostapowicz et al., 1998) and that increased virus load often correlates with increased disease severity. In addition, the hepatotoxic effects of ethanol in the liver inhibit regeneration during CLD (Diehl, Chacon & Wagner, 1988) and ethanol may promote fibrogenesis by activating stellate cells in the liver, which then produce and secrete collagen (Mezey et al., 1977). Hence, the natural history of HCV infection is significantly influenced by a variety of genetic and environmental factors.

The chimpanzee model has contributed centrally to a better understanding of the natural history of NANBH and, later, HCV infection (Section 1.2 and Ch. 13). This is because the timespan of the infection, the characteristics of the inoculum, and the time of experimental infection are known in this system. In addition, HCV infection of chimpanzees has many of the same characteristics as HCV infection in human populations (Table 4.2). For example, years before the discovery of HCV, it was established that NANB-infected chimpanzees developed persistent viremia and disease (Bradley et al., 1981, 1982) similar to that observed in patients (Koretz, Suffin & Gitnick, 1976). Experimentally infected chimpanzees developed detectable intrahepatic HCV RNA by day 2 postinfection, followed by the consistent detection of HCV RNA in blood by day 7, then by acute hepatitis (elevated ALT) by day 14, and finally by histological resolution of disease (Shindo et al., 1992). Follow-up studies showed that acute hepatitis remained resolved for 2–3 years in some animals, but intermittent or persistent ALT elevations indicated chronic infection in others. Further work showed persistent viremia in chimpanzees in the absence of elevated ALT (Tabor, Seeff & Gerety, 1980; Bradley et al., 1981, 1982). The transmission of NANBH from chimpanzees who had been infected but had normal transaminases to other "naive" chimpanzees demonstrated that virus could be transmitted from a "disease free" animal. The development of a "silent" infection in some of the recipients confirmed that the NANBH agent could establish subclinical infections in chimpanzees (Bradley, 2000) similar to that in people (Lee, 1993). The reappearance of disease in chimpanzees that had recovered from acute hepatitis showed that the resolution of disease was not necessarily predictive of the outcome of infection (Bradley et al., 1981). Infected chimpanzees were also susceptible to the same or heterogeneous virus inoculum, suggesting that the immunity generated during infection was not protective (Section 1.2 and Ch. 14). These observations not only outline the challenges for vaccine development but also, in combination with other results, demonstrate that variability in outcome is a hallmark of NANBH and HCV infections.

The natural history of acute exposure to HCV results in two major outcomes

Table 4.2. Features of hepatitis C (HCV) infection shared between experimentally infected chimpanzees and naturally infected patients

Aspects of infection	Common features
Acute infection	Necroinflammation in liver
	Elevated serum alanine aminotransferase (ALT)
	Ultrastructural alterations in hepatocytes (proliferation of endoplasmic reticulum)
	Focal degeneration of hepatocytes
	Bile duct alterations
	Portal tract inflammation (possible lymphoid aggregates)
	Hepatic inflammation and injury occur prior to elevations in ALT
Chronic infection[a]	Hepatitis in chimpanzees resembles chronic persistent hepatitis in humans, with sinusoidal cell proliferation, focal necrosis, and portal inflammation
	Frequency of persistent infection is 70% of acutely infected humans and chimpanzees
Virus replication and gene expression	Virus replication precedes the onset of acute hepatitis by several weeks (virus replication detected by in situ hybridization in liver and by reverse transcriptase/polymerase chain reaction in serum within days of experimental infection; acute hepatitis usually takes 7–10 weeks to appear)
	Immunohistochemical detection of viral antigens in the liver during the acute phase
	Decrease in viremia at the onset of elevations of ALT
	Virus titers vary over a 4–6 log range
	Virus circulates as quasispecies
	HCV mutation rates 1.44×10^{-3} to 1.92×10^{-3} base substitutions/genome site/year
Virus-associated immune responses	Seroconversion to C 100 (clone located in nonstructural proteins 3 and 4) several weeks to months postinfection
	Seroconversion in third-generation antibody test occurs at 15–20 weeks postexposure
	Persistent infection established despite appearance of antibodies to most viral proteins
	Envelope antibodies that appear during infection are partially neutralizing
	Both chimpanzees and patients are susceptible to reinfection or superinfection even by homologous strains of HCV; this implies that cell-mediated immune responses are weak

Table 4.2. (cont.)

Aspects of infection	Common features
	No relationship between virus replication and elevation in ALT values
	Concentrations of virus in blood increase upon treatment with cytotoxic or immunosuppressive drugs
	CD8$^+$ T cells have been detected in peripheral blood and liver in chronically infected humans and chimpanzees; these are usually detected against one or two virus epitopes in a given infection
	Cytotoxic T cell (CTL) clones to HCV antigenic determinants are few (i.e., low frequency) and do not correlate with disease
	Strong CTL responses sometimes observed transiently during acute infection

From Walker (1997)

[a] The natural history is such that liver pathology progresses in human infections (from chronic persistent hepatitis and chronic active hepatitis to cirrhosis to hepatocellular carcinoma) but not in chimpanzees (mostly chronic persistent hepatitis). In human infections, progression has been observed to occur over as long a period as several decades to as short a period as 5 years (Seeff, 1995).

(Fig. 4.1). In most patients, acute infection results in the appearance of HCV in the blood by 1–2 weeks postexposure (Alter et al., 1990; Farci et al., 1991). In these cases, the HCV RNA genome is detected by RT/PCR (Houghton et al., 1991; Gretch et al., 1995b). By 7 weeks postexposure, up to 30% of infected patients develop clinical symptoms (Ch. 8), while the rest are subclinical, although nearly all have elevated serum ALT levels, reflecting liver cell damage. Anti-HCV usually develops during the peak of ALT and persists for many years. Acute hepatitis usually resolves in 2–12 weeks and is signaled by clearance of HCV RNA from blood, the return of serum ALT to normal levels, and the disappearance of symptoms (Hoofnagle, 1997). Unfortunately, the resolution of acute infection occurs in only about 15% of patients (Fig. 4.2 and Ch. 8).

In up to 85% of acutely infected patients, ALT levels remain elevated and HCV RNA persists in blood (Alter et al., 1989a; Farci et al., 1991; Mattsson et al., 1993) (Figs. 4.1 and 4.2). However, the persistence of HCV viremia, rather than elevated ALT, best predicts the development of histologically proven CLD among chronically infected patients (Alberti et al., 1992). Symptoms usually resolve in acutely symptomatic patients, but liver disease often progresses and becomes more severe with the passage of time (Ch. 8). Most patients remain asymptomatic for 10–30 years, even though they have persistently elevated ALT levels and moderate or severe CLD (Hoofnagle, 1997; Sharara, 1997). For this reason, chronic HCV

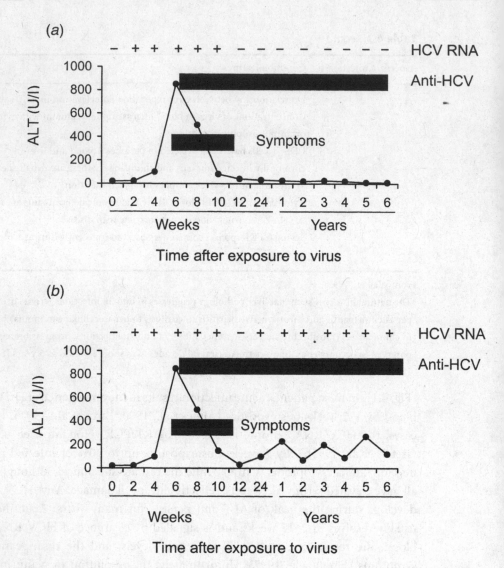

Fig. 4.1.   Natural history of acute (*a*) and chronic (*b*) hepatitis C (HCV) infections. Additional details
are explained in the text. ALT, alanine aminotransferase. (From Hoofnagle (1997) with
permission from W. B. Saunders.)

infection has been dubbed the "silent epidemic" (Lee, 1993). Interestingly, up to
one-third of chronically infected patients with persistent viremia have consistently
normal ALT levels, while ALT levels in others are intermittently elevated (Barrera
et al., 1995a; Conry-Cantilena et al., 1996). Among chronically infected patients
with elevated ALT who become symptomatic (Ch. 8), up to 35% develop cirrhosis
by year 20 after infection, while almost a quarter of chronically infected patients

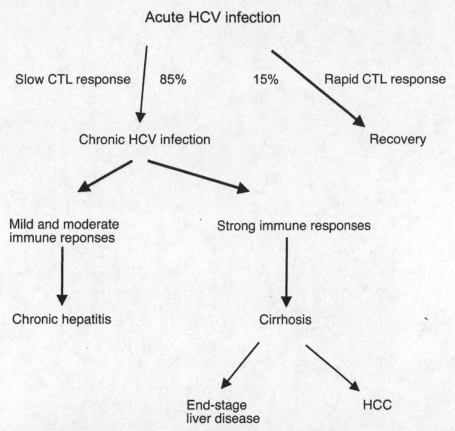

Fig. 4.2.   Hepatitis C (HCV) infection: spectrum of disease and kinetics of immune response. CTL, cytotoxic T lymphocyte; HCC, hepatocellular carcinoma. (Modified from Hoofnagle (1997) with permission from W. B. Saunders.)

develop HCC by year 30 (Kiyosawa et al., 1990; Tong et al., 1995; Sharara, 1997) (Fig. 4.2). Cirrhosis, for example, develops in 10–20% of chronically infected patients over a period of 20–30 years, while HCC appears in 1–5% of patients with cirrhosis per year (Di Bisceglie et al., 1991; Seeff et al., 1992; Fattovich et al., 1997). Factors that predict the severity of CLD have recently been established, with liver disease being more severe among infected alcoholics and when infection occurs in men over the age of 40 years (Poynard et al., 1997) (Table 4.1). There is now strong evidence that even moderate alcohol intake ($>10\,g/day$) promotes the progression of liver disease and the development of HCC (Koff & Dienstag, 1995). These observations underscore the variability in the natural history of infection and highlight the difficulties in assessing the risk that chronically infected patients will develop liver cancer (see Ch. 12 and the related question 10 in Ch. 24).

Pathogenesis of infection

5.1 Is hepatitis C cytopathic?

There are a number of mechanisms whereby HCV could trigger liver cell injury during infection (Table 5.1). Injury could be triggered directly by the virus (i.e., a cytopathic effect) and/or by immune responses against virus-infected cells. HCV-associated liver cell injury could also result from the interactions of HCV with a variety of environmental agents, some of which are mentioned below. Flaviviruses are often cytopathic (Chambers et al., 1990) in that they damage or destroy the cells in which they are growing; consequently it was initially thought that the related HCV might also be cytopathic (Table 5.2). Some evidence has supported such a cytopathic effect whereas other studies have suggested that HCV is not cytopathic. Cell damage was observed with a minimal inflammatory response in monkeys experimentally infected with selected flaviviruses (Monath, 1990). Early studies with NANBH showed cell rounding, shrinkage, and nuclear pyknosis, which are characteristic, cytopathic effects. Damage was also observed in the membranes of mitochrondria and ER (Omata et al., 1981; Dienes et al., 1982). Following the discovery of HCV, it was shown that HCV RNA in the liver, but not in serum, was associated with severe inflammation (Lau et al., 1993). The likelihood that HCV maturation and replication is membrane associated may provide an explanation for the membrane alterations in HCV infection. However, the fact that some chronically infected patients and chimpanzees develop little or no evidence of liver disease despite the persistent replication of virus for many years, and that there is no correlation between virus in the blood and ALT levels, suggests that HCV is not cytopathic (Villa et al., 1991; Sakamoto et al., 1994). This is further supported by the finding that there is no correlation between the presence of virus antigens in the liver and localization or extent of disease activity (Hiramatsu et al., 1992; Krawczynski et al., 1992b). In contrast, other studies have shown a high frequency of histopathology in asymptomatic patients with normal ALT, suggesting that HCV is cytopathic or that underlying immune-mediated liver disease is subclinical (Esteban et al., 1991; Alberti et al., 1992). In addition, tissue culture systems replicating HCV produce low, inconsistent levels of virus, which could be a consequence of HCV-triggered cytopathic effects, leaving only

Table 5.1. Some mechanisms by which liver cell injury can occur in infections with hepatitis C virus (HCV)

Immune mediated killing of HCV-infected cells

Killing of uninfected cells by immune responses to infected cells

Direct cytopathic effects (CPE) of HCV

HLA haplotype of infected host

Virus genetic variation

Multiple viral infections in liver (hepatitis B (HBV) and HCV and human immunodeficiency virus)

Viruses altering sensitivity of liver to drugs, alcohol, etc.

Viruses altering sensitivity of liver to cytokines

Drugs (e.g., ethanol) altering liver cell sensitivity to viruses (e.g., HBV and HCV)

Autoaggressive immune responses triggered by HCV

Drug-induced immunosuppression

Modified from Feitelson (1996) with permission from W. B. Saunders.

cells replicating little or no virus persisting in culture (Table 5.2 and Ch. 11). However, increased levels of HCV are observed in the blood of chimpanzees treated with cytotoxic or immunosuppressive drugs (Krawczynski et al., 1992b) and similar data have been published from patients after liver transplantation (Rice & Walker, 1995; Fukumoto et al., 1996). This would suggest that virus load is, in part, controlled by corresponding antiviral immune responses. During the incubation phase of acute infection, virus replicates in the liver in the absence of abnormal histopathology or elevations in transaminases, suggesting that replication is not directly cytopathic. Yet HCV-associated CLD appears to be more severe in HIV-coinfected hemophiliacs (Eyster et al., 1993; Zylberberg & Pol, 1996), despite the fact that CD4$^+$ T cells, which make up an important component of antiviral immunity (Section 5.4), are depressed in many coinfected individuals. In fact, there appears to be an inverse correlation between CD4$^+$ T cell counts and severity of liver disease among some HCV/HIV-coinfected hemophiliacs (Rockstroh et al., 1996). While this may be a result of variable antiviral immune responses, HCV may be directly cytopathic under these conditions. The finding of severe cholestatic hepatitis in a subset of HCV-infected liver transplant recipients (Schluger et al., 1996; Collier & Heathcote, 1998) is also consistent with the idea that HCV may be directly cytopathic in certain circumstances (Table 5.2). This is also implied by a report that hepatic decompensation occurred more than 20 times more frequently in HCV-infected patients who were coinfected with HIV than in patients who were HIV seronegative (Telfer et al., 1994). Independent observations have also linked HIV/HCV coinfection to the accelerated appearance of cirrhosis and liver failure (Makris et al., 1996). A subset of pathological changes common in chronic HCV infection, including fatty changes (steatosis) (Dienes

Table 5.2. Characteristics of the pathogenesis of hepatitis C (HCV) infection

Effects	Evidence for effects	Evidence against effects
Cytopathic effects	Flaviviruses produce disease by direct cytopathic effects (CPE) Infected immunosuppressed patients sometimes develop severe cholestatic liver disease, which may result in liver failure and death HCV may induce apoptosis in tissue culture cells under certain conditions	There are chronically infected patients with little or no hepatitis Transplant recipients with high virus titers often have normal transaminases More than 60% of infectious volunteer blood donors have normal transaminases Several transgenic mouse models expressing one or more HCV genes do not develop acute or chronic liver injury There is no correlation between intrahepatic HCV antigen expression and disease activity There is no apparent correlation between cytotoxic T lymphocyte (CTL) responses, virus markers, and clinical course of infection
Immune-mediated effects	Recovery from acute infection is associated with a more vigorous proliferative response (from peripheral blood mononuclear cells (PBMC)) to HCV antigens than seen in PBMC from patients who develop chronic infection and disease There is a risk of developing fulminant hepatitis after withdrawal of chemotherapy Immunopathological changes are seen: intralobular and portal inflammation, bile duct damage, activation of macrophages and Kupffer cells, spotty necrosis, cholangitis, cholestasis Intrahepatic lymphoid aggregates correlate with the severity of liver disease HCV-specific CTL can be identified and cloned from liver and PBMC; the combined response to multiple HCV epitopes inversely correlates with virus load In vitro autocytotoxicity is seen using T cells (or T cell clones) as effectors and autologous infected hepatocytes (or HLA-restricted target cell lines) as targets Increased levels of inflammatory cytokines tumor necrosis factor α and β, and interferon α are associated with and may contribute to hepatocellular injury in chronic HCV Strong anti-HCV responses plus poor T helper proliferative responses to HCV antigens are common in patients with chronic hepatitis (T helper type 2); the opposite is common in patients who clear HCV (T helper 1)	

et al., 1982; Lefkowitch & Apfelbaum, 1989) and the development of Mallory bodies within the cytoplasm of periportal hepatocytes (Lefkowitch & Apfelbaum, 1989; Lefkowitch et al., 1993) are also consistent with virus induced cytopathology. The development of steatosis in HCV core transgenic mice (Moriya et al., 1997) (Ch. 11) is also consistent with virus-induced cytopathology, since such mice are tolerant and do not mount immune responses to the HCV core protein. On the cellular level, expression of HCV core antigen alone in several tissue culture cell lines appears to trigger apoptosis (Ruggieri et al., 1997; Zhu et al., 1998; Lu et al., 1999) (Section 5.4), although it is not clear whether this occurs in infected liver. Hence, it is uncertain whether HCV is cytopathic, and if so, under what circumstances.

5.2 Immunopathology

Extensive immunopathological analysis of liver sections from chronically infected patients suggested early on that the pathogenesis of chronic NANBH, and later HCV infection, were likely to be immune mediated (Table 5.2). These features include lymphoid follicles or aggregates, especially within the portal tract region (Lefkowitch & Apfelbaum, 1989; Lefkowitch et al., 1993), bile duct damage (Poulsen & Christoffersen, 1969; Lefkowitch et al., 1993), and activation of sinusoidal inflammatory cells (Dienes et al., 1982). Interestingly, the development of lymphoid follicles or aggregates have also been observed in a variety of autoimmune diseases, some of which are associated with chronic HCV infection (Lefkowitch et al., 1993) (Table 5.2 and Ch. 7). These changes occur early during infection and blur the distinction between acute and chronic HCV infection (Schmid et al., 1982). Additional early lesions, which include macrophage and Kupffer cell activation, cholestasis, spotty necrosis, and cholangitis, also suggest immune-mediated damage (Goodman & Ishak, 1995). Among patients that progress to chronic infection, the histopathology varies from normal liver and nonspecific reactive hepatitis to chronic persistent (periportal) or chronic active (lobular) hepatitis, and either active (progressive) or inactive cirrhosis (Bronkhorst & ten Kate, 1998). From those with chronic hepatitis, who make up the majority of patients, most liver biopsies have evidence of mild piecemeal and focal necrosis, mild cholangitis, steatosis, and lobular infiltrates, as well as moderate portal infiltration (Bronkhorst & ten Kate, 1998). Hence, many of the lesions that are prevalent in acute and chronic HCV infection have immunological components. However, it is not clear from these studies whether the immune responses associated with the liver diseases are the cause or the result of the pathology. In other words, it is not clear whether liver disease results from virus-induced cytopathic effects that trigger immune responses or whether the virus gene products directly prime immune responses that are then directed against infected hepatocytes (Table 5.2). It is clear that immune responses to HCV contain but do not eliminate the virus.

The nature of the immune responses that mediate acute and chronic liver disease (Fig. 4.1), however, remain the subject of intense study. Following acute exposure to the virus, the first line of defense is thought to consist of natural killer (NK) cells, neutrophils, and professional antigen-processing cells such as macrophages (Moretta et al., 1994). If the hepatocyte is the initial cell type that supports HCV replication, then antigen and virus particles shed early in the incubation phase of infection are likely to be picked up and processed by professional antigen-presenting Kupffer cells (fixed macrophages) within the liver. NK cells with T cell markers, or NKT cells, may also play an important role soon after infection (Matsuura et al., 2000). NKT cells are abundant in the liver and are activated by host-encoded glycolipid antigens (Gumperz et al., 2000), which may be present in the envelope of HCV. Activated NKT cells then secrete large amounts of cytokines (e.g., IFN-γ and interleukin (IL) 4) that may have direct antiviral effects and trigger the development of specific immune responses against virus-infected cells (Kennedy et al., 2000). Glycolipid-activated NKT cells also exhibit perforin- and/or Fas ligand (FasL)-mediated cytotoxicity (Cui et al., 1997; Kawamura et al., 1998), which may contribute importantly to inflammatory liver disease. Cytotoxicity may also occur following the activation of NKT cells by IL-12, which is made by Kupffer cells following the processing of viral antigen (Diepolder et al., 1998) (Fig. 5.1). Although these arguments suggest important roles for NK and NKT cells in the early stages of HCV infection, there is little evidence supporting the contribution of these cell types at this time.

The uptake and processing of virus antigens by macrophages and Kupffer cells in the liver is very important for the priming of virus-specific CD4$^+$ T cells early after infection (Fig. 5.1). CD4$^+$ T cells are activated by recognizing virus epitopes presented in the context of major histocompatibility complex (MHC) class II antigens on the surface of the professional antigen-presenting cells (Murray et al., 1992). T cell activation is also triggered by the presence (or absence) of costimulatory molecules on the surface of the antigen-presenting cells (Kuchroo et al., 1995) and by the production of IL-12 from these cells (Sypek et al., 1993) (Fig. 5.1). These considerations, combined with the affinity of the T cell receptor (TCR) for each peptide–MHC antigen complex, determine whether CD4$^+$ T cell activation results in the development of T helper cells of types 1 or 2 (Th1 and Th2, respectively). Th1 cells secrete IL-2, tumor necrosis factor alpha (TNFα), and IFN-γ (Ramsay, Ruby & Ramshaw, 1993), which then stimulate the development of NK cells and CD8$^+$ CTLs (Zinkernagel et al., 1993) (Fig. 5.1). As an immunomodulator, IFN also contributes to macrophage activation (Young &

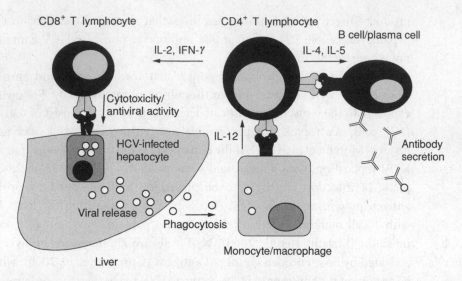

CD8$^+$ T lymphocyte   CD4$^+$ T lymphocyte

IL-2, IFN-γ IL-4, IL-5

B cell/plasma cell

Cytotoxicity/
antiviral activity

HCV-infected
hepatocyte

IL-12

Antibody
secretion

Viral release

Phagocytosis

Monocyte/macrophage

Liver

Fig. 5.1.   Cellular and humoral immune responses involved in the pathogenesis of hepatitis C infection. IL, interleukin; IFN-γ, interferon γ. (From Diepolder et al. (1998) with permission from S. Karger, New York.)

Hardy, 1995) and recruitment of T cells (Shields et al., 1999), NK cells (Salazar-Mather, Orange & Biron, 1998), and/or NKT cells (Kaneko et al., 2000). The impact of IFN in vivo is underscored by the finding that transgenic mice overexpressing IFN-γ develop chronic active hepatitis (Toyonaga et al., 1994). Interestingly, the finding that the majority of T cells isolated from the livers of patients with chronic HCV infection are Th1 cells, which produce IFN-γ but not IL-4 or IL-5 (Bertoletti et al., 1997), is also consistent with a causal role of Th1 cells in chronic liver cell damage. IFN-γ also upregulates the expresson of MHC class I molecules on hepatocytes and bile duct cells (Ballardini et al., 1995b). The association on the surface of liver cells of virus antigen peptides with MHC class I molecules is recognized by virus-specific CTLs, which then mediate the lysis of the virus-infected hepatocytes (Fig. 5.1). This is supported by the finding that enhanced patterns of class I MHC expression correlate with the severity of liver disease (Mossier et al., 1994). Alternatively, or in addition, antigen-presenting cells stimulate CD4$^+$ T cells to differentiate into Th2 cells. Th2 cells secrete IL-4, IL-5, and IL-10, which promote the development of virus-specific antibody-producing B cells (Doherty, Allan & Eichelberger, 1992) (Fig. 5.1). Th2 cytokines also downregulate Th1 cytokine production, CTL activity, MHC expression, and the degree of antigen presentation by macrophages, Kupffer cells, and infected hepatocytes (Abbas, Murphy & Sher, 1996). These observations support the hypothesis that the balance between Th1 and Th2 responses in the early phase of acute infection may be central in determining the outcome of infection. This is now empirically supported by evidence that patients who develop an early, strong proliferative response to multiple HCV antigens, accompanied by high levels of IFN-γ production (i.e., a Th1 response), are likely to eliminate virus and recover from a bout of acute hepatitis. In contrast, a strong Th2 response was observed in the majority of patients who developed chronic infection (Lechmann et al., 1996; Gerlach et al., 1999; Takaki et al., 2000) (Table 5.2). CD4$^+$ T cells were also dominant in HCV-infected patients following liver transplantation (Carucci et al., 1997; Rosen et al., 1999). The presence of predominantly CD4$^+$ T cells in portal areas (Weiner et al., 1992), and of mostly CD8$^+$ T cells in the hepatic lobules (Koziel et al., 1992), implies that both T cell types mediate hepatocellular damage. This is further supported by the observation that their numbers correlate with ALT levels and with the histological severity of liver disease. These findings suggest that T cells are critically important in the pathogenesis of liver disease. In addition, the development of a vigorous, early, polyspecific Th1 response appears to be associated with the resolution of acute infection (Section 5.4).

In addition to timely Th1 activation, the outcome of acute infection is influenced by the HLA antigens of the host (Murray et al., 1989), the presence of appropriate costimulatory molecules (Cai & Sprent, 1996), as well as the quality and quantity of viral antigens. Several studies have documented a statistically significant relationship between HLA class II haplotype and outcome of infection (Congia et al., 1996; Tibbs et al., 1996; Mangia et al., 1999), although this has not been consistently found (Czaja et al., 1995). In this regard, peptide–class II complexes that bind strongly to the TCR favor a Th1 response, whereas those complexes that bind poorly are likely to trigger a Th2 response (Pfeiffer et al., 1995). With regard to appropriate costimulation, the finding of differences in the virus variants between the liver and periphery implies that costimulation of immune responses generated in the periphery (i.e., in lymph nodes) to virus may not efficiently target overlapping but distinct viral epitopes in the liver. Unlike the serum, the liver contains both replicating and defective virus variant proteins. In addition, the virus load is likely to influence the nature of the immune response generated, since different T cell activities are triggered by different levels of virus antigens. Finally, the Th1 : Th2 ratio may be partially dependent upon the activity of NKT cells during the very early period of infection (Bendelac et al., 1995). Hence, there are multiple factors that influence the nature of the T cell response after acute infection. Variability of these factors among individuals may contribute importantly to the variability in the natural history of HCV infection.

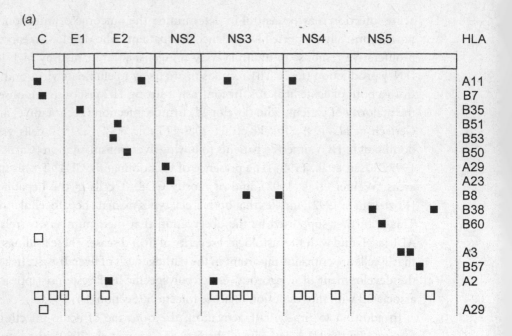

(a)

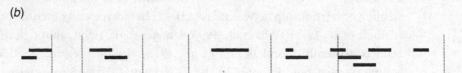

(b)

Fig. 5.2.   Antigenic determinants in hepatitis C (HCV) infection. (a) Epitopes detected in chronic HCV
infection in cytotoxic T lymphocytes derived from liver (■) and peripheral blood
mononuclear cells (□). (b) Horizontal lines show the positions of HCV cDNA clones scoring
positive in antibody-binding assays. (Modified from Choo et al. (1990) with permission
from Williams & Wilkins, from Chang, Rehermann & Chisari (1997a) with permission from
Springer-Verlag, and from Koziel (1997) with permission from Blackwell Science, Inc.)

5.3 Virus-specific B cell responses

One of the consequences of HCV infection is the appearance of specific antibodies
to viral antigens among infected patients and chimpanzees (Table 4.2). Although
antibody responses to most of the virus proteins have been detected (Fig. 5.2), and
have been useful in the diagnosis of HCV infections (Fig. 1.1 and Section 1.5), the
significance of these responses to the pathogenesis and outcome of infection
remain to be firmly established. For example, the development of anti-HCV in
chimpanzees, which is similar in its range of antiviral specificities and its time of

appearance to that in human infections, did not predict whether an acute infection would resolve or become chronic. In particular, IgM anti-NS3, an early marker of HCV infection, is more common during acute infections, although it does not seem to have any predictive value (Quinti et al., 1995). Similar considerations hold for antibody responses against other HCV-encoded epitopes in core (Nasoff et al., 1991), E2 (Mink et al., 1994), NS3 (Mondelli et al., 1994), and NS4 (Bhattacherjee et al., 1995). In addition, persistent infections were established in chimpanzees (as in humans) despite the presence of antibody responses to multiple virus antigens (Abe et al., 1991; Farci et al., 1992b) (Table 4.2 and Ch. 14). This is further supported by the finding that antibodies collected from chimpanzees years after acute infection often failed to neutralize either homologous virus from the original inoculum or heterologous virus (Farci et al., 1994). While neutralization may depend upon the binding of viral antibodies to multiple epitopes, most attention has been based upon the envelope glycoproteins (E1/E2) and, in particular, the HVR1 sequences near the amino-terminus of E2. This is because envelope antibodies have been shown partially to protect chimpanzees against infection (Choo et al., 1994). High titers of anti-E2 were also found among patients who resolved acute HCV but were absent from those who developed chronic infection (Ishii et al., 1998) (Ch. 14). In addition, anti-E2 has been shown to block the in vitro binding of recombinant E2 and HCV to MOLT-4 cells (Rosa et al., 1996; Ishii et al., 1998). This assay has been used to test whether chimpanzee sera from animals immunized with recombinant HCV E1/E2 antigens developed potentially neutralizing antibodies (Choo et al., 1994). Similar assays have also been used to detect potentially neutralizing antibodies in human sera (Zibert, Schreier & Roggendorf, 1995). The existence and evolution of virus quasispecies within the HVR1 sequence suggests that envelope antibody responses neutralize only subsets of virions containing corresponding HVR1 sequences. It has been proposed that the neutralization and clearance of these HCV subsets permits the outgrowth of the remaining quasispecies (Weiner et al., 1992; Taniguchi, Okamoto & Sakamoto, 1993; Kato et al., 1994). Hence, antibody-mediated clearance of major quasispecies results in the expansion of minor quasispecies to which there is no corresponding neutralizing antibody. This process results in the persistence of HCV, with different major quasispecies sequences at different times during chronic infection. Neutralizing antibody responses to only a portion of the virus particles from an inoculum, therefore, may actually contribute significantly to chronic HCV infections (Section 3.2). In support of this model, recent results have shown that rabbit antisera raised to a specific HVR1 synthetic peptide sequence protected chimpanzees from challenge with the homologous, but not a heterologous, HCV isolate (Farci et al., 1996b). This "immune selection" is also supported by the finding that in a chronically infected agammaglobulinemic patient

Table 5.3. Characteristics of hepatitis C virus and cytotoxic T lymphocytes (CTL) specific for hepatitis C in immunopathogenesis

Infectious stage	Viral characteristics	Virus-specific CTL characteristics
Acute resolving infection	A low initial inoculum	Strong, multispecific CTL response
	Low replication efficiency	CTLs migrate efficiently to targets
	No mutations in relevant CTL epitopes	CD4$^+$ T cell activation/expansion
Chronic infection	High initial inoculum	Monospecific, weak CTL response
	High replication efficiency	CTLs do not migrate to targets
	Mutations in relevant CTL epitopes	Poor CD4$^+$ T cell activation/expansion

Modified from Bertoletti & Maini (2000) with permission from Elsevier Science, Ltd.

followed for 2.5 years, no mutations in the HVR1 were detected (Kumar, Monjardino & Thomas, 1994a). HVR1 quasispecies also failed to appear in immunosuppressed patients who were agammaglobulinemic (Booth et al., 1998) and were coinfected with HIV (Toyoda et al., 1997) or had undergone orthotopic liver transplantation (Lawal et al., 1997). Although it is not clear why the infected host makes a limited repertoire of HVR1 antibodies during infection, the elimination of some viral antigen-specific B cells by cytotoxic T cells may occur (Barnaba et al., 1990). This could occur if B cells are infected with HCV (Ch. 11) and/or if B cells are sensitized to viral antigens through cell surface immunoglobulin. The recent finding that anti-HCV becomes undetectable as chronic infection progresses supports this hypothesis (Takaki et al., 2000). Hence, the kinetics and strength of the antiviral CTL response, and the genetic predisposition of the host, may limit the titer and specificity of neutralizing antibodies throughout infection, permitting the selection and persistence of various HCV quasispecies. If this occurs, then the nature of the T cell response to virus may influence pathogenesis, in part, by altering the patterns of viral antibody during the course of acute and chronic infection (Table 5.3).

In addition to envelope antigens, antibody responses to other HCV gene products have also been detected. In chronic HCV infection, these include antibody responses to core, NS3, NS4, and NS5, which were present in more than 80% of infected patients. Closer examination, however, showed that most of these responses were restricted to the IgG1 isotype, suggesting a widespread but rather limited humoral response to HCV (Chen et al., 1999). Antibody responses to multiple virus antigens were also detected in patients who resolved acute infection, but at significantly lower titers (Chen et al., 1999; Takaki et al., 2000). Since the production of antibodies, including IgG1, are stimulated by Th2 cells, while cell-mediated immune responses are stimulated by Th1 cells, an important difference between an HCV infection that resolves and another that develops into a chronic infection may be the balance between Th1 and Th2 activities (Table 5.2). In this context, an acute, resolving infection would be characterized by the predominance of a Th1 response, while a chronic infection would be characterized by predominantly a Th2 response. Recently, there has been experimental evidence that supports this hypothesis (Tsai et al., 1997; Takaki et al., 2000).

The relatively high frequency of anti-HCV in chronic infections, and the fact that most chronically infected people develop liver disease, both imply that viral antibodies may contribute importantly to the pathogenesis of chronic infection. However, hypo- or agammaglobulinemic patients who acquired HCV infection following treatment with pooled, contaminated immunoglobulin developed chronic hepatitis at a high frequency, and this progressed on to cirrhosis within a few years (Thomson et al., 1987; Bjorkander et al., 1988). These observations imply that viral antibodies may contribute both to the persistence of virus (through quasispecies selection) and the progression of liver disease (possibly by partially blocking the elimination of virus-infected cells). A clearer understanding of the role of viral antibodies in the pathogenesis of infection will have to await the development of an animal model in which the humoral and cellular arms of the antiviral immune response can be individually evaluated (Ch. 13).

5.4 Virus-specific T cell responses

As indicated in Section 5.2, the priming of Th cells within the first few weeks of infection may determine the outcome of HCV infection. In this context, it is proposed that a strong, multispecific Th1 response early after infection will stimulate sufficient CTL responses to result in the clearance of virus and resolution of acute infection. In support of this hypothesis, recent work has documented the presence of virus-specific CTL activity more than a year following the resolution of acute infection (Cooper et al., 1999). In contrast, it has been proposed that a weak or impaired Th1 response early on in infection will permit the development of chronic infection and liver disease (Battegay, 1996) (Tables 5.2 and 5.3). This immune-mediated nature of HCV pathogenesis is highlighted by the lack of correlation between virus load in blood and extent of histological disease in the liver among both immunocompetent (Lau et al., 1993; Shindo et al., 1995; Romeo et al., 1996a; Rodriguez-Inigo et al., 1999) patients and organ transplant recipients under immunosuppression (Chazouilleres et al., 1994). Similar observations have been reported with experimentally infected chimpanzees (Negro et al., 1992). In contrast, independent observations have shown an apparently direct relationship between HCV RNA titers in blood and histological evidence of liver disease (Alberti et al., 1992; Prieto et al., 1995). In addition, there is some evidence that

HCV RNA in the liver, as detected by in situ hybridization, colocalizes with mononuclear inflammatory cells (Tanaka et al., 1993). Although the last study is consistent with the possibility that HCV may be cytopathic, it may also reflect the possibility that more virus antigens may generate broader and/or stronger immune responses, which mediate a more severe liver disease. In support of this hypothesis, CD8[+] T cells have been shown to predominate in the intrahepatic inflammatory infiltrate of those with HCV-associated CLD (Autschback et al., 1991). This observation is similar to the situation in HBV-associated CLD, which is known to be immune mediated (Yang et al., 1988; Lau, Alexander & Alberti, 1991).

A general measure of CD4[+] T cell responses during HCV infection has been documented using T cell proliferation assays, in which peripheral blood T cells from infected patients are stimulated to uptake and incorporate [^{3}H]-thymidine into their DNA upon stimulation with one or more virus antigens. These proliferation assays reflect antigen recognition and expansion of T cell clones, implying the presence of antiviral immune responses in vivo. Among acutely infected patients who resolved infection (i.e., cleared HCV RNA), strong T cell proliferative responses were observed in all patients against NS3, NS4, and NS5, which persisted for years after infection (Diepolder et al., 1995, 1997; Missale et al., 1996). The response to NS3 appeared to be immunodominant. This was supported by the finding of an NS3 epitope spanning positions 1251–1259 that was conserved among isolates of genotypes 1 and 2 and was shown to bind with high affinity to multiple HLA alleles (Diepolder et al., 1997). In parallel, immunodominant CTL epitopes from conserved regions of the HCV polyprotein were demonstrated in HLA-A2 transgenic mice (Wentworth et al., 1996). Further analysis has shown that the NS3 response is persistent in recovered patients, and that it consists of mostly a Th1 cytokine profile. In contrast, generally less than half the patients who develop chronic HCV infection generate a response to core or NS4, and there is only a transient response to NS3 (Botarelli et al., 1993; Ferrari et al., 1994; Leroux-Roels et al., 1996). Further characterization of the PBMCs from chronically infected patients has demonstrated a Th2 cytokine profile (Cacciarelli et al., 1996; Tsai et al., 1997). These results suggest that a strong, persistent T cell proliferative response to multiple antigens may be important for resolution of acute infection, while weak or absent responses are characteristic of patients who develop chronic infections. This picture, however, may not tell the whole story, since most of the data is based upon analysis of T cells isolated from peripheral blood, while the effector cells that are also important to pathogenesis are likely to be sequestered in the liver (see related question 11 in Ch. 24).

One of the potentially protective Th1 immune responses involves the generation of HCV-specific CTLs. CTLs to multiple virus antigens have been detected in both peripheral blood and in the livers of patients with chronic HCV infection (Koziel et al., 1992, 1993; Cerny et al., 1995). Among patients repeatedly exposed to virus occupationally or sexually, persistent NS3 Th responses developed in the absence of antibody, suggesting that T cell memory could be established by periodic exposure to virus in subclinical infections (Schupper et al., 1993). T cell memory was also observed in patients and chimpanzees who recovered from acute infection (Cramp et al., 1999). In populations of chronically infected humans (Battegay et al., 1995; Cerny et al., 1995; Koziel et al., 1995) and chimpanzees (Erickson et al., 1993), CTL specificities to a variety of epitopes in all virus proteins have been documented (Fig. 5.2). This has helped to identify immunodominant epitopes in chronic infections (Koziel et al., 1992). While this suggests that HCV is immunogenic, the restricted and variable CTL reactivity observed in individual infections suggests that only a small number of epitopes are actually targeted in a given individual. In addition, the frequency of CTL precursors in the peripheral blood of chronically infected patients has been estimated to be 1 in 10^5–10^6 PBMC (Cerny et al., 1995). Although the CTL precursor frequencies are likely to be higher in the liver, they are far below that of other viruses (e.g., lymphocytic choriomeningitis virus) (Byrne & Oldstone, 1984). This low precursor frequency is not a result of generalized immunosuppression, since CTL activities to recall antigens are normal in HCV-infected patients (Rehermann et al., 1996a), suggesting that chronic infections are often characterized by weak CTL responses (Table 5.3). A possible basis for this weak response has to do with the characteristics of the infection itself. If 1–10% of the total number of hepatocytes in the human liver become infected, then it is estimated that 10^9–10^{10} cells are potential targets for cell-mediated immune responses. If the precursor frequency of HCV-specific CTL is 10^{-5}, based upon a total population of ~10^{12} lymphocytes in the human body, then at most 10^7 virus-specific CTLs would be generated, which would provide one CTL for every 100–1000 infected hepatocytes (Chang, Rehermann & Chisari, 1997a). Although these CTL responses do not eliminate virus, there is an inverse correlation between the magnitude of the CTL responses and virus load (Rehermann et al., 1996b, Nelson et al., 1997), suggesting that HCV CTL responses could exert some control over virus production (see related question 12 in Ch. 24). The relatively strong CTL responses that partially control the levels of virus, however, also contribute to the development and progression of CLD, suggesting that such responses in the long run may do more harm than good (Cerny & Chisari, 1999; Bertoletti & Maini, 2000) (Table 5.2).

There is now considerable evidence suggesting that CTLs are major effector cells in the pathogenesis of chronic viral hepatitis (Chisari, 1997) (Table 5.3). This was realized even prior to the discovery of HCV: in experiments where PBMCs lysed autologous hepatocytes presumably infected with the NANBH agent in an HLA-restricted manner (Poralla, Hutteroth & zum Buschenfelde, 1984; Mondelli et al., 1986). Parallel results were obtained in later work with HCV-infected patients (Liaw et al., 1995). These effectors were identified as CD4[+] and CD8[+] T cells, suggesting that these are major effectors in the pathogenesis of HCV infection. One of the mechanisms whereby virus-specific CD8[+] T cells mediate cytotoxicity involves the direct binding of CTLs to virus-infected hepatocytes. This binding is mediated through FasL on the lymphocyte (Suda et al., 1995) and the Fas receptor on infected hepatocytes. Receptor binding results in the activation of the Fas signal transduction pathway, which then triggers a form of programmed cell death known as apoptosis (Patel & Gores, 1995; Depraetere & Golstein, 1997). The susceptibility of hepatocytes to Fas-mediated killing is illustrated by the massive hepatocellular necrosis triggered by anti-Fas treatment of mice. Intraperitoneal injection of anti-Fas into mice resulted in the binding of antibody to the Fas receptor on hepatocytes, which was rapidly followed by massive hepatocellular necrosis that resembled fulminant hepatitis, and finally by death of the animals (Ogasawara et al., 1993). This histopathology was also observed in an HBV transgenic mouse model of fulminant hepatitis following adoptive transfer of HBV-primed CTLs (Ando et al., 1993), implying the participation of direct Fas-mediated killing. This was directly shown by further work in which injection of soluble Fas, which neutralizes the FasL function of CTLs, prevented the development of fulminant hepatitis and loss of animals following adoptive transfer (Kondo et al., 1997). Among patients with chronic HCV, there is an upregulation in Fas expression on hepatocytes, especially in periportal regions near areas of piecemeal necrosis (Hiramatsu et al., 1994; Jin et al., 1997) (see related question 13 in Ch. 24). Interestingly, the level of Fas expression in the liver was significantly reduced in patients who developed a sustained response to IFN treatment compared with nonresponders (Okazaki et al., 1996) (Ch. 9), again suggesting a correlation between Fas expression and inflammation. Moreover, human hepatocytes have been shown to produce soluble Fas (Krams et al., 1998). Further work showed that serum levels of soluble Fas were significantly higher in patients with chronic HCV infection compared with uninfected controls (Iio et al., 1998). The levels of soluble Fas in serum correlated with Fas expression on hepatocytes, with the severity of chronic hepatitis (Iio et al., 1998), and with cirrhosis (Seishima et al., 1997), suggesting that soluble Fas does not effectively block CTL activity in natural human infections. Although it is not known with certainty, the discrepancy between the studies in mice and the observations in humans may be explained if the levels of soluble Fas in mice are higher than those seen in chronic human infections. Still, the question remains as to why there is an upregulated expression of Fas receptor expression on HCV-infected hepatocytes. In this regard, recent work has shown that HCV core polypeptide could sensitize the human hepatoblastoma cell line HepG2 (Knowles, Howe & Aden, 1980) to Fas-mediated killing by stimulating the Fas-associated signal transduction pathway leading to apoptosis (Ruggieri et al., 1997). Interestingly, the finding that HCV core is a transcriptional regulatory protein (Ray et al., 1995; Shih et al., 1995) that induces p53 expression under certain conditions (Ray, Meyer & Ray, 1996a), and that p53 enhances Fas expression (Owen-Schaub et al., 1995), may provide at least a partial explanation for the increased Fas expression in infected cells within areas of piecemeal necrosis. Although it is uncertain whether these correlations reflect an underlying mechanism in vivo, the promotion of Fas-mediated apoptosis is consistent with the release of virus particles from cells undergoing turnover and the rapid appearance of newly dominant quasispecies of HCV (Fukumoto et al., 1996) (Section 3.2). The promotion of Fas-mediated hepatocellular turnover by HCV may also be important for the development of fibrosis and cirrhosis, which accompany hepatocellular turnover, and for the propagation of genetic changes in surviving hepatocytes, which contributes to the pathogenesis of HCC (Ch. 6).

Although T cells represent a major inflammatory cell type in chronic HCV infection, the majority of intrahepatic T cells are not HCV specific, although they produce cytokines characteristic of Th cells (Bertoletti et al., 1997). The IFN produced by these Th1 responses, in turn, appears to contribute significantly to the recruitment of T, NK, and NKT nonantigen-specific effectors (Salazar-Mather et al., 1998; Shields et al., 1999). In addition, both antigen-specific and nonspecific inflammatory cells may contribute to target cell killing by other pathways in addition to Fas. For example, the observation that activated CD4[+] T cells stimulate antigen nonspecific inflammatory cells (Mosmann et al., 1986) suggests a mechanism whereby immune responses could be amplified even in the absence of strong antigen-specific T cell responses. Activated NK and NKT cells, which are effectors for nonspecific viral antigens, mediate Fas killing (Leite-de-Moraes & Dy, 1997; Tsutsui et al., 2000) but are also capable of causing cell destruction using the perforin/granzyme system (Shresta et al., 1998). In this pathway, perforin made by effector cells causes the formation of pores in target cell membranes, which permits the penetration of a battery of proteases (granzymes), resulting in target cell destruction. Both the Fas and perforin systems have been shown to kill hepatocytes in HBsAg transgenic mice (Nakamoto et al., 1997), and in woodchucks infected with the HBV-like woodchuck hepatitis virus (Hodgson, Grant & Michalak, 1999). Interestingly, the perforin system was activated in animals that developed acute hepatitis, compared with those who developed chronic infection, suggesting that the perforin system may contribute importantly to the resolution of acute infection. In HCV infection, immunohistochemical observations have shown elevated expression of Fas receptor in hepatocytes and increased expression of FasL in liver-infiltrating mononuclear cells in tissues from chronically infected patients (Hiramatsu et al., 1994; Mita & Hayashi, 1997). Independent work using RT/PCR has shown an increase in perforin mRNA in the liver of chronically infected patients, but not in uninfected liver or in PBMCs from infected patients (Fukuda et al., 1995), suggesting that the perforin system is active in chronic HCV infection. Together, these data suggest that both pathways play important roles in the pathogenesis of HCV infection, although their relative contributions to acute versus chronic liver disease remain to be closely examined.

Given the opportunities for immune amplification of antigen-specific and nonspecific immune responses, it is not easy to understand how as much as 85% of acute HCV infections become chronic (Fig. 4.2; Ch. 14). One of the potential mechanisms of virus-persistence involves the suboptimal activation and proliferation of virus-specific T cells in response to very low levels of virus gene expression and replication (Cai & Sprent, 1996). In addition, the replicative 'fitness' of different quasispecies or virus variants may elicit qualitatively and quantitatively different immune reponses, since various T cell functions are turned on only above different thresholds of virus antigen concentrations (Valitutti et al., 1996) (Section 3.2). This probably relates to the fraction of TCRs on each cell that is occupied by peptide. Low peptide concentrations, for example, stimulate CTL activity, while intermediate peptide concentrations elicit IFN-γ and IL-2 production, and very high peptide concentrations are required to trigger T cell proliferation. This hierarchy of T cell activation helps to explain why chronic infections are accompanied by weak T cell reponses to few virus antigens. In addition to the extent of TCR occupancy, the affinity of viral peptides for each TCR will influence the nature of the immune response generated, with low-affinity binding peptides inducing a Th1 response and high-affinity binding peptides inducing a Th2 response (Pearson, van Ewijik & McDevitt, 1997) (Section 5.2). Hence, the nature of the immune response generated to HCV in any given infection will depend, in part, on the concentration and ratio of high-affinity to low-affinity epitopes.

Immune reactivity for immunodominant peptides will also depend, in part, upon the HLA haplotypes of the infected host. For example, several groups have reported an association between certain HLA class II alleles and viral clearance or persistence (Congia et al., 1996; McKiernan & Kelleher, 2000) (Section 5.2). As indicated above, HLA haplotypes have also been associated with disease severity (Chang et al., 1999; Mangia et al., 1999). Interestingly, viral persistence also appears to be promoted by the development of quasispecies and viral variants (Section 3.2) that antagonize CTL activity (Kaneko et al., 1997; Tsai et al., 1998) at the level of TCR binding (Lanzavecchia, 1997). Recent evidence in chronically infected patients, for example, showed that intrahepatic CTLs inefficiently recognized autologous virus sequences relative to prototype sequences from the same subtype (Kaneko et al., 1997; Giuggio et al., 1998). In this setting, antagonist sequences block TCR internalization of both wild-type and antagonist peptides, resulting in suppressed responses to both. Virus genetic variation could also lead to the appearance of neutralization and CTL escape variants, which are also likely to contribute to virus persistence (Farci et al., 1992a; Weiner et al., 1995). Escape variants have been found in acutely infected chimpanzees (Weiner et al., 1995) and in chronically infected patients (Chang et al., 1997b), suggesting that they contribute importantly to persistent infections. Even so, it is not clear whether these or other mutants are the cause or the consequence of virus persistence. Moreover, the finding of a poorly immunogenic escape or antagonistic mutant does not invariably signal a central role of this mutant in persistence, since the epitope involved is one of many that make up the host–virus relationship (Chang et al., 1997b). Other epitopes could lead to the production of IFN-γ and IL-2, for example, which partially compensate for the anergy (nonresponsiveness) of T cells to an escape mutant or antagonistic epitope. It is also possible that HCV infection interferes with antigen processing and/or that the virus is not susceptible to partial or complete elimination by cytokines. While there is no evidence to suggest that either of these mechanisms is operative, the partial activation of HCV-specific cell-mediated immune responses may cause prolonged liver damage but will not be effective in eliminating virus. These immune responses may do more harm than good and, along with virus genetic variation, may enable virus persistence (Table 5.3).

Many viruses that establish persistent infections make one or more gene products that block the elimination of virus or virus-infected cells. HCV-encoded NS5A (Gale et al., 1997, 1998a; Gale, Korth & Katze, 1998b) and, possibly, E2 (Taylor et al., 1999) appear to play important roles in blocking the antiviral effects of IFN. However, there is also increasing evidence that the HCV core polypeptide may contribute importantly to pathogenesis. Interestingly, while HCV core polypeptide normally assumes a structural role in virus replication/assembly by oligomerization in the cytoplasm (Matsumoto et al., 1996), truncated forms of core polypeptide have been detected in the nucleus (Lo et al., 1995; Suzuki et al., 1995a). During the virus life cycle, core polypeptide is cleaved from E1 at the cytoplasmic side of the ER membrane by one or more cellular signal peptidases (Santolini et al., 1994) (Sections 2.4 and 2.5). Some of the mature core is further processed in cultured cells (Lo et al., 1994; Hussy et al., 1996; Liu et al., 1997) to yield truncated polypeptides that accumulate in the nucleus. This truncation results in the elimination of the hydrophobic carboxy-terminus, which anchors the core polypeptide to the ER membrane, and leaves a hydrophilic molecule to which several functions have been ascribed. These include binding to RNA, DNA, and ribosomes (Santolini et al., 1994). While the significance of these properties remains to be understood, the finding of exclusively cytoplasmic core antigen in the hepatocytes from infected humans and chimpanzees calls into question the significance of core protein in the nucleus of transfected cells. Perhaps where all virus gene products are available for viral replication, HCV core is retained in the cytoplasm, whereas when it is expressed alone in transfected cells or with the envelope polypeptides of HCV in transgenic mice (Kawamura et al., 1997), some nuclear localization is observed. However, in natural infections, it is not clear whether core is expressed in a context other than virus maturation and replication.

Despite these uncertainties, it is well documented that HCV suppresses the replication of HBV in coinfections (Liaw et al., 1998); this activity has been mapped to the HCV core polypeptide and seems to require phosphorylation of HCV core (Shih et al., 1993). Further work showed that HCV core polypeptide was phosphorylated at Ser-116 by protein kinase A and at Ser-99 by protein kinase C (Shih et al., 1995). Although phosphorylation of full-length and truncated forms of core were observed, this post-translational modification did not correlate with the appearance of truncated core polypeptides in the nucleus. While the mechanism of inhibition of HBV replication is not known, it may involve the direct binding of HCV core to cellular promoters and/or to transcription factors. In this context, it has been reported that HCV core upregulates the expression of c-*myc* and c-*fos* (Chang et al., 1998) while it downregulates the promoters of p53 and p21$^{WAF1/CIP1/SDI1}$ (Ray et al., 1997, 1998a). Core protein has also been shown to suppress nuclear factor kappa B (NF-κB) activation (Ch. 6), which is usually stimulated by a number of cytotoxic cytokines (such as TNF), thereby promoting apoptosis (Shrivastava et al., 1998). In contrast, core protein has been shown to stimulate activation protein 1 (AP-1), which occurs through activation of Jun amino-terminal kinase (JNK) and mitogen-activated protein kinase kinase (Shrivastava et al., 1998). Both NF-κB and AP-1 regulate the growth and survival response of infected cells to antiviral immune activity; consequently their differential activation by HCV core may alter the fate of infected cells relative to uninfected cells in the liver. The recent demonstration that HCV core binds to heterogeneous nuclear ribonucleoprotein K (Hsieh et al., 1998), which regulates the promoters of c-*myc* and c-*fos* (Tomonaga & Levens, 1995), not only suggests a mechanism where core protein may contribute to hepatocarcinogenesis (Ch. 6), but also a way whereby core-mediated alterations in host gene expression may favor virus replication. The additional finding that HCV core significantly activates the mitogen activated protein kinase/extracellular signal-regulated kinase signal transduction cascade in cell lines (Hayashi et al., 2000), and that this pathway is also activated in HCC (Schmit et al., 1997), further suggests that core expression is important for hepatocellular transformation. This is further supported by the finding that activation of the extracellular signal-related kinase induces the expression of c-*myc* (Kerkhoff et al., 1998) and cell cycle progression, both of which contribute to the development of HCC (Ch. 6).

The case that HCV core protein causes cellular injury by direct cytopathic effects is not settled (Section 5.1). For example, some core transgenic mice develop liver steatosis (Moriya et al., 1997) while other similarly constructed mice do not (Kawamura et al., 1997; Pasquinelli et al., 1997) and some HCV core-expressing cell lines do not appear to develop abnormalities consistent with cytopathic effects (Moradpour et al., 1996; Zhu et al., 1998). The ability of core either to inhibit or to enhance apoptosis seems to be dependent upon the experimental conditions used. While the inhibition of apoptosis may promote virus persistence and the development of HCC (Ray et al., 1996a,b), the core-mediated enhancement of apoptosis induced by lymphotoxin $\alpha\beta$, TNF, or Fas (Chen et al., 1997; Ruggieri et al., 1997; Zhu et al., 1998) may promote both hepatocellular turnover and the propagation of mutations that also contribute importantly to the development of HCC. The balance of these outcomes is likely to depend upon the nature of the core polypeptides produced (full length versus truncated), their subcellular localization (cytoplasmic versus nuclear), phosphorylation state, and the cellular proteins to which they bind during infection.

The alteration of cellular phenotype by HCV core in tissue culture cells and in some strains of transgenic mice, combined with its putative *trans*-regulatory function, suggest that it may act, in part, by binding to selected cellular proteins. Work directed to this end has shown that HCV core binds to members of the TNF family of receptors, including the lymphotoxin β receptor (Chen et al., 1997; Matsumoto et al., 1997) and the TNF receptor-1 (Zhu et al., 1998). There are also preliminary data suggesting that HCV core protein may bind other members of the TNF receptor family, including Fas (Lai & Ware, 2000). Although the biological implications of these relationships remain to be determined, receptor activation mediates cell death, and binding to HCV core may alter the sensitivity of infected cells to TNF- and Fas-mediated killing. The difficulty at present seems to stem from not knowing whether HCV core increases or decreases the sensitivity of infected cells to apoptotic signals, since both effects have been reported. The effect of core may depend upon which TNF family member(s) it is binding to and the state (growing or quiescent) of the infected cell at the time of signaling (Lai & Ware, 2000). The extent of signal transduction pathway crosstalk may also influence the outcome of these interactions (Ray et al., 1998b; Zhu et al., 1998). If core enhances the sensitivity of infected hepatocytes to apoptosis, then it would be expected to accelerate the development of hepatitis and/or facilitate viral spread within apoptotic bodies (which would not be susceptible to antibody-mediated neutralization). In contrast, if core suppresses the sensitivity of infected hepatocytes to TNF killing, then this would promote virus persistence. In addition, if the functional integrity of infected lymphocytes is affected by core expression, then it may result in altered antiviral immune responses (von Boehmer, 1997; Lai & Ware, 2000) that could contribute importantly to the high rate of chronicity. Knockout mice that no longer make lymphotoxin α or β show altered trafficking of lymphocytes, which, in HCV infection, may prevent appropriate targeting from the place of priming (probably peripheral lymph nodes) to the place of effector function (the liver) (Alimzhanov et al., 1997). The lungs and liver of such knockout mice develop T cell infiltrates as a result of altered trafficking, although this has not been observed in the HCV core transgenic mice described so far. However, this does raise the question as to whether the lymphoid follicles that develop in chronically infected human livers reflect altered lymphocyte trafficking.

HCV core polypeptide has also been shown to bind a putative RNA helicase in transfected cells (You et al., 1999). In addition to colocalization, which was observed mostly in the nuclei of transfected cells, HCV core was shown to stimulate the activity of the RNA helicase by stimulating the activity of a reporter gene that was responsive to the helicase. It turns out that cellular RNA helicase activity is dependent upon a helicase-encoded ATPase activity, which is itself stimulated by HCV core (You et al., 1999). Although it is not known whether these events occur in infected liver, it is striking that HCV NS3 is also a helicase, with activity dependent upon an NS3-encoded NTPase activity (Section 2.4). If the latter is stimulated by core polypeptide, then core may contribute importantly to the virus life cycle by stimulating the unwinding activity of NS3 upon the double-stranded RNA replication intermediate of HCV. It would also be of interest to see whether the cellular RNA helicase that binds to core is incorporated into the replication complexes of HCV, where it may augment NS3 activity.

Hepatitis C and hepatocellular carcinoma

6.1 Prevalence and risk factors

The association between HCV and HCC predates the discovery of the virus, since early on it had been shown that there was a close relationship between NANBH and the development of HCC (Kiyosawa et al., 1982, 1984, 1990; Sakamoto et al., 1988). However, once HCV was discovered (Choo et al., 1989) and serological assays became available for its detection (Kuo et al., 1989) (Sections 1.4 and 1.5), a close association was established between anti-HCV and HCC all over the world (Bruix et al., 1989; Colombo et al., 1989; Hasan et al., 1990; Kew et al., 1990; Saito et al., 1990; Vargas, Costella & Esteban, 1990; Yu et al., 1990; Sulaiman et al., 1991). In southern Europe and Japan, for example, more than half of the reported HCC has been associated with HCV (Bruix et al., 1989; Colombo et al., 1989) whereas the prevalence of anti-HCV in Alaskan patients with HCC is nearly zero. Intermediate frequencies of anti-HCV have been reported among patients from Greece, Austria, and Taiwan (Jeng & Tsai, 1991; Baur et al., 1992; Hadziyannis et al., 1993), indicating geographic variation in this association. Worldwide, there are an estimated 170 million people who are chronically infected with HCV (Bradley et al., 1983; Choo et al., 1989; Houghton, 1996; Delwaide & Gerard, 2000; Wild & Hall, 2000) (Section 3.1), and the annual incidence rate of newly diagnosed HCC associated with HCV infection ranges from 1 to 7% in different populations (Di Bisceglie, 1997). This high incidence, however, does not always take into account the contribution of other important risk factors, such as age, gender, alcohol intake, long-term aflatoxin consumption, and coinfection with HBV. In addition, most of these observations have been made at about 20 years postinfection, suggesting that they do not represent the true incidence of HCV-associated HCC in chronically infected patients.

Most HCV-associated HCC arises from a background of cirrhosis. This implies that chronic HCV infection may contribute importantly to HCC by stimulating a long-term necroinflammatory response that promotes the development of fibrosis and cirrhosis (Kiyosawa et al., 1984, 1990; Hasan et al., 1990; Booth et al., 1998). Other factors also contribute to the development of cirrhosis in HCV-infected patients (Table 4.1). The centrality of cirrhosis is illustrated by the finding that between 5 and 28% of chronically HCV-infected patients with cirrhosis also had HCC (Craig et al., 1991). Hence, chronic HCV infection and the development of cirrhosis are major risk factors for the development of HCC, although it does not shed much light on the associated mechanisms of tumor development.

The persistence of HCV during chronic infection is not only important for the appearance and progression of CLD but also for the development of HCC. Indeed, HCV RNA has been detected in both tumor and surrounding nontumor liver tissue of patients with HCC (Gerber et al., 1992; Haruna et al., 1994; Di Bisceglie, 1995). Independent observations have also recently shown the presence of both virus RNA and antigens in HCC cells (Sansonno et al., 1997). Although the levels of HCV RNA in tumor tissue is generally lower than in surrounding nontumor liver (Takeda et al., 1992; Tang et al., 1995), tumor cells appear to support virus replication (Section 2.5), since both plus and minus strand RNAs were observed in HCC (Horiike et al., 1993). In addition, HCV gene expression has been detected in HCC cells (Uchida et al., 1994), further suggesting an association between virus and tumor. However, the HCV genome does not seem to integrate into the host DNA (Fong et al., 1991b; Di Bisceglie, 1995) and, therefore, the mechanism(s) that support(s) persistence of the viral genome in cells during chronic infection remain(s) to be identified.

6.2 Putative direct mechanisms of hepatitis C-mediated hepatocarcinogenesis

There are a variety of possible mechanisms whereby HCV gene products contribute to the pathogenesis of CLD and HCC. For example, the HCV core protein sensitizes the human hepatoblastoma cell line HepG2 to anti-Fas and TNFα-mediated apoptosis (Ruggieri et al., 1997; Zhu et al., 1998). In addition, HCV core protein has been shown to bind to and stimulate the *trans*-activation properties of the tumor suppressor p53, which also promotes apoptosis (Lu et al., 1999). HCV core has also been shown to promote apoptosis by downregulation of NF-κB (Shrivastava et al., 1998). If this occurs in the chronically infected liver, it would promote hepatocellular turnover and may promote the accumulation of mutations in rapidly regenerating cells that have limited time for lesion recognition and repair. Expression of HCV core protein in human cervical epithelial cells, however, inhibited cisplatin-mediated apoptosis (Ray et al., 1996a). Independent observations have also shown that HCV core protein has antiapoptotic properties (Ray et al., 1998b; Marusawa et al., 1999). This may involve the downregulation of the p53 and p21$^{WAF1/CIP1/SDI1}$ promoters, as indicated in Section 5.4 (Ray et al., 1997, 1998a). If this occurs in infected liver, it would help to sustain the survival of infected hepatocytes replicating HCV, thereby promoting chronic infection. These observations also imply that the function of HCV core protein may depend upon the type or state of the cell in which it is expressed, and perhaps whether core protein is expressed in the context of HCV replication or independent of it.

The finding that HCV core protein may alter the response of cells to apoptotic stimuli suggests a direct role for HCV in the development of HCC. This is further supported by the finding that HCV core protein activates the human c-*myc* promoter gene (Ray et al., 1995; Chang et al., 1998) (Section 5.4). Interestingly, c-*myc* gene amplification has also been detected during tumor progression (Abou-Elella et al., 1996), suggesting that the sustained elevation of Myc expression may be an important component in the pathogenesis of HCC. This is further supported by the finding that overproduction of Myc and TGFα in transgenic mice strongly stimulates tumor formation (Santoni-Rugiu et al., 1996, 1999). HCV core protein also transforms the rat embryo fibroblast cell line Rat-1 (Chang et al., 1998) and appears to cooperate with an activated *ras* oncogene in transformation of rat embryo fibroblasts (Ray et al., 1996b), although this latter observation has not been confirmed (Chang et al., 1998). Strikingly, at least one strain of transgenic mice overexpressing the HCV core antigen developed HCC in the absence of inflammatory liver disease (Moriya et al., 1998) (Ch. 13). This not only underscores the potentially direct contribution of high levels of HCV core protein to the development of HCC but also suggests that necroinflammatory liver disease and hepatocellular turnover are not absolute requirements for the pathogenesis of this tumor (see related question 15 in Ch. 24).

The integrity of *p53* and the function of its protein product appear to be important in the pathogenesis of HCC, since *p53* mutations occur in high frequency during tumor progression (Murakami et al., 1991; Mishida et al., 1993; Nose et al., 1993). As indicated above, the HCV core gene appears to bind and stimulate the *trans*-activating activity of p53 (Lu et al., 1999); however, other studies suggested that the HCV core protein transcriptionally represses *p53* (Ray et al., 1997) (Section 5.4), suggesting decreased p53 expression. The levels of exogenous *p53*, combined with the use of different cell lines in these contrasting studies, may account for the differences. HCV core protein has also been shown to repress the $p21^{WAF1/CIP1/SDI1}$ in several cell types in a p53-independent manner (Ray et al., 1998a) (Section 5.4). Downregulation of $p21^{WAF1}$ expression may perturb cell cycle checkpoint control at G_1/S phase and contribute to the escape of HCV-infected cells from senescence. Recently, HCV core has also been shown to bind to and functionally inactivate a bZIP nuclear transcription factor by cytoplasmic sequestration; these events correlated with cellular transformation (Jin et al., 2000). This suggests that inactivation of multiple negative growth regulatory pathways by HCV core may contribute importantly to the development of the transformed phenotype. Interestingly, it has also been reported that HCV-encoded NS3 also binds to p53 (Ishido & Hotta, 1998). Although the consequences of NS3/p53 complex formation is uncertain, NS3 has been shown to transform NIH 3T3 cells (Sakamuro, Furukawa & Takegami, 1995) and inhibit actinomycin D-induced apoptosis (which is p53 dependent) (Fujita et al., 1996), suggesting that NS3 may inactivate p53. However, in the context of the virus life cycle, NS3 acts as a serine proteinase in the cleavage and maturation of the HCV nonstructural proteins (Bartenschlager et al., 1993) (Section 2.4), and as a helicase and NTPase, which is likely to play an important role in virus replication (Suzich et al., 1993) (Section 2.5). Since the transformation of NIH 3T3 cells mapped to the proteinase domain of NS3 (Sakamuro et al., 1995), it is possible that NS3 activates oncogene proteins or inactivates tumor suppressor proteins by cleavage. Alternatively, or in addition, the NS3 helicase activity may promote genetic instability in cellular DNA by stimulating DNA recombination (Takamizawa et al., 1991). However, the contribution of these mechanisms to the development and/or progression of HCC remain to be evaluated.

Prolonged IFN therapy in responders with CLD (Mazzelia et al., 1996; Onodera et al., 1997), or successful retreatment of partial responders (Toyoda et al., 2000), has shown a statistically significant decrease in the incidence of HCC. In addition, the frequency of HCC appeared to be lower among responders after 20 years of follow-up (Ikeda et al., 1999) (Ch. 9). Among nonresponders, the most common HCV sequence found corresponds to genotype 1 (Martinot-Peignoux et al., 1995). Closer examination has shown that sequence variability within the NS5A of HCV subtype 1b correlates with IFN resistance (Bruno et al., 1997; Fernadez et al., 1997). NS5A binds and functionally inactivates double-stranded RNA-induced protein kinase (PKR) (Ch. 10), which has also been identified as a tumor suppressor (Meurs et al., 1993) that regulates stress-induced apoptosis in dividing cells (Clemens & Elia, 1997). If apoptosis is blocked by the action of NS5A upon PKR, then it may contribute to the development of HCC. However, other possible HCC risk factors may not have been consistently controlled for in these studies, including the severity of liver disease, alcoholism, viral load, and underlying ("occult") HBV infection during the time of treatment, the dose and duration of treatment, and the definition of "responder" and "nonresponder" to treatment. According to the NIH consensus panel statement, for example, the risk of developing exacerbated CLD and accelerating the appearance of HCC in chronically infected patients who are also chronic alcoholics is so great that the panel has recommended total abstinence from alcohol among patients with HCV infection (NIH, 1997). In addition, the presence of HBsAg-negative HCC with or without HCV markers is often associated with underlying or "occult" HBV infections. Over the years, the latter has been demonstrated by the presence of HBV DNA integrated into the livers and tumors of patients with HBsAg-negative or anti-HCV-positive HCC (Brechot et al., 1981; Lai et al., 1990b; Urashima et al., 1997), and by HBV X region mRNA overexpression in tumors (Diamantis et al., 1992).

More recently, it has been shown that the HBV X protein, which is involved in hepatocellular transformation both in vitro (Hohne et al., 1990) and in vivo (Kim et al., 1991), is also detectable in many HBsAg-negative HCC (Zhu et al., 1993; Greenblatt et al., 1997). Given that it often takes 10–40 years between the time of HCV infection and the appearance of HCC, the answer to the question of whether a favorable response to IFN results in the delayed appearance or prevention of HCC may have to await longer-term follow-up studies in which additional risk factors are either excluded or randomized in the treated and untreated groups. The latter may not be possible, since it would involve withholding medication that is known to be effective in a fraction of patients in the placebo group.

The role of NS5A in the biology of HCV is poorly understood, although its presence in complexes with other HCV nonstructural proteins suggest that NS5A may be a cofactor in virus replication (Pawlotsky & Germanidis, 1999) (Section 2.5). Removal of the amino-terminal one-third of NS5A yields a truncated polypeptide that has been shown to have *trans*-activation activity (Fig. 2.3) (Chung, Song & Jang, 1997; Kato et al., 1997; Tanimoto et al., 1997). Consistent with these roles is the finding of full-length NS5A in the perinuclear cytoplasm, which is the site of virus replication, and of amino-terminally truncated NS5A in the nucleus, where it can act as a *trans*-regulatory protein (Ide et al., 1996; Moradpour et al., 1998). It is thought that, in infected cells, the amino-terminal region of NS5A blocks the *trans*-regulatory and nuclear localization domains located in the carboxy-terminal two-thirds of the molecule. A conformational change, promoted by binding of NS5A to other proteins or by the phosphorylation of NS5A, may result in the nuclear translocation of a protein with *trans*-regulatory activities (Han et al., 1997) (Section 2.5). The translocation of NS5A to the nucleus may repress the transcription of the cyclin kinase inhibitor $p21^{WAF1/CIP1/SDI1}$ and stimulate the expression of proliferating cell nuclear antigen (Ghosh et al., 1999), resulting in stimulated cellular growth (Section 2.5). In addition, NS5A has recently been shown to interact with a cellular protein containing SH3 domains, which may be a tumor suppressor (Herion et al., 1998). Further, NS5A appears to bind to growth factor receptor bound protein 2 adaptor protein and may inhibit signal transduction that normally regulates cell growth (Tan et al., 1999). The functional consequences of these interactions remain to be studied. NS5A stimulates anchorage-independent growth of NIH 3T3 cells in soft agar and promotes tumor formation of these cells in nude mice (Ghosh et al., 1999), suggesting that NS5A may contribute to increased cellular growth and to tumor formation. However, it is not clear whether the behavior of NS5A in NIH 3T3 cells accurately reflects the effects of this protein upon hepatocytes, nor whether any of the molecular based mechanisms mentioned above contribute to malignant transformation.

6.3 Subtypes of hepatitis C and hepatocellular carcinoma

Based upon genome sequence heterogeneity, HCV clones have been divided into at least 6 genotypes (Section 3.2) and heterogeneity within virus genotypes further subdivided into a total of more than 50 subtypes (Section 3.2) (Bukh et al., 1995; Simmonds, 1998). Among these, HCV subtype 1b appears to be more commonly associated with HCC than other subtypes (Hatzakis et al., 1996; Zein et al., 1996; Bruno et al., 1997). The enhanced oncogenicity of subtype 1b compared with other subtypes is in doubt, since 1b is the predominant subtype in many infected populations (Lopez-Labrador et al., 1997) and not all studies see a close association between subtype 1b and HCC (Benvegnu & Alberti, 1996; Naoumov et al., 1997; Reid et al., 1999). The correlation between 1b infection and CLD may reflect the increased propensity of subtype 1b to establish chronic infections (Kao et al., 1996; Bruno et al., 1997) and to be associated with CLD (Bruno et al., 1997; Fernadez et al., 1997). However, other work has shown no correlation between subtype of infection and CLD (Benvegnu & Alberti, 1996; Han et al., 1997), suggesting that cirrhosis is the dominant risk factor for tumor development (Tarao et al., 1999). These results suggest that the pathogenic potential of HCV subtypes may be variable in different populations, and that other risk factors also contribute to the development of HCC to varying extents throughout the world.

6.4 Other mechanisms that may contribute to hepatocellular carcinoma associated with hepatitis C

The development of HCC involves epigenetic changes in host gene expression, some of which are likely to be mediated by the action of one or more HCV gene products, as indicated above. However, there are additional changes in gene expression that have not been assigned to the actions of one or more HCV proteins. For example, the development of HCC in chronically infected patients often involves the activation of insulin-like growth factor II and TGFα (Nardone et al., 1996; Tanaka et al., 1996), both of which contribute importantly to tumor development (Lee, Merlino & Fausto, 1992; Schirmacher et al., 1992). In addition, a number of genetic mutations appear during tumor progression. The most common genetic alterations observed in HCC involve the loss of heterozygosity (LOH) in chromosome arms spanning portions of 1p, 4q, 6q, 8p, 9p, and 17p (Nagai et al., 1997). Independent studies, however, have reported LOH at 5q, 11p, 13q, 16q, and 17p (Sheu et al., 1999), suggesting that tumor progression may arise from multiple, different genetic alterations in individual patients. LOH in these regions suggests the presence of multiple tumor suppressor genes that are lost during tumor progression. Interestingly, LOH at 1p was commonly found in small, well-differentiated HCCs, while LOH at 16p and 17p was prevalent in advanced, metastatic tumors (Nishida et al., 1992; Boige et al., 1997). An increased loss at 8p was also associated with tumor metastasis (Qin et al., 1999). Interestingly, LOH at chromosome 4q was associated with the presence of p53 mutations (at 17p13) (Rashid et al., 1999), with LOH of the retinoblastoma tumor suppressor gene (*Rb*) (in 13q14), and with LOH of the breast cancer susceptibility 2 (*BRCA2*) gene (Wooster et al., 1995) in HCC, suggesting that the inactivation of multiple tumor suppressor genes contribute importantly to tumor formation. *p53* point mutations have also been found among 25–45% of HCCs examined (Montesano, Hainaut & Wild, 1997), suggesting that the LOH at one *p53* allele is accompanied by mutation in the other in a large percentage of cases. In some studies, the *p53* codon 249 mutation was associated with chronic aflatoxin exposure, while the origin of other *p53* mutations was not clear. While LOH of *Rb* has been detected in advanced HCC, the downregulation of *Rb* in the absence of mutation is associated with the upregulated expression of gankyrin oncogene product (Higashitsuji et al., 2000), which acts by binding to the Rb gene product and promoting degradation in the proteasome. Decreased expression of E-cadherin (which is involved in cell–cell adhesion) associated with methylation of its promoter or LOH has also been documented in about 60% of HCCs (Kanai et al., 1997; Hirohashi, 1998). Amplification of c-*myc* (Peng, Lai & Hsu, 1993) and the gene for the cell cycle modulator cyclin D_1 (Nishida et al., 1994) has also been observed in a small percentage of patients. More recently, mutations affecting β-catenin have been found in almost half the cases of HCV-associated HCC (Huang et al., 1999; Hsu et al., 2000). Mutation often results in the stabilization of β-catenin, which then constitutively activates the Wnt signal transduction pathway and, finally, gives rise to alterations in cell fate that are characteristic of malignant transformation. In addition, given that E-cadherin sequesters wild-type β-catenin, reduced E-cadherin expression could also result in increased β-catenin-associated Wnt signal transduction, which activates the genes for Myc, Jun, and cyclin D_1 (Behrens, 2000). Changes in the expression patterns of other tumor suppressor genes and oncogenes have also been recently documented in HCC, but their role in the development and progression of HCV-associated HCC remains to be firmly established (Buendia, 2000). Hence, both epigenetic and genetic events are likely to contribute to hepatocarcinogenesis, although it is not known whether they are the cause or an effect of hepatocellular transformation.

7

Hepatitis C and autoimmune diseases

Soon after the discovery of HCV, high frequencies of anti-HCV ($>$ 50%) were reported among patients with autoimmune hepatitis (Esteban et al., 1989; Lenzi et al., 1990) and, later, among patients with other autoimmune diseases (Table 7.1 and Section 1.5). Further work among patients with HCV-associated autoimmune hepatitis showed that many anti-HCV results were caused by false positives generated by hypergammaglobulinemia (McFarlane et al., 1990) and by immune complexes (McFarlane et al., 1983), which interfered with first-generation anti-HCV ELISAs. False-positive anti-HCV results were also noted in patients with other autoimmune diseases (Fusconi et al., 1990), although the frequency of anti-HCV correlated directly with the levels of gammaglobulin in sera (Schwarcz, von Sydow & Weiland, 1990) (Section 1.5). The introduction of second-generation anti-HCV testing and RT/PCR, however, still showed that 20–40% of patients with autoimmune hepatitis had detectable markers of HCV infection (Cassani et al., 1992; Nishiguchi et al., 1992). Independent work showed that the frequency of anti-HCV among patients with primary biliary cirrhosis or primary sclerosing cholangitis was low ($<$ 5%) and similar to that of the general population (Lohse et al., 1995), suggesting that HCV infection is not closely linked with autoimmune diseases. Likewise, anti-HCV was found in 3–5% of patients with liver–kidney microsomal autoantibodies (Abuaf et al., 1993), a non-organ specific marker of autoimmunity, although the titers in patients with HCV-associated hepatitis are usually much lower than in patients with autoimmune hepatitis (Strassburg et al., 1996). Other autoantibody specificities, such as anti-nuclear and anti-smooth muscle antibodies, also appear during the course of chronic HCV infection (Cassani et al., 1992) (Table 7.1). Consequently, the role of HCV in autoimmune hepatitis remains controversial.

There is considerable evidence linking HCV infection with essential mixed cryoglobulinemia (EMC), which is a lymphoproliferative disorder resulting in the production of rheumatoid factors (usually IgM) against IgG (Lunel & Musset, 1998). This is evidenced by a number of studies showing a high frequency of anti-HCV in patients with EMC (Cacoub et al., 1994; Zignego et al., 1997a), although much of this work was originally conducted with the first-generation anti-HCV assays. HCV sequences have also been detected in PBMC and in

Table 7.1. Autoimmune diseases and autoantibodies associated with chronic hepatitis C infection

	Examples
Liver diseases	Autoimmune hepatitis
Lymphoproliferative disorders	Essential mixed cryoglobulinemia, Waldenström's macroglobulinemia, other monoclonal gammopathies
Malignancies	NonHodgkin's lymphoma, chronic lymphocytic leukemia, multiple myeloma
Dermatological autoimmune diseases	Lichen planus, porphyria cutanea tarda
Other autoimmune diseases	Autoimmune thyroiditis, idiopathic pulmonary fibrosis, Sjögren's syndrome, membranous glomerulonephritis, polyarthritis, polyarteritis nodosa
Autoantibodies[a]	Liver-kidney microsomal autoantibodies (target antigen is cytochrome P450), rheumatoid factor (IgM anti-IgG), anti-GOR, anti-nuclear antibodies, anti-smooth muscle antibodies, anti-thyroid antibodies, anti-asialoglycoprotein receptor antibodies

From Strassburg et al. (1996) and Zignego & Brechot (1999).
[a]With the exception of anti-GOR, most of these antibodies have also been readily detected in corresponding autoimmune diseases that are not associated with hepatitis C infection

bone-marrow derived mononuclear cells from patients with EMC, although this is often associated with a lack of viremia (Ferri et al., 1993). Interestingly, more than 50% of patients with anti-HCV and EMC are responsive to IFN treatment, which results in a reduction in HCV viremia and serum cryoglobulin levels (Misiani et al., 1994), suggesting a pathogenic link between HCV and EMC. The fact that 5–10% of EMC evolve into nonHodgkin's lymphoma implies that there may also be an association between HCV and this neoplasm. Studies have verified this association not only among patients with EMC (La Civita et al., 1995) but also in patients without a prior history of EMC (Ferri et al., 1997a; Zignego et al., 1997a). HCV has also been implicated in other B cell malignancies (e.g., chronic lymphocytic leukemia and multiple myeloma) (Table 7.1), but not in non-B cell lymphoproliferative disorders nor in T cell nonHodgkin's lymphoma (Zignego & Brechot, 1999), although whether these constitute cause and effect relationships remain to be established. Although HCV core, NS3, and possibly NS5A proteins have been associated with transformation (Sakamuro et al., 1995; Moriya et al., 1998; Ghosh et al., 1999) (Ch. 6), and HCV appears to replicate in lymphoid cells (Ch. 11), the limited number of transgenic mice expressing one or more of these proteins do not develop B cell-related lymphoproliferative disorders or tumors. Hence, it is difficult to say whether HCV is strongly associated with tumor types other than HCC (see related question 16 in Ch. 24).

Seroprevalence studies have also suggested a link between HCV and several skin disorders, such as EMC-associated purpura, sporadic porphyria cutanea tarda (Navas et al., 1995), and lichen planus (Nagao et al., 1995). These associations have not been consistently found among patients from different parts of the world. Combined with the finding that IFN treatment for HCV triggers lichen planus in some cases (Nagao et al., 1996), these observations imply that HCV may trigger these diseases by as yet unknown mechanisms.

There is also evidence that HCV may be associated with other autoimmune diseases (Table 7.1). For example, some studies describe a high prevalence of thyroid dysfunction and anti-thyroid antibodies in up to 30% of patients with chronic HCV infections (Zignego & Brechot, 1999), although other independent work has found no such association (Wong et al., 1996). A high prevalence of HCV markers has also been found associated with Sjögren's syndrome (i.e., autoimmune sialadenitis or inflammation of the salivary glands) (Haddad et al., 1992). Unlike some of the other proposed associations above, the appearance of a Sjögren's-like syndrome in transgenic mice expressing HCV envelope protein provides a direct link between HCV gene expression and extrahepatic pathology (Koike et al., 1997). Interestingly, Sjögren's syndrome is commonly found among HCV-infected patients with EMC (Haddad et al., 1992). Given that EMC is a lymphoproliferative disorder that may evolve into B cell nonHodgkin's lymphoma, it is possible that the appearance of Sjogren's syndrome among infected patients reflects one aspect of HCV-associated lymphoproliferation (Zignego and Brechot, 1999). Finally, there is also a high frequency of HCV markers in some patients with idiopathic pulmonary fibrosis (Ohta et al., 1993), although other work has found no relationship (Irving, Day & Johnston, 1993). The finding of pulmonary fibrosis in patients with EMC (Ferri et al., 1997b) suggests that HCV may trigger autoimmune responses that indirectly mediate extrahepatic pathology.

The likely lymphotrophism of HCV may not only contribute to B cell lymphoproliferative disorders, ranging from EMC to nonHodgkin's lymphoma, but may also promote the development of chronic infection and disease in a high frequency of infected patients. For example, HCV-infected patients with EMC develop an IgM specific for a cryptic epitope of the CD4-like LAG-3 protein. This may be triggered by abnormal processing of the LAG-3 protein in the infected lymphocyte

(Mecchia et al., 1996). It has also been shown that PBMCs isolated from chronically infected patients produce anti-HCV in vitro, while uninfected cells did not (Lohr et al., 1995). Interestingly, it has recently been shown that viral antibody responses predominate and persist in patients who develop chronic infection, while CD4[+] proliferative and CD8[+] CTL responses predominate and persist in patients who resolve acute infections (Takaki et al., 2000) (Sections 5.2 and 5.3). Hence, HCV infection of lymphocytes may alter their function and, as a consequence, the relative strengths of humoral versus cellular immunity following acute infection. If these functional alterations occur in vivo, then it would serve as an important example of how an extrahepatic infection could influence the pathogenesis of both liver and extrahepatic diseases.

8

Clinical aspects of the disease

Much of what is known about the clinical course of HCV infection comes from retrospective studies of patients with acquired NANB PTH and from prospective studies of those who were acutely exposed to HCV (Prince et al., 1974; Alter et al., 1975; Feinstone et al., 1975; Knodell et al., 1975; Esteban et al., 1990; Tremolada et al., 1991). Overall, the clinical presentation of acute hepatitis is similar in patients infected with HAV, HBV or HCV, although acute HCV infection tends to be milder than acute HBV infection. In fact, 70–95% of HCV-infected people do not recall an episode of acute hepatitis, suggesting a subclinical course is very common (Meyers et al., 1977; Koretz et al., 1993b; Hoofnagle, 1997). Apart from the fact that the average incubation period for acute HCV infection (Seeff, 1991; Koretz et al., 1993b) is between that of HAV and HBV (Table 1.1), acute cases of sympto-matic HCV infection are indistinguishable from severe acute HBV or HAV infections. Symptoms of acute HCV infection, which vary in duration and inten-sity, span 2–12 weeks (Ch. 4) and often include malaise, nausea, and upper right quadrant pain, followed by jaundice and dark urine (Hoofnagle, 1997). Loss of appetite may also occur (CDC, 1998). These symptoms occur weeks after the appearance of HCV RNA in blood and overlap in time with the elevation of transaminases (Fig. 4.1). ALT elevations often reach a peak 10-fold or more above normal, independent of whether patients develop symptoms. Acute infection is also characterized by the appearance of HCV RNA in blood 1–2 weeks after infection, which may peak at concentrations of 10^8–10^9 genomes/ml prior to the onset of elevated ALT (Farci et al., 1991; Alter et al., 1995). This is followed by the appearance of anti-HCV at 8–9 weeks (Alter et al., 1991) and clearance of virus from blood as the bout of acute hepatitis resolves. Long-term normalization of serum ALT values is characteristic of a truly acute HCV infection (Fig. 4.1 and Ch. 4). Hence, while biochemical and virological markers define acute HCV infection, there is considerable variability in the intensity and duration of accompanying symptoms, with the majority of patients not developing symptoms at all.

The outcome following acute infection differs among viruses. HAV, for example, is not associated with chronic infection, and essentially 100% recovery follows acute hepatitis. In contrast, about 10% of adults with acute HBV infection become chronic carriers of the virus, which is characterized by the persistence of virus and viral antigens in the blood for years or decades. Up to 30% of HBV carriers later develop CLD (Hoofnagle, Shafritz & Popper, 1987). By comparison, up to 85% of patients with acute HCV infections go on to develop chronic infections, which are characterized by the persistence of anti-HCV and virus in the blood (Esteban et al., 1991; Seeff et al., 1992) (Fig. 4.2). More than half of the latter group (60–70%) develop liver disease (Aach et al., 1991; Esteban et al., 1991; Seeff et al., 1992; Alter, 1993a; Koretz et al., 1993b; Hoofnagle, 1997). In the remaining 30–40% of chronically infected individuals, ALT values remain persistently normal (Ch. 4). At the present time, there are no characteristics of acute infection that predict which patients will develop chronic infection or CLD. Hence, a high frequency of HCV-infected patients go on to develop chronic infections and CLDs, making this virus especially burdensome with regard to both morbidity and mortality.

An important difference that distinguishes CLD in HBV from that in HCV infections is that the onset of symptomatic CLD occurs within the first few years in HBV infections while symptomatic disease occurs some 10–20 years after the onset of HCV infection. Additional comparisons between HAV, HBV, and NANB (HCV) infections are outlined in Table 1.1. A phenomenon that commonly occurs in both acute and chronic infections consists of episodic fluctuations in ALT. These fluctuations may peak at 10–15-fold above normal and alternate with either normal or near normal transaminase values over many weeks or months (Fig. 4.1). Characteristically, the amplitude of these relapsing ALT spikes decreases over several years (Di Bisceglie et al., 1991). Other patterns of ALT have also been documented in chronic HCV infections, although they are less frequent. For example, some patients develop a sustained plateau of elevated ALT following acute infection, while others experience a bout of acute hepatitis that resolves, followed by a relapse months or years later (Alter et al., 1989a). Each of these ALT patterns is accompanied by persistent viremia (Farci et al., 1991; Puoti et al., 1992; Mattsson et al., 1993). This variability has made it very difficult to know whether ALT values have prognostic value either during the natural history of infection or during treatment (Dienstag, 1983; Esteban et al., 1990; Mattson, Weiland & Glaumann, 1990; Di Bisceglie et al., 1991; Wejstal, Hermodsson & Norkrans, 1991). Even normal transaminases during the first 20 years of chronic infection can be misleading, with some studies reporting a range of histopathology from normal or nonspecific changes through chronic active hepatitis and cirrhosis (Naito et al., 1994; Healey, Chapman & Fleming, 1995), while other studies report mostly periportal or lobular hepatitis (Alberti et al., 1992; Alter et al., 1992; Kodama et al., 1993). Blood donors who test anti-HCV positive are also asymptomatic and in most cases unaware of being infected, although they readily transmitted HCV through transfusions prior to anti-HCV testing and often developed symptoms of chronic HCV infection years later. Consequently, although sustained elevated levels of transaminases are usually indicative of underlying CLD, they are not predictive of long-term outcome.

As noted above, the symptoms most commonly associated with chronic HCV infection are fatigue and right upper quadrant pain. These are nonspecific and are most often intermitant and mild. These and other symptoms are rarely incapacitating but can significantly decrease the quality of life. Unfortunately, because of the indolent nature of chronic hepatitis, a diagnosis of HCV is often not made until patients present with cirrhosis or HCC. Anti-HCV and HCV RNA appear to correlate poorly, or not at all, with disease severity and stage as determined by histological examination of needle biopsy specimens. Even monitoring ALT levels has not been reliable as a prognostic marker of CLD, since there appears to be no correlation between ALT levels, the presence and severity of symptoms, and liver histopathology (Desmet et al., 1994). However, among patients with cirrhosis, a large percentage were symptomatic, suggesting that symptoms may help in the identification of late-stage liver disease. Further observations have shown that elevated ALT values were often, but not always, indicative of underlying fibrosis and inflammation, while patients with normal transminases rarely had evidence of advanced disease or cirrhosis (Haber et al., 1995; Healey et al., 1995; McCormick et al., 1996). Given the nonspecificity and late onset of symptoms, and that ALT appears to have limited utility as a prognostic indicator, there is a great need to find more reliable serum or tissue markers to assess the risk for disease progression and the efficacy of therapeutic approaches.

9

Current therapeutic approaches

Therapeutic decisions in chronic HCV infection have been made difficult by the subclinical nature of most acute and chronic infections. This is because, in many cases, infections are not even detected unless anti-HCV or HCV RNA tests are performed (Section 1.6 and Ch. 19). This does not lessen the danger of chronic HCV, which often does not become symptomatic until the development of cirrhosis some 20 years following infection. Given the high morbidity and mortality associated with cirrhosis, combined with the insidious nature and variable progression of CLD, it is not surprising that so many chronically infected patients are not treated until liver disease is fairly advanced and considerable permanent damage is done. For example, patients that become symptomatic and then present with cirrhosis may already be in end-stage liver disease. Such patients are also at very high risk for the development of HCC (Chs. 4 and 6). Given these considerations, HCV is often not diagnosed for a long period after virus exposure, since patients are "well" and do not seek medical help. This represents one of the major challenges in treating HCV infection.

IFN-α is one of a family of naturally occurring glycoproteins that have both direct antiviral and immunomodulatory activities. Initially, IFN-α was obtained from leukocyte cultures in very limited quantities, but the availability of recombinant IFN-α in the 1980s finally permitted large-scale, controlled trials of its utility. The activity of IFN-α against a wide range of DNA and RNA viruses prompted its use among patients with chronic NANBH, where it was shown to reduce the mean ALT levels in 8 of the first 10 treated patients (Hoofnagle et al., 1986). Among responders, the treatment was well tolerated, and ALT levels decreased within a few weeks after the start of treatment. Treatment for up to a year resulted in reduced inflammatory liver disease. Based upon these encouraging results, a number of larger clinical trials were initiated. The combined results showed a reduced or normalized ALT in up to 50% of treated patients, but that only 25% of treated patients had a sustained suppression of ALT after the end of treatment (Tine et al., 1991). These results were independent of IFN dose ($1 \times$ to 3×10^6 units three times a week) or duration of treatment (6 or 12 months). When assays for HCV RNA were developed, the sustained virological response (i.e., a loss of HCV RNA from blood) was seen in 6–12% of treated patients after a 6 month course of therapy, while the response was seen in 13–25% after 12 months (Poynard et al., 1996). The finding that a histological response correlates much more closely with the virological response than does a biochemical response (i.e., a decrease or normalization of ALT) (Alberti et al., 1992; De Alava et al., 1993) suggests that a virological response is more indicative of the efficacy of IFN in chronically infected patients. Even so, the fact that only one in four or fewer patients derive sustained benefit from IFN therapy suggests that IFN monotherapy is inadequate in the majority of patients with chronic HCV. Additional studies show similar findings (Damen & Bresters, 1998). However, higher doses of IFN for greater durations have initially shown sustained response rates of 40–50% (Gretch et al., 1996; Koff, 1997). In the relatively few studies carried out with children, the sustained virological response to IFN appears to be higher (38–69%) than in adults (Bortolotti et al., 1995; Iorio et al., 1996). Histological improvement in the liver was also observed (Iorio et al., 1996). Hence, IFN monotherapy is effective against HCV, although the sustained response rates among chronically infected adults is low (see related question 17 in Ch. 24).

The low sustained response rate from a single course of IFN monotherapy prompted the design of trials in which retreatment was performed among chronically infected patients who relapsed after the first course of IFN. The results of several trials showed that retreatment, especially for more than 6 months, resulted in a virological response in up to 50% of the patients. However, relapse was common after the end of retreatment (Weiland, Zhang & Widell, 1993; Gerken et al., 1995). Among trials using a single course of therapy where follow-up liver biopsies were performed, the histological activity improved significantly by the end of treatment, especially in patients who also had a virological response (Hopf et al., 1996; Rumi et al., 1996). Several other studies showed that IFN treatment resulted in reduced fibrosis independent of virological or biochemical response (Manabe et al., 1993; Hiramatsu et al., 1995). Some studies have even showed a decreased incidence of HCC among IFN responders (Nishiguchi et al., 1995; Mazzella et al., 1996), although this has not been consistently observed (Blendis, Wong & Sherman, 2000) (Ch. 6). Given that more than 80% of acute infections become chronic, several trials of acutely infected patients have been performed. In one trial, IFN treatment of patients at various times after acute infection brought about a sustained virological response in 52 of 100 treated patients, while only 8 of 70 untreated patients cleared virus RNA from blood (Camma, Almasio & Craxi, 1996). Independent observations also showed that IFN treatment of acutely infected patients resulted in normal liver histology 1–2 years post-treatment (Ohnishi, Nomura & Nakano, 1991). Given the high frequency in which acute infection becomes chronic, it will be very important to see whether IFN treatment more consistently prevents the acute-to-chronic transition.

In assessing criteria that would predict the outcome of treatment, it appears that a lower pretreatment viral load is much more common in IFN responders than in nonresponders (Yamada et al., 1995). Additional observations suggested that the response rate is significantly higher among patients infected with genotypes other than 1 (Kanai, Kako & Okamoto, 1992; Chemello et al., 1995a), although this finding has not been confirmed in all studies (Picciotto et al., 1997) (Section 3.2). Part of the problem is the differential distribution of genotype 1 in various human populations worldwide, and the fact that the success of IFN therapy may also be related to factors such as age at treatment and duration of infection, as well as the extent of liver damage and the quasispecies diversity present at the beginning of treatment (Lam et al., 1994; Davis & Lau, 1997). In addition, there is evidence suggesting that subtype 1b may be more pathogenic than other subtypes in that it is found in a high percentage of patients with HCC (Hatzakis et al., 1996; Zein et al., 1996) (Chs. 3, 4, and 6). However, genotype 1 may not be inherently more pathogenic, as suggested by the fact that subtype 1b is the most common subtype among populations in which many of the HCC studies were conducted. Its association with more severe liver pathology may also reflect the possibility that genotype 1 infections persist longer in chronically infected patients than other genotypes (Benvegnu et al., 1997).

Studies examining the effect of quasispecies diversity on the response to treatment have had mixed results. In one series, the more heterogeneous the pretreatment genome sequences in serum (i.e., the greater the quasispecies complexity), the less likely it was that a patient would respond to IFN treatment (Kanazawa et al., 1994; Koizumi et al., 1995; Zeuzem, 2000) (Section 2.5). In natural infections, a high complexity of quasispecies following acute infection is also associated with progression to chronicity (Ray et al., 1999). The link between these observations is that immunostimulation mediated by IFN or during natural acute infection could clear virus if the quasispecies complexity is limited. In addition, the divergence in sequence among quasispecies, and not the number of quasispecies per se, has been implicated as being important in IFN responsiveness, with HCV having a greater divergence of sequences being less responsive (Polyak et al., 1997). Other groups, however, have found no relationship between pretreatment complexity of quasispecies and the outcome of therapy (Shindo et al., 1996). In fact, in a 5 year follow-up of two chimpanzees inoculated with an infectious clone of HCV, no changes in the sequence of the HVR1 region was noted, even though both animals developed chronic infections (Major et al., 1999). It may be relevant that infected chimpanzees do not often develop chronic hepatitis, suggesting that immune responses to the virus are weak, resulting in little change in the complexity of quasispecies. Pretreatment HCV subtype also appears to play a role in predicting the response to IFN, with genotype 1 infections being much less responsive to IFN

(8–26% responders) than genotype 2 (54–83% responders). Pretreatment virus load is also important, with a lower virus load generally more responsive to therapy than a high load (Bell et al., 1997) (Section 1.6). In terms of the characteristics of quasispecies post-treatment, successful IFN therapy appears to be associated with a decrease in the number of quasispecies and in the sequence heterogeneity of these variants in some (Shindo et al., 1996; Gonzalez-Peralta et al., 1997) but not all (Sandres et al., 2000) studies. An increase in complexity quasispecies appears to occur among patients who fail to respond to IFN therapy (Pawlotsky et al., 1999) (Section 2.5). While these results suggest that IFN treatment may have a profound effect upon the number and complexity of quasispecies in chronically infected patients, they also imply that mutations at other sites within the HCV genome may be important either pre- or post-treatment (Pawlotsky et al., 1998). However, a low frequency of mutation within the NS5A HVR2 was observed in IFN nonresponders who were successfully retreated (Gerotto et al., 1999). Similar results were obtained for the NS5A HVR2 independent of IFN treatment response (Sarrazin et al., 2000a). In fact, no amino acid sequence within NS5A has turned out to be predictive of responsiveness to IFN therapy, nor is there any evidence that mutations are selected during treatment (McKechnie, Mills & McCruden, 2000) (Ch. 10). Since successful IFN therapy is associated with decreased virus load, work was conducted to determine whether it was associated with the appearance of mutations in the IRES and/or NS5B. No correlation was found between the number of mutations within the IRES, serum HCV RNA levels, and the outcome of IFN treatment (Yamamoto et al., 1997). However, there was a direct correlation between the development of NS5B quasispecies and the effectiveness of IFN treatment (Tao et al., 1998), implying that such mutations may render the polymerase less effective in the support of HCV replication, although this needs to be demonstrated. A more thorough analysis of other regions of the HCV genome will reveal whether other mutations exist and correlate with the outcome of IFN treatment.

Despite the benefits of IFN therapy, especially where retreatment or prolonged courses of treatment are provided, IFN has many side effects. These include a "flu-like" illness that generally resolves soon after the start of treatment (Di Bisceglie et al., 1989). Other side effects that have been reported include irritability, lethargy, dizziness, nausea, diarrhea, seizures, fatigue, depression, vomiting, and weight loss. In addition, pruritus, retinal abnormalities, cutaneous necrosis at the injection sites, alopecia, leuko- and thrombocytopenia, the appearance of anti-IFN, and, in some cases, autoantibodies have also been documented (Marcillin et al., 1991; Davis, 2000). Thrombocytopenia and leukopenia result from IFN-mediated bone marrow suppression. Antibodies to thrombocytes have also been detected and may contribute to thrombocytopenia (Hoofnagle, 1991).

Among autoantibodies, antithyroid microsomal antibodies and antithyroglobulin antibodies have been described and may lead to thyroid gland dysfunction (Burman et al., 1985; Di Bisceglie et al., 1989). Although IFN treatment may result in the appearance of anti-nuclear and anti-smooth muscle autoantibodies, these are not associated with corresponding autoimmune disease (Fattovich et al., 1991). Likewise, although anti-IFN has been detected in treated patients, its presence does not seem to alter the efficacy of treatment (Antonelli et al., 1992). These side effects suggest that treatment with IFN must be monitored closely and that appropriate counseling should be provided to patients and families of patients considering such treatment.

The side effects of IFN, combined with high cost and the fact that only a minority of chronically infected patients benefit from IFN monotherapy, suggest that other therapeutic approaches need to be developed. Over the past few years, the guanosine nucleoside analog ribavirin (1-β-D-ribofuranosyl-1,2,4-triazole-3-carboxamide) has been shown to be active in combination with IFN among patients with chronic HCV. Unlike other nucleoside analogues, ribavirin has a modified base instead of a modified sugar. Although its mechanism(s) of action are uncertain, it appears to affect the phosphorylation of guanosine into the trisphosphate nucleotide, resulting in a depletion of intracellular GTP, which is required for virus replication. It is also possible that ribavirin may directly suppress the action of the HCV-encoded RdRp (NS5B) (Damen & Bresters, 1998). It has also been suggested that ribavirin augments virus-specific CTL activity by inhibiting IL-4, which inhibits CTL activity, and preserving IFN-γ and IL-2 production, which sustains CTL activity (Patterson & Fernandez-Larson, 1990). Regardless of the mechanism(s) involved, ribavirin monotherapy resulted in a decrease or normalization in ALT values during treatment in up to 40% of treated patients (Reichard et al., 1991; Dusheiko et al., 1996), followed by a relapse after the end of treatment. Decreases in viral load during therapy were not consistently observed when untreated or IFN nonresponders were given ribavirin (Reichard et al., 1993; Di Bisceglie et al., 1995). Hence, the utility of ribavirin as an effective monotherapy has not been established.

Among drug-naive patients, combination IFN/ribavirin therapy resulted in a sustained virological response in 37–60% (Chemello et al., 1995b; Lai et al., 1996; Reichard et al., 1998). Retreatment of IFN relapsers with combination therapy resulted in an end-of-treatment response of approximately 75–90% and a sustained virological response of about 50%, while retreatment of IFN nonresponders yielded a response in up to 30% of patients (Chemello et al., 1995b; Lai et al., 1996; Davis, 2000). Histological activity in patients treated by combination therapy was also significantly improved (Lai et al., 1996). Close examination of patients on IFN monotherapy compared with combination therapy showed that the addition of ribavirin prevented the high rate of relapse observed with IFN monotherapy, thereby increasing the fraction of patients with a sustained response (Bellobuono et al., 1997; Reichard et al., 1998). A sustained response from combination therapy was most effective in patients with a low titer of virus prior to a 6 month treatment ($< 2 \times 10^6$ copies/ml HCV RNA), and among infections with genotypes 2 or 3 ($\sim$66% responded) compared with genotype 1 (17–29%). For patients with a higher virus titer and/or genotype 1 infections, 12 months of treatment increased the sustained response to 38% (McHutchison & Poynard, 1999). Twelve months of combination therapy was also effective in patients with pretreatment fibrosis or cirrhosis (Schalm et al., 1999), suggesting the efficacy of combination therapy in a wide range of patients. Unlike IFN, the side effects of ribavirin consist mostly of mild hemolytic anemia accompanied by a rise in the serum concentration of bilirubin and uric acid. Other side effects include upper respiratory tract inflammation, mild skin disorders (e.g., rash, alopecia, and dry skin), and nervous system disorders (e.g., depression, nervousness, insomnia) (Reichard et al., 1993; Chemello et al., 1995b; Di Bisceglie et al., 1995; Lai et al., 1996). All in all, however, ribavirin has been well tolerated and appears to be quite effective in combination therapy against hepatitis C. In patients with low virus titer ($< 2 \times 10^6$ copies/ml) and infections with genotypes other than 1, a 6 month course of treatment is currently recommended. Among patients with high titers of virus, genotype 1 infections, or with underlying fibrosis/cirrhosis, a 12 month course of treatment is recommended. These recommendations apply to both drug-naive and retreated patients, provided there are no contraindications (see related question 18 in Ch. 14).

Because of the experimental nature of these therapies, it is very important to monitor the progress of the patient during treatment. Once a patient is selected for therapy, HCV RNA levels prior to and periodically during treatment must be determined. Although many physicians treat for 6 months before making a decision about continuing or discontinuing therapy, patients who are going to be responders often show a 100-fold drop in virus titer within the first 2–3 months of therapy. The possibility of making a decision at this earlier time may save money and the morbidity associated with treatment side effects among patients who are likely to be nonresponders. If ALT values normalize during treatment, and are still normal 6 months after the end of treatment, it is consistent with a sustained response. This is confirmed if a HCV RNA determination at 6 months after the end of treatment is also negative.

10

Nonstructural protein 5A and interferon resistance

The observation that a poor IFN response in clinical trials correlated with a high degree of variability of quasispecies (Kanazawa et al., 1994; Chayama et al., 1995; Koizumi et al., 1995) (Ch. 9) implies that mutations in one or more HCV gene products may alter the sensitivity of the virus to IFN. Further work revealed the presence of an IFN sensitivity-determining region (ISDR) within the carboxy-terminal region of the NS5A polypeptide that spans amino acid residues 2209–2248 (Enomoto et al., 1995, 1996), which may be selected for during the course of IFN therapy (Enomoto et al., 1994). Patients that failed to respond to IFN therapy had one sequence within this region, while patients that were IFN responders had a ISDR sequence that differed in 4–11 amino acid residues. Among HCV sequences reported in the literature, the NS5A sequence associated with IFN resistance was identical to that of subtype 1b (Kato et al., 1990), implying that subtype 1b was associated with IFN resistance. The existence of an ISDR was confirmed by independent studies in Japan (Chayama et al., 1997; Kurosaki et al., 1997), but the correlation broke down when similarly designed studies were reported from other countries (Hofgartner et al., 1997; Squadrito et al., 1997). Further work showed that there were no intrinsic properties of the putative ISDR that conferred sensitivity or resistance to IFN; instead, the data showed that a low viral load and a limited quasispecies (genetic) diversity are the most important features that correlate with IFN responsiveness (Pawlotsky et al., 1998). Alternative, or additional, explanations for differences in reports for the existence of an ISDR may be variations in IFN dosage and/or the possibility that other mutations within HCV may contribute importantly to IFN sensitivity or resistance. For example, mutations within E2 have been shown to contribute importantly to the IFN-resistant phenotype (Taylor et al., 1999; Sarrazin et al., 2000a). It is not known how the putative ISDR in NS5A confers IFN resistance, although NS5A has several actions that could be involved. It appears to be part of the replication complex of HCV, which would suggest that mutations within NS5A could result in decreased levels of virus replication, thereby conferring greater "sensitivity" to the actions of IFN. NS5A also binds and functionally inactivates PKR and 2',5'-oligoadenylate synthetase (OAS), both of which are important mediators of the IFN response. In addition, there is evidence that NS5A may be a transcriptional *trans*-regulatory protein (Ghosh et al., 1999; Pawlotsky & Germanidis, 1999) (Section 2.5) that may either inhibit the expression of IFN-inducible genes or promote the expression of genes that block the function of IFN-responsive genes. Interestingly, the *trans*-activating domain of NS5A (Section 2.5) has been mapped between amino acids 2135 and 2331, which completely encompasses the putative ISDR region (Fig. 2.3).

As discussed in Ch. 9 only 20–25% of chronically infected patients with HCV respond to IFN treatment, as measured by clearance of viral RNA and normalization of transaminases, within one year after the start of therapy (Tanaka et al., 1998). The observation that NS5A of genotype 1, which is common among IFN nonresponders (Martinot-Peignoux et al., 1995), can directly bind to and block the function of PKR (Gale et al., 1997, 1998a,b), provides a molecular basis for NS5A-associated IFN nonresponsiveness. PKR phosphorylates eIF2α, thereby inhibiting viral mRNA translation and replication (Clemens & Elia, 1997). It also regulates cellular gene expression through the activation of NF-κB by phosphorylating the natural NF-κB inhibitor IκB (Kumar et al., 1994b). PKR also stimulates the expression of IFN-inducible genes (Kirchhoff et al., 1995). Although many viruses make proteins that inhibit PKR activity by a variety of mechanisms, NS5A appears to inhibit PKR function by preventing the formation of active PRK dimers (Korth & Katze, 2000). Independent observations have shown that the HCV-encoded E2 glycoprotein from most subtypes also inhibits PKR (Taylor et al., 1999; Sarrazin et al., 2000a), and the combined action of NS5A and E2 may result in sustained virus replication, which promotes chronicity. NS5A, as well as other virus encoded proteins, may also inhibit IFN-induced signalling through the Jak/Stat pathway, which is upstream of PKR (Heim et al., 1998), suggesting an additional mechanism whereby the virus could dampen the natural IFN response. The inhibition of IFN-mediated responses is also important in the context of virus replication, since without this inhibition the double-stranded viral RNA formed during HCV replication would strongly induce a natural IFN response, which would sharply decrease the frequency whereby acute lapses into chronic HCV infection. Hence, inhibition of the IFN response appears to link virus replication to chronicity.

There is now indirect evidence that the inactivation of PKR by HCV may be relevant to the natural history and pathogenesis of chronic infection. The finding that the majority of intraheptic T cells in chronic HCV infection are Th1 cells, which secrete IFN-γ but not IL-4 or IL-5, suggests that IFN-γ is an important cytokine produced during chronic infection (Bertoletti et al., 1997). If not enough IFN-γ is made soon enough during acute infection, it may contribute to liver cell damage instead of virus clearance. This idea is supported by the finding that IFN-γ-overproducing transgenic mice develop hepatitis (Toyonaga et al., 1994).

In addition, the recent finding of elevated PKR mRNA (Yu et al., 2000) and protein (Shimada et al., 1998) in the livers of patients with chronic HCV infections suggests that the expression of this IFN effector is actually upregulated during CLD. Interestingly, these elevated PKR levels correlate with elevated serum ALT levels (Yu et al., 2000), implying that PKR may trigger cell death. Independent results have shown that tissue culture cells overexpressing PKR undergo apoptosis (Lee & Esteban, 1994) and are also especially sensitive to Fas-mediated cell death (Balachandran et al., 1998). Although the binding of NS5A and E2 to PKR has not been directly demonstrated in vivo, the resulting functional inactivation of PKR appears to be an important mechanism whereby HCV neutralizes intracellular antiviral mechanisms and prevents the destruction of cells replicating HCV.

Part II

Recent advances

11

Cell types supporting hepatitis C replication in vivo and in vitro

The replication of HCV in various lymphoid and hepatocellular cell lines suggests that these cell types are permissive for HCV replication. Lymphotrophism has been further documented by the finding of HCV in PMBCs (Meller et al., 1993; Gunji et al., 1994; Cribier et al., 1995; Lerat et al., 1996) and bone marrow (Gabrielli et al., 1994). HCV has also been found at higher titer in lymph nodes than in sera from individual infected patients (Sugiyama et al., 1997), although it is not known whether this reflects replication and/or immune-based accumulation of HCV in vivo. The transmission of NANBH to a chimpanzee using PMBCs from a patient with NANBH implies that either HCV is transmitted passively upon transfer of the lymphoid cells or that these cells actually support replication (Hellings et al., 1985). The high frequency of HCV markers in selected lympho-proliferative disorders (Strassburg et al., 1996; Zignego & Brechot, 1999), in EMC (Gabrielli et al., 1994), and in nonHodgkin's lymphoma (Luppi et al., 1996) is also consistent with an etiologic role for HCV in these lymphoid diseases, although these correlative studies do not establish cause and effect. HCV replication has also been reported in primary biliary epithelial cells isolated from infected patients and in a gall bladder epithelial cell line (Ahmed et al., 1995; Loriot et al., 1999), although at the present time there is no known association between the infection of this cell type and biliary disease. The reported replication of HCV in a porcine embryonal kidney cell line (Deriabin et al., 1997) and in African green monkey kidney (Vero) cells (Valli et al., 1997) suggests that the kidney may also support HCV replication. Regardless of whether infection of these extrahepatic sites gives rise to pathogenesis in other organ sites, extrahepatic infection may certainly provide sources of virus that can infect susceptible hepatocytes following a bout of chronic hepatitis or can infect a new liver following transplantation. In this context, extrahepatic infection would provide HCV with additional replicative "space" (i.e., additional susceptible cells) at sites other than the liver. Hence, the virus provided by extrahepatic sites of viral replication may not only promote the persistence of virus in the blood and liver but may also influence the pathogenesis of CLD.

Table 11.1 lists most of the primary cells and cell lines that appear to support HCV replication. Among primary cells, HCV replication has been detected in

Table 11.1 Tissue culture systems that support replication of hepatitis C (HCV)

Culture type	System
Lymphoid cell cultures susceptible to HCV infection	Molt-4, a human T cell line, had detectable minus strand HCV RNA and virus antigens (core and NS4) for up to 7 days (Shimizu et al., 1992)
	HPB-Ma, a subclone of Molt-4, had detectable viral RNA and antigens for more than 2 months (Shimizu et al., 1993) and, more recently, for more than a year (Nakajima et al., 1996)
	CE and TOFE, human B cell lines, had detectable viral RNA and antigens for more than 2 months (Bertolini et al., 1993; Valli et al., 1995)
	HCV infects human T cell leukemia virus 1-infected MT-2 cells for more than 6 months (Mizutani et al., 1996a,b)
	Peripheral blood mononuclear cells (PBMC) from HCV infected patients have detectable HCV RNA for up to a month in culture (Cribier et al., 1995)
Liver cell cultures susceptible to HCV infection	Primary (adult) human hepatocytes had detectable minus strand HCV RNA for up to 2 weeks (Fournier et al., 1998)
	Human (primary) fetal liver cells had detectable minus strand HCV RNA and viral antigens for up to 2–3 weeks (Carloni et al., 1993; Iacovacci et al., 1993)
	Primary chimpanzee hepatocytes were susceptible to infection by HCV, with minus strand of HCV RNA detectable for up to a month (Lanford et al., 1994)
	Human gall bladder (biliary) epithelial cells replicated HCV at low levels for up to 35 days (Loriot et al., 1999)
	PH5CH8, a human liver cell line immortalized with Simian virus 40 (SV40) T antigen, had detectable plus strand of HCV RNA for up to 30 days (Kato et al., 1996); growth at 32°C instead of 37°C yielded replication that persisted for 70–100 days (Ikeda et al., 1998)
Cell lines that support HCV replication after transfection with HCV cDNA or RNA	Huh7, a human hepatoma cell line, was transfected with HCV RNA; minus strand RNA persisted for many weeks (Yoo et al., 1995; Seipp et al., 1997) and tissue culture supernatants were capable of infecting fresh cultures
	HepG2, a human hepatoblastoma cell line, transfected with HCV RNA had detectable viral RNA for up to 2 months (Dash et al., 1997; Hiramatsu et al., 1997) or 4 months (Seipp et al., 1997) in culture; tissue culture supernatants were capable of infecting susceptible cultures
	UHCV, a human osteosarcoma cell line transfected with HCV cDNA under control of the inducible *tet* promoter, expressed HCV structural and nonstructural proteins (Moradpour et al., 1998)
	HeLa G cells transiently transfected with full-length HCV cDNA produced virus proteins, viral RNA and virus-like particles (Mizuno et al., 1995)
	Huh7 cells transfected with HCV subgenomic constructs had replication that was viral polymerase (NS5B) dependent (Lohmann et al., 1999; Blight, et al., 2000)
	Stably integrated HCV cDNA in HepG2 cells generated viral RNAs that supported virus replication (Sun et al., 1999)

Table 11.1 (*cont.*)

Culture type	System
Replication from already infected cells	HCV has been produced in primary hepatocyte cultures from infected patients (Ito et al., 1996)
	HCV replication was observed for about a week in primary biliary epithelial cells isolated from HCV-infected patients (Ahmed et al., 1995; Loriot et al., 1999)
Other cell lines	PK15 and STE are porcine liver cell lines that had detectable HCV RNA for more than 4 months after infection (Seipp et al., 1997); tissue culture supernatants were capable in infecting fresh cultures
	PS, a porcine embryonal kidney cell line, demonstrated persistent HCV RNA replication and viral protein expression (Deriabin et al., 1997)
	Vero, a kidney cell line isolated from an African green monkey, can be infected with HCV (Valli et al., 1997)

PBMC (Cribier et al., 1995), in chimp hepatocytes (Lanford et al., 1994), and in human adult and fetal hepatocytes (Carloni et al., 1993; Iacovacci et al., 1993; Fournier et al., 1998). A variety of lymphoid cell lines, including several T cell (Shimizu et al., 1992, 1993; Mizutani et al., 1996a,b) and B cell (Bertolini, Lacovacci & Carloni, 1993; Valli et al., 1995) lines also support HCV replication. Among liver-related cell lines, HCV replication has been reported in the human liver cell line PH5CH8 and other related clones (Kato et al., 1996; Ikeda et al., 1998), in the human hepatoblastoma cell line HepG2 (Dash et al., 1997; Hiramatsu, Dash & Gerber, 1997; Seipp et al., 1997; Sun et al., 1999), and in the human hepatoma cell line Huh7 (Yoo et al., 1995; Seipp et al., 1997). Although many of these in vitro synthesized systems are susceptible to HCV, the levels of virus are low and can only be detected by RT/PCR. An exception is the recent reports of Huh7 cells transfected with expression plasmids that have episomal replication dependent upon expression of the HCV-encoded RdRp (Lohmann et al., 1999). These "minireplicons" encode a subset of HCV proteins that are detectable by conventional Western blotting. This system has recently been significantly improved using a subgenomic clone that carries a mutation (S1179I) within NS5A, so that viral proteins are produced in roughly 1 in 10 cells, compared with 1 in 10^6 (Blight, Kolykhalov & Rice, 2000). However, neither of these systems support replication of the intact virus, and other systems expressing one or more HCV proteins from stably integrated cDNA constructs have already been described (Moradpour et al., 1998). Even with these limitations, the NS5B dependence of minireplicon replication will be useful in that such a system will be able to screen inhibitors of the viral polymerase. Transfection of HCV RNA into Huh7 (Yoo et al., 1995; Seipp et al., 1997) or HepG2 (Dash et al., 1997; Hiramatsu et al., 1997; Seipp et al., 1997) cells also resulted in high levels of HCV replication, but the levels of both viral RNA and protein progressively decreased and became undetectable within a few weeks, thereby limiting the utility of these systems. Consequently, there has been considerable difficulty in maintaining high levels of virus production in tissue culture systems. It is possible that these limitations result from HCV-associated cytopathic effects (Section 5.1), although if true, this needs to be better documented (see related question 19 in Ch. 24).

In addition to the low levels of virus made, most of the primary cells and cell lines that are susceptible to HCV infection do not produce consistent levels of virus for a long enough period to establish a baseline from which therapeutic manipulations could be judged (Table 11.1). In most cases, long-term virus production was assayed by asking whether tissue culture supernatant collected at different cell passages infected susceptible cells, and not by assaying viral RNA by semiquantitative RT/PCR. While this followed the production of infectious virus in culture, it did not address whether there were consistent levels of virus made by the tissue culture system over time. The latter is quite important, since in tissue culture systems where HCV RNA levels were monitored, consistent baseline levels of virus production were not observed. Even with these limitations, when the T cell line HPB-Ma clone 10-2 infected with HCV-positive serum was treated with IFN-α and IFN-β, effective inhibition of HCV replication was observed (Shimizu and Yoshikura, 1994). In the human T cell line MT-2C, HCV replication was inhibited by treatment with IFN-α and by an antisense oligonucleotide that included sequences complementary to the translation start site of the core gene (Mizutani et al., 1995, 1996b) (Chs. 15 and 16). In both cell lines, treatment was short, partly because of the failure to achieve consistent virus production by these cells. In this context, a HepG2 cell line stably transfected with a full-length infectious cDNA clone of HCV was recently shown to produce stable levels of virus for more than a year (Sun et al., 1999), although it is not yet known how much viral RNA is transcribed from the integrated HCV cDNA and how much from authentic replication.

12

Understanding the natural history of hepatitis C

In order to study the natural history and pathogenesis of acute and chronic HCV infections in more detail, infectious clones of HCV RNA have been constructed and used for experimental infection of chimpanzees. A number of lessons have been learned from these experiences. Initially, a full-length viral RNA was constructed from fragments of liver-derived material, but when a full-length cDNA was used for intrahepatic injection of chimpanzees, it was not infectious (Major & Feinstone, 2000). Since the intrahepatic viral RNA originally cloned for this work may have been shorter than a genome length replication intermediate, cloning was done again using a patient's serum as starting material. Compared with the liver-derived material, the serum-derived clone had an additional 98 bp at the 3' end, within an UTR that was highly conserved among HCV isolates at the primary and secondary structural levels (Tanaka et al., 1995; Kolykhalov et al., 1996), suggesting that these sequences may be important for replication. This was confirmed by showing that some mutations within the 3' 98 bp untranslated region rendered an otherwise infectious clone uninfectious in chimpanzees (Yanagi et al., 1999). Another striking observation was that RT/PCR amplification of full-length clones from serum were also noninfectious, in all probability because of point mutations introduced during the amplification procedures. Based upon this assumption, a "consensus" clone was made, and only this proved to be infectious. Experimental infection of two chimpanzees with the "consensus" RNA by intrahepatic infection resulted in the establishment of chronic infections with mild (periportal) hepatitis. Sequence analysis of the HCV RNA from the serum of these animals showed no changes in the HVR1 region but instead showed consistent mutations in other regions of the envelope gene as well as within NS2, NS3, and NS5 (Major & Feinstone, 2000). Although it is not clear which of these mutations, singly or in combination, contribute to chronicity, the development of an infectious clone in this study, and independently in other laboratories (Hong et al., 1999), should allow these issues to be addressed experimentally.

13

Animal models

The narrow host range of HCV infection has limited animal studies to chimpanzees (Section 1.2), even though numerous attempts have been made experimentally to infect a wide variety of both laboratory and wild animals (reviewed in Bradley, 2000), including several primates other than chimpanzees (Abe et al., 1993). The success in transmitting HBV to primates other than chimpanzees prompted additional attempts with HCV. In this regard, several reports showed successful transmission of HCV to tamarins (Dienes, Feinstone & Popper, 1980; Feinstone et al., 1981; Watanabe et al., 1987), although their lower susceptibility to the virus, combined with the variable incubation periods of infection in different animals (Feinstone et al., 1981), has made this primate model less attractive than the chimpanzee for further development and application. Recently, HCV has been successfully transmitted to tree shrews, which are plentiful and much less expensive than chimpanzees (Xie et al., 1998). Although transient viremia, seroconversion to anti-HCV, and mild hepatitis were observed in many tree shrews, it was not clear whether the liver disease was associated with HCV infection. Much more work needs to be done on this interesting model to assess its future utility properly. As outlined in Sections 1.2 and 1.4, chimpanzees are readily infected with HCV, and their use was central to the discovery of this virus. Chimpanzees have also been very useful for studying various aspects of the natural history of infection, including the immunity that develops after infection and cross-challenge, and the development of CTLs during the course of chronic infections. Although they only develop the mild chronic disease, HCC has been reported in HCV-infected chimpanzees (Muchmore et al., 1988) (Ch. 4). Given that HCV antigens and RNA have been found in chimpanzee livers (Krawczynski et al., 1992a; Negro et al., 1992), these animals are currently being used for testing of protective and therapeutic vaccine candidates.

HBV, like HCV, has a very narrow host range. However, transgenic mice constructed with subgenomic fragments of the HBV genome can support virus gene expression (Babinet et al., 1985; Chisari et al., 1985; Burk et al., 1988), while animals constructed with full-length HBV DNA support virus replication (Farza et al., 1988; Araki et al., 1989; Choo et al., 1991a). These observations show that the livers of animals that are not susceptible to virus infection are clearly permissive for virus gene expression and replication. This raises the possibility that the limited host range of HBV infection may be (at least in part) at the level of the host-encoded receptor for virus infection: animals that are not susceptible to HBV do not encode a recognizable virus receptor. If the narrow host range for HCV infection is also associated with lack of a host-encoded receptor for the virus, then transgenic mice containing HCV sequences may also be useful for exploring HCV gene expression and replication in vivo. However, studies with transgenic mice have produced conflicting results. When subgenomic sequences encoding the HCV core and envelope polypeptides were used for the construction of transgenic mice, virus gene expression was observed, but no histological changes developed in the liver, suggesting that the structural proteins of HCV did not directly damage the cells (i.e., they were not cytopathic) (Koike et al., 1995; Kawamura et al., 1997; Pasquinelli et al., 1997). However, another transgenic model mouse expressed the HCV core protein and developed fatty liver (steatosis) (Moriya et al., 1997) and, later, HCC (Moriya et al., 1998) (Ch. 6). Hepatitis was observed in yet another line of transgenic mice expressing the core and envelope proteins under the control of the mouse MHC class I gene regulatory region (Honda et al., 1999a). The basis for these differences has yet to be explained, although the different constructs used and the corresponding levels of virus gene expression in the various transgenic mice reported, may exceed thresholds for triggering phenotypic changes in hepatocytes in some cases but not others. This certainly seems to be the case in HBx transgenic mice, where high levels of sustained HBxAg expression was associated with the development of HCC (Ueda et al., 1995), while low levels of expression did not result in tumors (Lee et al., 1990), although the latter mice were more susceptible to the action of hepatocarcinogens than nontransgenic littermates (Slagle et al., 1996). For HCV, the development of HCC in HCV core transgenic mice is provocative (Moriya et al., 1998), but it is not clear whether this occurs in chronically infected patients.

Many other attempts have been made to develop a small animal model for HCV. For example, transgenic mice made with a full-length HCV cDNA have been shown to express HCV core protein in hepatocytes and to develop anti-HCV, but it is not clear whether they produce virus particles (Matsuda et al., 1998). Other transgenic mice have been made that conditionally express HCV E1, E2, and core; upon induction of antigen expression, transient hepatitis was observed (Wakita et al., 1998). Anti-HCV core was also observed after the induction of transgene expression. When the transgenic mice were depleted of T cells, transient hepatitis did not follow induction of transgene expression. These results suggest that HCV core and envelope proteins are not directly cytopathic, and that the acute hepatitis observed in transgenic mice with intact T cells is immune mediated (Wakita et al., 1998). An HCV core and E1 expression plasmid was also introduced into the liver of rats through the asialoglycoprotein receptor (Yamamoto et al., 1995). HCV core antigen expression was detected by immunohistochemistry and viral RNA detected by RT/PCR within two days of injection, although the levels of expression were both transient and low (Yamamoto et al., 1995). The transient expression of HCV core protein was also observed in rats injected with complexes of full-length HCV cDNA and cationic liposomes. HCV RNA was detected in the liver by RT/PCR by two days postinjection, and HCV core antigen was detected in scattered hepatocytes up to day 7 postinjection (Takahara et al., 1995). In both cases, HCV gene expression was obtained in a host that was not tolerant to the virus antigens, which correctly mimics the case when people are exposed to HCV for the first time. The construction of a small laboratory animal model supporting sustained virus gene expression and replication in a nontolerant setting is not yet available for HCV, although such a model has recently been published for HBV (Larkin et al., 1999). The key to making the HBV model consisted of using a full-length HBV DNA clone of known infectivity as the transgene, and severe combined immunodeficient (SCID) mice as hosts. The SCID phenotype is deficient in the production of mature T and B cells (Bosma, Custer & Bosma, 1983), meaning that virus-specific cell-mediated and humoral immune responses cannot be generated in the transgenic host. These HBV transgenic SCID mice had consistent baseline levels of virus gene expression and replication, confirming that HBV is not cytopathic. However, upon adoptive transfer of these mice with unprimed, syngeneic splenocytes, they partially cleared virus markers and developed chronic hepatitis that persisted for months. The recent development of a HCV transgenic mouse (in a normal, not SCID, host) that appeared to produce HCV stably (Matsuda et al., 1998) is an important step on the way to establishing a small animal model for HCV that will be amenable for drug testing and eventually for the development of a model of CLD.

The ability of SCID mice to accept tissue xenografts readily has prompted their use as recipients of human liver fragments from HCV-infected or HCV-negative individuals. Liver tissue fragments introduced either subcutaneously or intraperitoneally into SCID mice survived 1–2 months. Transplanted tissues from susceptible individuals were capable of being infected with HCV, while tissues obtained from infected individuals produced virus for up to 10 weeks after engraftment. While it is not clear that the levels of virus are stable in such mice over the course of many weeks, this approach may be useful for the short-term testing of compounds with putative antiviral activity (Schinazi et al., 1999). Recently, human hepatocytes in Matrigel transplanted under the kidney capsule of nonobese diabetic/SCID mice have been shown to survive for more than 3 months (Ohashi et al., 2000). Combined with the successful infection of these cells with HBV, this approach will likely be useful in the future development of an HCV model. In a variation of this approach, SV40 (simian virus 40) immortalized human hepatocytes stably transfected with full-length HBV DNA were transplanted by intrasplenic injection into the livers of mice lacking *rag-2* (a recombinant activating gene) (Brown et al., 2000). These mice, like SCID mice, do not have functional T and B cells (Shinkai et al., 1992). Intrasplenic injection of human hepatocytes permitted migration of individual cells into the liver, where they survived and supported virus replication of up to 3×10^8 virus genome equivalents/ml blood for 8 months following transplantation. Unlike transgenic mice, human hepatocytes carry out the complete life cycle of HBV and HCV, which is particularly important in the screening compounds that target virus replication.

Independent attempts to establish a reproducible animal model of HCV have also involved the use of human–mouse radiation chimerae (Lubin et al., 1991). In this system, normal mice subjected to lethal whole body irradiation are reconstituted with SCID mouse bone marrow cells, and then further engrafted with human liver fragments (Galun et al., 1995). Transplantation of HCV- (or HBV-) infected human liver fragments under the kidney capsule has been successful in up to 85% of mice, with replication (minus strand HCV RNA in the liver) detected in nearly all of the successfully engrafted animals. Although HCV RNA became detectable by day 8, and peaked by days 18–25, no stable baseline of HCV RNA was achieved, and HCV RNA as well as replicative forms in the engrafted tissue became undetectable after a few weeks (Galun et al., 1995). The recent successful use of this trimeric mouse model to examine the treatment of HBV-infected liver grafts with lamivudine (Ilan et al., 1999), which is highly effective against HBV in infected patients (Jarvis & Faulds, 1999; Malik & Lee, 2000), helps to validate this system for the further evaluation of drug candidates against HBV, and with additional experience, against HCV.

In summary, chimpanzees are the only animals that can be readily infected with HCV. They have been very important in the discovery of HCV and in characterizing the natural history and pathogenesis of infection. Unfortunately, because of too limited numbers and expense, chimpanzees have not been utilized for antiviral drug discovery. Instead, a variety of small animal models supporting HCV gene expression or replication have been constructed, which are presently being refined so that they can be used to screen putative antiviral drugs in vivo. Among the challenges for the future is the establishment of a small animal model that develops acute liver disease and CLD, and which progresses to HCC. This will permit the preclinical evaluation of drug candidates not only against virus but also against liver disease.

Vaccine research

The development of a protective HCV vaccine has been among the most difficult challenges since the discovery of the virus for a number of reasons. First, despite the consistent efforts of many laboratories, there is still no permissive system that consistently replicates HCV at high enough levels to evaluate antibodies that may be neutralizing (Table 11.1 and Ch. 11). Second, with the exception of the chimpanzee, which is expensive, endangered, and difficult to work with, there are no convenient animal models that are susceptible to HCV and that could be used for candidate vaccine challenge studies (Section 1.2). Third, the genotype, subtype and quasispecies nature of HCV (Weiner et al., 1992; Bukh et al., 1997; Simmonds et al., 1993, 1997) (Section 3.2) may require the construction of polyvalent vaccines that would protect against a large number of closely related epitopes. The fact that the genetic heterogeneity of the virus can change rapidly in an infected individual (Ogata et al., 1991), and that antiviral immunity may select for neutralization escape mutants (within HVR1) (Martell et al., 1992; Weiner et al., 1992; Shimizu et al., 1994) as well as CTL escape mutants (Weiner et al., 1995), may limit the effectiveness and utility of any vaccine. Fourth, it is not clear whether the envelope polypeptides contain all of the antigenic determinants required for effective neutralization (Chien et al., 1993). Even though envelope antibodies have been shown to be neutralizing in chimpanzees (Choo et al., 1994; Farci et al., 1996b), reinfection of convalescent animals with the same isolate readily occurs and may result in the development of chronic infection and liver disease (Farci et al., 1992a; Prince et al., 1992). Reinfection and a renewed bout of hepatitis has also been documented in human studies (Feitelson et al., 1994; Lai et al., 1994). Fifth, HCV tends to persist in the great majority of infected people (Alter, 1993b) even though cellular and humoral immune responses have been observed against nearly all of the virus-encoded polypeptides (Chien et al., 1993; Battegay et al., 1995; Rehermann et al., 1996a; Wong et al., 1998) (Fig. 5.2; Section 5.3). Sixth, the association of virus particles with immunoglobulin and/or β-lipoprotein may "mask" the virus in blood, thereby greatly reducing the efficiency of neutralization (Thomssen et al., 1992, 1993) (Section 2.1). This situation is compounded by the apparent lack of consistent and persistent antiviral immune responses among patients who recover from acute HCV infection. This list is incomplete but represents some of the concerns that need to be addressed in vaccine development (see related question 20 in Ch. 24).

The case for vaccine development is a strong one, with an estimated 170 million chronically infected people who are at high risk for the development of hepatitis, cirrhosis and HCC (Section 3.1 and Ch. 6). In addition, the tendency of acute exposures to develop into chronic infections, the fact that the available treatments for chronically infected patients are few, and that the outcomes of treatment are often not satisfactory in the majority of patients further underscore the need to develop a protective vaccine. In addition, the past use of nondisposable injection needles/syringes in developing countries for vaccination campaigns against other infectious agents (for example, against schistosomiasis in Egypt) has recently given rise to HCV outbreaks at "epidemic" levels (Frank et al., 2000) (Ch. 3). The observation that HCV-associated CLD is exacerbated in people coinfected with HIV (Eyster et al., 1993; Soto et al., 1997) (Ch. 4) identifies yet another population in which protective vaccination would have made all the difference. In developed countries like the United States, the cost of HCV-related morbidity and mortality is of the order of hundreds of millions of dollars annually (CDC, 1998). In such a setting, vaccination of high-risk populations would further reduce the incidence of HCV, while the universal vaccination of newborns or children will go far to stem the transmission of HCV by later intravenous drug abuse and by high-risk sexual practices.

The chimpanzee has been used almost exclusively to evaluate potential approaches to prevent HCV infection, since they could be challenged with live virus to evaluate the efficacy of any protective vaccine. A suitable protective vaccine would prevent the establishment of HCV infection when administered prior to infection. In addition, the chimpanzee model can also be exploited for the development of a therapeutic vaccine, which would bring about resolution of liver disease but would not necessarily result in the clearance of the virus. In the context of protective vaccines, high levels of antibodies against the envelope glycoproteins of HCV (anti-HVR1) have been shown to be completely protective in chimpanzees against challenge with the same isolate (Choo et al., 1994; Farci et al., 1996b; Section 5.3). Animals that developed lower titers of envelope antibodies became infected, but the infections were mild and self limited, suggesting some protective effect even after infection. Partial protection was also independently observed when a subunit vaccine containing E1 and E2 was used for immunization of chimpanzees, and the animals then challenged with the strain of HCV from which the vaccine was made (Rosa et al., 1996). These observations, however, were tempered by the independent finding that experimental challenge of convalescent chimpanzees with the original isolate of HCV resulted in reinfection and the development of another bout of liver disease (Farci et al., 1991; 1992a; Prince et al.,

1992). Hence, antibodies against HCV E1 and E2 appear to be important for neutralization, although the reasons why they are not consistently protective remain to be fully understood.

In the absence of a convenient laboratory animal model that is susceptible to HCV infection (Chs. 13 and 15), immune responses against HCV antigens in protective and therapeutic vaccine candidates have been evaluated in mice. For example, intramuscular injection of mice with a plasmid expressing the HCV core protein resulted in the development of a Th1 response, as characterized by the production of IL-2 and IFN-γ (Inchauspe et al., 1997a). Genetically immunized mice also developed a Th2 response (IL-4 and IL-10) as well as antibodies to viral antigens (Inchauspe et al., 1997b; Howard et al., 1998). These antibody and CTL responses were shown to be mediated by CD4$^+$ and CD8$^+$ T cells, respectively (Hu et al., 1999). The titers of envelope antibodies obtained were dependent upon the route of injection, with intraepidermal injections giving statistically significant higher titers of antibodies than intramuscular or gene gun injections (Nakano et al., 1997). It was also observed that addition of the gene encoding granulocyte-macrophage colony-stimulating factor (GM-CSF) to a bicistronic plasmid expressing the HCV E1/E2 gene significantly boosted antibody titers and lympho-proliferative responses among immunized animals (Lee, Cho & Sung, 1998). The inclusion of the murine gene for IL-2 in a bicistronic expression plasmid also provided a similar simulatory role (Papa et al., 1998). Inclusion of an IL-12-producing vector has been shown to shift the resulting immunity to a predominantly Th1 response, as shown by enhanced CTL and depressed viral antibody responses (Shan, Liu & Fang, 1999). Specific viral antibody and CTL responses were also shown to be stimulated by DNA vaccination (for example, to E2), followed by boosting using E2 protein (Song et al., 2000). Strong polyspecific humoral and cellular immune responses were also obtained in mice vaccinated with a polycistronic plasmid expressing HCV core/E1/E2/NS2/NS3 followed by a nonreplicating canarypox booster encoding the same HCV antigens (Pancholi et al., 2000). Subunit peptide vaccines containing known Th and CTL epitopes against HCV core antigen have also been used successfully to produce corresponding CTL responses in mice (Hiranuma et al., 1999). Collectively, the importance of this work is underscored by the fact that acute resolving HCV is characterized by strong, rapid, multispecific immune responses (Section 5.4). If therapeutic DNA vaccination is going to work, protocols need to be developed that emulate these characteristics, and the above work in mice will provide some of the clues whereby this might be accomplished.

Genetic immunization has also resulted in the development of CTL responses against the HCV nonstructural proteins that could eliminate tumor cells stably expressing HCV NS5 (Encke et al., 1998). Further characterization of the CD8$^+$

CTL responses to HCV core showed them to be MHC restricted (Hu et al., 1999). Moreover, in HLA-A2.1 transgenic mice immunized with a DNA vaccine expressing HCV core, and then challenged with recombinant vaccinia virus expressing HCV core, the core-specific CTL generated by DNA immunization significantly reduced the levels of recombinant vaccinia in the mice (Sarobe et al., 1998; Arichi et al., 2000). These results showed that HCV core epitopes that bind to the human HLA-A2.1 determinant can serve as a target for therapeutic vaccination. While these results are provocative, it is not known whether HCV core is an important immunological target in acute or chronic human infections. However, the testing of several potential therapeutic vaccines in mice will provide the foundation for future evaluation of the most promising candidates in chronically infected chimpanzees and, ultimately, in human clinical trials.

The development and increasing availability of virus vectors capable of expressing one or more cloned genes means that there is now the potential to use these vectors to express high levels of one or more HCV proteins in vivo. This may be able to trigger cellular immune responses that could contribute importantly to eliminating virus in the chronically infected liver. For example, therapeutic vaccines could result from DNA immunization using classical expression vectors (Inchauspe, 1997; Houghton, 2000) or from self-replicating RNA vectors (Ying et al., 1999), which potentially yield high levels of antigen expression for a sustained period of time. In some studies, intrahepatic and intramuscular injection of DNA vectors encoding HCV antigens resulted in the development of corresponding CTL responses, which may be useful in studying immune-mediated pathogenesis in the liver (Kamei et al., 2000) and will be very important in the design of appropriate therapeutic vaccine candidates.

Part III

Experimental approaches

15

New systems to understand hepatitis C biology

The development of HCV subgenomic replicons that produce high levels of one or more HCV polypeptides (Lohmann et al., 1999; Blight et al., 2000), in contrast to the very low and inconsistent levels of wild-type virus produced in tissue culture cells infected with HCV (Table 11.1 and Ch. 11), suggests that there are properties of wild-type HCV that normally attenuate virus gene expression and replication, and that when these constraints are removed, much higher levels of expression could be achieved. One of these constraints may be the complex secondary structural features within the 5' and 3' UTRs of the virus. Many laboratories are developing additional self-replicating replicons that are capable of persisting, and some at high copy number, within transfected or infected cells. These include replicons made from alphavirus (Garoff & Li, 1998; Ying et al., 1999), pestivirus (Moser et al., 1999), other flavivirus (Varnavski & Khromykh, 1999), and coronavirus (Thiel, Siddell & Herold, 1998) vectors. Whether the entire HCV polyprotein could be expressed from such constructs remains to be seen. In addition, since the HCV would be produced from artificial templates, it is not clear whether the sensitivity of virus gene expression and replication to putative antiviral agents would be the same or different to that of virus made from native HCV templates in an infected cell. However, this does not limit the use of such recombinant vectors to screen compounds against individual HCV proteins (Lohmann et al., 1999) and, in fact, such efforts are underway for NS5B (Baginski et al., 2000).

In addition to generating new tissue culture systems using subgenomic replicons (Ch. 11), there have been attempts to increase the efficacy of existing treatments. As outlined in Ch. 9, IFN has been used effectively against both HBV and HCV. However, the sustained response rate is low (less than 20% of treated patients) and side effects could be serious. In addition, treatments are expensive and consist of up to three injections per week for 6–12 months. Recently, it has been shown that polyethylene glycol-modified IFN, referred to as pegylated IFN, is more stable in the bloodstream that unmodified IFN, and that this modification does not alter the properties of IFN. Clinical trials with pegylated IFN are now underway in patients who are chronically infected with HCV. Initial findings have shown that up to 30% of treated patients with cirrhosis treated in this way have a sustained virological response, compared with less than 10% of patients treated with standard IFN therapy. Transaminase levels normalized in twice the number of patients treated with pegylated IFN compared with standard IFN (Heathcote et al., 2000). Similar results were obtained among patients with an entry diagnosis of chronic hepatitis (Zeuzem et al., 2000). In both trials, pegylated IFN was better tolerated and only required one weekly injection instead of three. Clinical trials using pegylated IFN in conjunction with ribavirin are currently underway, and preliminary results suggest that the majority of patients may benefit (Glue et al., 2000). However, it will be very important to document carefully the sustained virological and histological response to this new combination therapy in current and upcoming clinical trials.

Liver disease associated with chronic HCV infection is a major target for the development of future therapeutics, although there is no laboratory-based animal model that develops HCV-associated CLD (Ch. 13). Certainly, the inducible expression of HCV core in vivo has led to the development of a transient or acute hepatitis (Wakita et al., 1998), which strongly suggests that, in a nontolerant host, the pathogenesis of HCV is immune mediated. A model for HBV-associated CLD has recently become available (Larkin et al., 1999), but an analogous model for HCV is yet to be developed (Ch. 13). However, recent work has shown that when a vaccinia virus recombinant containing the HCV IRES sequences cloned just upstream from the luciferase reporter gene was used to infect mice, they became strongly positive for luciferase gene expression in the liver. Treatment of these animals with antisense oligonucleotides against the HCV IRES significantly reduced reporter (luciferase) gene expression (Zhang et al., 1999) (Ch. 17), indicating that such an approach may be important for the development of reagents that block the production of virus gene products in vivo. Alternatively, it has recently been demonstration that human hepatocytes can survive for months in a matrix under the kidney capsule of mice treated with anti-Met. These hepatocytes are susceptible to HBV and hepatitis delta virus infection (Ohashi et al., 2000), suggesting that such a model could readily be used to screen for drugs against HBV and delta. If, as expected, this model is susceptible to HCV, it may also be adaptable for drug screening.

16

New antiviral screening assays

The lack of tissue culture systems that consistently support HCV replication (Ch. 11) has prompted the development of other assays with individual virus gene products that may be converted into high throughput screens for drug screening and discovery. A powerful tool in the design of such assays has been the development of cell lines and cell-free systems that express one or more HCV proteins (Table 11.1). For example, the recent development of HCV subgenomic replicons in Huh7 cells provides opportunities to test antiviral compounds against the virus polymerase, which is responsible for the replication of the subgenomic plasmids in this system (Lohmann et al., 1999; Blight et al., 2000). In addition, the development of cell lines or chimeric viruses with replication dependent upon HCV NS3 expression (Hirowatari, Hijikata & Shimotohno, 1995; Hahm et al., 1996; Song et al., 1996; Filocamo, Pacini & Migliaccio, 1997) will allow screening against the NS3 protease and helicase. Another important contribution has been the publication of the crystal structure for several HCV proteins. This information will be central to the rational design of inhibitors based upon the three-dimensional active sites of the corresponding virus proteins. For example, the recent crystallographic structure of the NS3 helicase domain (Yao & Weber, 1998; Kwong, Kim & Lin, 2000) (Sections 2.4 and 2.5), which recognizes and unwinds double-stranded RNA in an NTP-dependent reaction during virus replication, has revealed amino acid residues that could be sites for inhibitor design and interaction. Comparison of the crystal structure of the NS3 helicase domain with that of other helicases (Korolev et al., 1998), coupled with site-specific mutagenesis and functional characterization of the NS3 helicase by in vitro assays (Yao & Weber, 1998; Paolini, DeFrancesco & Gallinari, 2000a; Paolini et al., 2000b; Preugschat et al., 2000), has resulted in identification of the HCV residues that are critical for activity. This information will now provide for structure-based or rationale drug design aimed at inhibiting NS3 binding to RNA, inhibiting hydrolysis of ATP by NS3-encoded NTPase, and inhibiting helicase (unwindase) activity (Ch. 22).

In addition to the helicase, NS3 exhibits a serine protease activity that is responsible for the successive cleavage of most HCV nonstructural polypeptides

(Section 2.4). Inactivation of the NS3 serine protease encoded by other flaviviruses results in the production of noninfectious virus particles (Chambers et al., 1990). This suggests that this activity may be a good target for the screening and discovery of new anti-HCV drugs. However, the NS3/NS4A cleavage site can tolerate many amino acid substitutions, suggesting that cleavage depends upon an extended network of interactions between enzyme (NS3 plus NS4) and substrate and less upon a particular amino acid sequence. This implies that it will be very difficult to design low-molecular-weight inhibitors of NS3, since they would not mimic the multiple and extended network of interactions that exist in natural NS3 substrates. In addition, NS4A is an integral component of the NS3 protease (Section 2.4), as shown by crystal structure (Di Marco et al., 2000), and the two polypeptides make tight contacts at multiple sites, which implies that it will be difficult to disrupt these complexes by a dominant negative NS4A and/or small molecule inhibitors.

Although NS3/NS4A has serine protease activity, it is not inhibited by compounds that are highly effective against other serine proteases, suggesting that the active site of the NS3 protease is different from that of the cellular enzymes (D'Souza et al., 1995; Lin & Rice, 1995; Shoji et al., 1995). In addition, NS3/NS4A is not capable of cleaving most of the small peptide substrates that are readily cleaved by the corresponding cellular enzymes, although it reportedly cleaves a synthetic peptide substrate that mimics the NS5A/5B junction in vitro (Sudo et al., 1996). Interestingly, the affinity of NS3/NS4A for the cleaved substrates during polyprotein maturation is greater than for the reactants, meaning that the products of cleavage (especially the products of NS4A/B cleavage) inhibit further protease activity (Steinkuhler et al., 1998). This inhibition has been exploited for the design of short peptides with very high affinity and inhibitory activity (Ingallinella et al., 1998; Attwood et al., 1999), but the stable delivery of these peptides to infected cells in the liver remains a considerable challenge. Another approach to look for NS3 inhibitors is to use the NS3 protease domain as bait to screen random libraries of compounds for binding (Dimasi et al., 1997). This approach has resulted in the identification of several short RNA sequences (aptamers) that bind the NS3 active site and inhibit protease activity (Fukuda et al., 2000). In a similar way, two protease inhibitors have been identified. One is a thiazolidine-related compound (Sudo et al., 1997) and the other is phenanthrenequinone, which was isolated from *Streptomyces* sp. (Chu, Mierzwa & Truumees, 1996). More recently, another protease inhibitor isolated from *Penicillium griseofulvum* has been shown to inhibit NS3 protease activity (Chu et al., 1999). Peptide based α-ketoamides have also been shown to inhibit NS3 protease activity in vitro (Han et al., 2000). The clinical utility of these compounds, if any, is yet to be evaluated.

Other systems have been developed to screen for compounds with NS3 protease inhibitory activity. For example, two laboratories have stably expressed NS3 in tissue culture cells (Hirowatari et al., 1995; Song et al., 1996). Other laboratories have created a chimeric poliovirus (Hahm et al., 1996), Sindbis virus (Filocamo et al., 1997), or bovine viral diarrhea virus (Lai et al., 2000) so that virus replication was dependent upon expression of recombinant HCV NS3, with the idea that NS3 inhibitors would also inhibit replication of these viruses. Whether any compounds found using these assays will be effective against multiple HCV genotypes, and whether their eventual introduction into the clinic will result in the rapid appearance of virus resistance, remains to be seen.

HCV-encoded NS5B is an obvious target for antiviral intervention since it plays a central role in virus replication. The recent reports of the crystal structure of HCV NS5B (Ago et al., 1999; Bressanelli et al., 1999; Lesburg et al., 1999) (Ch. 23) have revealed features that will undoubtedly help in understanding enzyme template specificity and in the design of putative small molecule inhibitors. Additional reports of enzymatically active NS5B in mammalian cells (Heller et al., 1998; Baginski et al., 2000), combined with efforts to reconstitute all or part of an authentic virus replication complex in cells (Ishido et al., 1998), represent important strides in the development of systems that will permit the evaluation of antiviral compounds. The development of subgenomic plasmids with replication dependent on NS5B (Lohmann et al., 1999; Blight et al., 2000) (Ch. 11) represents another system that could be exploited for the preclinical screening of compounds with putative antiviral activity. An important feature of these tissue culture-based systems is that they metabolize the compounds that are being tested, permitting the assessment of antiviral activity under conditions that are similar to those in vivo. This is true, for example, with nucleoside analogs, which need to be converted into trisphosphates before they can be incorporated into viral nucleic acid as chain terminators. However, even with a good tissue culture system, it may not be easy to discover drugs that are effective in the majority of HCV-infected patients, since it is not clear what NS5B sequence among the many published clones actually replicates HCV. The microheterogeneity in NS5B sequence within one patient (infected with many quasispecies) and between patients (infected with different subtypes) means that a drug which is highly effective against a single HCV sequence in a tissue culture system may not be as effective in clinical trials. Although the need for the development of new HCV therapeutics is great, a problem that has plagued the development of new therapeutics for HBV and HIV is that monotherapies which show efficacy in some or most patients will probably lead to the development of drug resistance within a few years. This is already well documented for lamivudine monotherapy in chronic HBV infection (Richman, 2000) despite the fact that it is highly effective against virus and disease in the great majority of chronically infected patients. The RT of HBV and the RdRp of HCV both lack proofreading capabilities, suggesting that drug "escape" mutants could be rapidly generated and selected during therapy. Hence, the search for antiviral drugs will probably involve the development of combination therapies against mutiple virus targets, especially among those that are conserved and important to the virus life cycle.

In addition to NS3 and NS5B, there has been interest in targeting other sites in the HCV life cycle. For example, assays have been set up in which a reporter gene is under translational control of the HCV IRES (Klinck et al., 2000; Wang et al., 2000) so that potential inhibitors of reporter gene activity could be rapidly screened. The importance of the 5' UTR sequences in HCV as a potential antiviral target has also been demonstrated in experiments showing that antisense phosphorothioate oligodeoxynucleotides complementary to the 3' region of the 5' UTR strongly inhibited virus translation (Alt et al., 1997). Similar results were obtained with antisense oligonucleotides that targeted the adjacent sequences within the core region (Ch. 11). These combined results show that regulatory regions of HCV, in addition to HCV gene products, are potentially important targets in antiviral drug development. Other steps in the HCV life cycle, such as virus binding, uptake, and packaging, are also potential targets, but the development of drug candidates for these steps will probably have to wait for the development of a fully permissive, reproducible and robust tissue culture system that supports HCV replication.

Antiviral gene therapy

The anatomy of the normal liver is such that hepatocytes are closely accessible to the bloodstream without intervening basement membranes (Gumuncio & Berkowitz, 1992). Combined with the fact that the liver is a major organ of detoxification, and that it takes up foodstuffs, hormones, chemicals, asialoglycoproteins, metal ions, and a wide variety of other molecules, it is no surprise that the liver is a good candidate for the development of antiviral gene therapy against HCV. The goal of antiviral gene therapy is to make cells resistant to viral infection and/or block the virus life cycle at multiple steps. Antiviral gene therapy could supplement immunotherapy and/or the administration of small molecule inhibitors of NS3, NS5B, or other viral targets. However, the lack of a good animal model in which to study HCV pathogenesis (Chs. 13 and 15) and evaluate various forms of antiviral gene therapy represents a major challenge (see related question 21 in Ch. 24).

Despite these limitations, some progress has been made. For example, HCV-specific ribozymes against the 5' UTR and core region have been shown partially to inhibit virus translation in vitro and in cells transfected with a reporter gene cloned downstream from the HCV 5' UTR and core sequences (Sakamoto, Wu & Wu, 1996; Welch et al., 1996). In these experiments, ribozyme-mediated cleavage of the viral RNA was responsible for the decrease in the levels of virus gene expression. HCV RNA was also cleared from infected human hepatocytes treated with recombinant adenovirus encoding an HCV-specific ribozyme (Lieber et al., 1996). With these data as proof of principle, more recent studies have focused upon generating specific HCV ribozymes to several conserved regions of the viral genome, with the idea that their simultaneous use would greatly reduce the appearance of viral resistance (Welch, Yei & Barber, 1998). This would make it very difficult for a virus to develop mutations that would permit escape from an attack on several virus targets simultaneously.

Independent efforts have used intracellular antibody production (Baltimore, 1988) to inhibit one or more steps in the virus life cycle from within the infected cell. In a preliminary study, cells were transfected with an expression vector encoding a nonsecretable antibody fragment that strongly bound HCV core; this fragment bound HCV core expressed in the same cells (Heintges, zu Putlitz &

Wands, 1999). It will be important to test other intracellular antibody candidates (e.g., against NS3 and NS5B) in tissue culture systems expressing HCV proteins and, ultimately, in cells supporting HCV replication to determine whether "intracellular immunization" can significantly reduce virus load.

A number of groups have also explored the utility of antisense molecules against the 5' UTR and core regions in arresting HCV polypeptide synthesis. For example, several phosphorothioate or 2'-O-methoxyethyl-modified antisense oligonucleotides, which are more stable and bind more strongly to viral RNA than unmodified oligonucleotides, have been shown to inhibit HCV translation efficiently both in vitro and in HepG2 cells (Alt et al., 1997, 1999; Brown-Driver et al., 1999). In a number of studies, inhibition was not only associated with translation arrest but also with the induction of cellular RNase H, which degraded the viral RNA/antisense DNA complexes (Caselmann, Eisenhardt & Alt, 1997). In further work, when 5' UTR and core antisense oligonucleotides were complexed with asialoglycoprotein–polylysine conjugates, they were readily taken up by the asialoglycoprotein receptor in Huh7 cells (Wu & Wu, 1998). Since this receptor is found in high copy number only on hepatocytes (Ashwell & Morrell, 1974), and is important for removal of asialoglycoproteins from circulation, this approach may some day be used to target and concentrate therapeutic antisense oligonucleotides to the liver. In this regard, it has recently been shown that antisense oligonucleotides directed against the HCV core-encoding RNA region suppressed the ability of HCV core to stimulate cell growth and survival (Tsuchihara et al., 1999), suggesting that such an approach may be effective against the development of HCC. Alternatively, the IRES, which regulates polyprotein production (Section 2.3), is likely to be another important target for gene therapy. When a recombinant vaccinia virus in which luciferase reporter gene expression was under control of the HCV IRES was used to infect mice (as described in Ch. 15), high levels of luciferase activity was observed. However, when such mice were treated with phosphorothioate antisense oligonucleotides complementary to HCV IRES, there was a transient but significant inhibitory effect, indicating that antisense therapy was effective in vivo (Zhang et al., 1999). Given the complex secondary structure in the 5' UTR where antisense inhibition appears to be most effective, additional efforts have identified antisense HCV sequences from a combinatorial library that hybridize strongly with the viral sequences, thereby optimizing antisense inhibition (Lima et al., 1997). These sequences cluster around the stem–loop structure within the 5' UTR and sequences around the translation initiation codon for core (Fig. 2.1) (Hanecak et al., 1996; Lima et al., 1997), although the fine mapping of the 'best' viral sequences for antisense inhibition within the 5' UTR and core region vary among laboratories. If problems associated with delivery (liver targeting) and stability (within the infected hepatocyte) of antisense molecules could be solved, there may be a real chance that this approach will become useful in the future.

Other approaches to antiviral gene therapy have also been proposed but have largely not been put into practice (Ruiz et al., 1999). These include the use of dominant negative virus or host proteins that block the life cycle of HCV by competing for wild-type proteins and the production of decoy RNAs that bind to authentic virus proteins, thereby limiting the use of HCV RNA for packing, translation, or as a template for replication. Although appealing and highly specific, it is not clear whether any of the current vectors used for gene therapy are capable of delivering the therapy to a large enough fraction of liver cells for a long enough period of time to be effective in chronic HCV infections.

Among the vehicles used for antiviral gene therapy, both viral and nonviral-based vectors are currently being evaluated, or will be as appropriate cell culture and animal models continue to develop. Among the viral vectors, high titers of replication-deficient recombinant adenoviruses can deliver appropriate ribozymes or antisense molecules to a large proportion of quiescent hepatocytes (Kozarsky & Wilson, 1993), but the adenovirus vectors used so far are immunogenic, thereby limiting the number of effective treatment episodes. Immune elimination of adenovirus-infected cells (i.e., liver pathology) also limits expression of the therapeutic gene(s) (Yang et al., 1994). Recombinant adeno-associated viruses (AAV) are not immunogenic, are not pathogenic, infect nonreplicating cells in various tissues, and stably express the recombinant gene (Rabinowitz & Samulski, 1998), but their transduction efficiency in vivo is relatively low (Koeberl et al., 1997) and they persist by integration into host DNA, which risks the disrupted expression of one or more host genes (Xiao et al., 1998). Recently, however, the extent of AAV infection in the liver and the levels of recombinant protein expression have been boosted severalfold by exposure of rats to ethanol or other compounds in the diet, which creates oxidative stress in the liver (Wheeler et al., 2000). Further work along these lines may promote the widespread use of AAV vectors for gene therapy in a wide variety of applications. Replication-deficient retrovirus vectors can also be produced at high titers, infect most cell types, and confer long-term expression in the great majority of infected cells, although they only infect replicating cells (Grossman & Wilson, 1993). Increased efficiency of retrovirus-mediated gene transfer has been obtained when infection was carried out after a two-thirds partial hepatectomy, during the period of widespread liver regeneration (Kay et al., 1992). Recombinant adenovirus expressing exogenous urokinase, a protease that causes liver cell death, was later used in place of partial hepatectomy to trigger hepatocellular turnover. This increased retrovirus-mediated gene transduction by five- to tenfold in the liver (Lieber et al., 1995). Infusion of hepatocyte growth factor, which transiently stimulated liver growth, along with recombinant retrovirus also greatly increased the fraction of hepatocytes (up to 30%) that were stably transduced (Patijn et al., 1998). The development of replication-deficient recombinant lentivirus vectors has permitted infection of nonproliferating cells, including hepatocytes, either in vitro or in vivo (Naldini et al., 1996; Kafri et al., 1997). Recombinant, replication-defective SV40 has also recently been used to infect the majority of quiescent hepatocytes in vivo (Kondo et al., 1998). Despite the fact that the SV40 vector has a limited insert size, it can be produced at high titer, is stably expressed following integration into host DNA, is not immunogenic, and does not cause liver disease. Although not yet applied to HCV, each of these vectors could encode antiviral cytokines, prodrugs, ribozymes, antisense constructs, or virus-specific intracellular antibodies.

These same antiviral molecules could alternatively be packaged in nonviral liposomes that are efficiently endocytosed by the liver (Yao et al., 1994; Baru, Axelrod & Nur, 1995; Wu et al., 1998). Liposomes are often formed from cationic lipids, which encapsidate expression plasmids, drugs, or other therapeutically useful molecules. Another approach involves the design and use of bifunctional antibodies, in which the antibody binds to a cellular or viral antigen on infected cells and also to a drug that has therapeutic value, thereby concentrating the drug at the site where it will be most useful (Yuan, Baxter & Jain, 1991). The asialo-glycoprotein receptor has also been used for specific targeting of therapeutics to the liver, since the conjugation of drugs, prodrugs, or antisense oligonucleotides to an asialoglycoprotein ligand has been used successfully in inhibiting hepadnavirus replication both in vitro and in vivo (Ponzetto et al., 1991; Wu & Wu, 1992). It is likely that over time these and other forms of antiviral gene therapy (Zern & Kresina, 1997) may play important roles in combination therapy aimed at improving virological response in patients with chronic HCV infection. The importance of improving virological response is underscored by the fact that decreasing virus replication may help to limit quasispecies diversity and, hence, make it easier for specific immunotherapeutic approaches (e.g., IFN) to clear the remaining virus (Ch. 9).

In addition to directly targeting the virus, antiviral gene therapy may also encompass the introduction of selected cytokines that will contribute to the depression of virus gene expression and replication. Unlike the direct targeting of virus gene products, soluble cytokines made by one cell in the liver will have an effect upon virus in a number of neighboring cells. What this means is that vectors (such as AAV) that transfer the desired cytokine gene(s) to a small percentage of the cells in the liver may make enough cytokines to target virus in the entire liver. The problem is, of course, what cytokines to use. Since Th1 cytokines appear to be important mediators of virus clearance, it is likely that they will be chosen for antiviral gene therapy. This therapy may take the form of vectors that encode selected cytokines and/or genetic (DNA-based) immunization that promotes the development of the appropriate cytokine(s). However, it is not known which single or combination of cytokines will be most effective in reducing virus load and in resolving liver disease. Whatever the outcome, it is likely that antiviral gene therapy with cytokines will be used together with genetic or therapeutic immunization against one or more HCV gene products, as outlined elsewhere. In this way, cytokines could broaden and strengthen the resulting antiviral immune responses, thereby increasing the likelihood of virus clearance.

As discussed above, antiviral gene therapy may potentially contribute to the reduction in virus load and the resolution of CLD. These approaches may also be useful in the treatment of HCC and may complement the traditional treatment modalities of surgery, chemotherapy, radiation, and immunotherapy. For example, the transfer of the *E. coli* gene for purine nucleoside phosphorylase in recombinant adenoviruses to human hepatoma cells in culture, followed by treatment with the purine analog prodrug fludarabine, killed all of the cells expressing the microbial phosphorylase but not any of the vector-infected control cells (Mohr et al., 2000). Interestingly, activated drug was even cytotoxic to surrounding tumor cells that lacked purine nucleoside phosphorylase, indicating that only a small percentage of tumor cells needed to be infected with the recombinant adenovirus in order for treatment to be successful. *In vivo*, antitumor gene therapy may yield local high concentrations of cytotoxic drugs, thereby reducing the side effects commonly associated with cancer chemotherapy. The fact that tumors are composed of many replicating cells means that they are amenable to recombinant retrovirus-mediated gene therapy, and it has been shown that retroviruses preferentially target growing cells in preneoplastic and neoplastic lesions (Kimura et al., 1994). To increase specificity further, virus vectors have been constructed to express therapeutic genes from the α-fetoprotein promoter (Arbuthnot et al., 1995; Su et al., 1996), which is inactive in normal liver but is turned on in 60–70% of patients with HCC (Colombo, 1992). Interestingly, expression of IL-2 under the control of an α-fetoprotein promoter in a recombinant adenovirus significantly reduced tumor growth or eliminated HCC growth in mice (Bui et al., 1997). Other cytokines, such as TNFα (Cao et al., 1997), IL-4, IL-6, IL-7, IL-12, IFN-γ (Qin et al., 1998), and GM-CSF have also shown some antitumor effect. Tumor-infiltrating lymphocytes are detected in patients with HCC (Usuda et al., 1993), and their number directly correlates with an improved prognosis (Kawata et al., 1992) suggesting that the failure of immune-mediated tumor rejection may stem from the inability of HCC cells to stimulate effective immune responses (Chouaib et al., 1997) and that cytokine replacement therapy partially overcomes this deficiency. This may be a consequence of loss of MHC expression, decrease or loss of Fas receptor, increased expression of multidrug resistance, and/or secretion of immunosuppressive molecules by the liver. The ability of HCC to develop may also depend importantly upon alterations in signal transduction pathways and the appearance of mutations in oncogenes or tumor suppressor genes (Ch. 6). The importance of identifying the molecular changes that underlie the development of HCV-associated HCC is that this will permit the development of the approaches outlined above, or others (Zern & Kresina, 1997; Ruiz et al., 1999) to replace normal genes that are lost by epigenetic events (e.g., NS3 binding and presumably inactivating p53) or by mutation (e.g., of tumor suppressors). Gene therapy may also downregulate the expression of oncogenes and signal transduction pathways that contribute centrally to the abnormal growth and survival of virus-infected hepatocytes during chronic infection (Ch. 6). Whether the targets for gene therapy are virus gene products, host pathways, or a combination thereof, the outcome of such work will alter the outcome of chronic infection in an estimated 170 million people worldwide.

Part IV

Protocols and techniques

18

Sample collection, preparation, and storage

The low levels of HCV RNA in the blood requires sensitive template or signal amplification methods for detection. These procedures are highly sensitive and are prone to crossover contamination, especially when the procedures are carried out manually. To limit contamination, laboratories that are going to be doing amplification on a regular basis need to take a number of precautions (Table 18.1). One of the driving forces for automation of the amplification process is to eliminate virtually all contamination by reducing the number of steps that need to be performed manually. Even so, a major source of variability is sample collection, handling, and storage, especially prior to nucleic acid extraction and amplification. For HCV, it is very important to use a dedicated vacutainer tube that remains unopened until received by the molecular diagnostic laboratory. There does not seem to be a difference in HCV RNA levels between serum and plasma samples obtained from the same patient on the same day (Cuypers et al., 1992; Krajden et al., 1996). However, other independent observations have shown that fresh frozen plasma reproducibly yielded almost twofold higher levels of HCV RNA compared with a corresponding serum sample from the same patient (Busch et al., 1992). HCV RNA levels in clinical samples were also sensitive to storage at room temperature as well as to repeated freezing and thawing in some but not all studies (Busch et al., 1992; Wang et al., 1992; Fong et al., 1993; Quan et al., 1993; Halfon et al., 1996). Blood stored with EDTA (uncoagulated blood) at room temperature or at 4 °C before separation of plasma significantly decreased the levels of HCV RNA detected by RT/PCR (Cuypers et al., 1992) (Ch. 19). HCV RNA in serum decreased by nearly 50% when the time from clot formation until centrifugation was 24 hours (Davis et al., 1994; Halfon et al., 1996). Loss of HCV RNA was prevented if vacutainers containing a serum separator were used and centrifugation was conducted within 2 hours of serum collection. Long-term storage at −80 °C was found to be superior to storage at −20 °C (Halfon et al., 1996). Hence, the rapid separation of serum or plasma from a dedicated vacutainer, combined with storage at −80 °C until nucleic acid extraction, is probably the best way to prevent loss of HCV RNA from clinical samples.

Table 18.1. Precautions for preventing crossover contamination in clinical samples of hepatitis C virus

---

Physically separate pre- and postamplification areas of the laboratory

Use dedicated equipment and pipetmen etc. in each section of the laboratory

Use disposable supplies whenever possible in the preamplification area

Use positive displacement pipets and cotton plugged tips to avoid contaminating the pipets themselves

Use only dedicated clinical samples that have been collected in vacutainer tubes which are not opened until they reach the diagnostic laboratory

Use uracil-N-glycosylase in the clinical sample (Schmidt et al., 1996)

Always run positive and negative controls with each assay

Always run external controls to assess sensitivity of each assay run

Use only approved reagents if home-brew assays are being considered or appropriate commercially available kits, if possible

For home-brew assays, premix reagents and make "master-mixes" to limit the amount of pipetting; when a sample is prepared, add the nucleic acid from the sample last (just prior to amplification)

Separate reagents into portions, especially for home-brew assays, in order to limit contamination

Always use disposable gloves and wear laboratory coats in the pre-amplification area and discard them when leaving the area

---

From Kwok & Higuchi (1989)

19

Hepatitis C RNA in blood and tissue samples

There are several fundamentally different methods that have been developed to detect HCV RNA in blood. These include RT/PCR, branched chain signal amplification (bDNA), nucleic acid sequence-based amplification, ligase chain reaction, transcription-mediated amplification, and various postamplification hybrid capture systems (Hodinka, 1998; Allain, 2000). Northern blot analysis, in situ hybridization and RT/PCR have also been used to detect HCV RNA in tissue samples (Negro, 1998). However, RT/PCR has evolved as the most common method for viral RNA detection and quantification in clinical samples (Ch. 18). Briefly, total RNA is extracted and purified from clinical samples. The extraction procedure may involve pronase digestion in the presence of chaotrophic agents (e.g., guanidinium chloride) to release the RNA from the virion and with phenol extraction and ethanol precipitation to separate nucleic acids from protein. Alternatively, the clinical samples could be "lysed" by addition of detergent, and the released RNA purified and recovered from "mini-spin" columns, which bind nucleic acid and permit the removal of denatured proteins and potential inhibitors of PCR prior to RNA recovery. The HCV RNA in the resulting material is converted to DNA in a two-step procedure. Since HCV RNA is plus stranded, it is converted to minus strand DNA by addition of a complementary primer and by RT, which synthesizes the remaining minus strand. After minus strand synthesis, some protocols call for extraction and purification of the minus strand DNA followed by addition of plus and minus strand primers together with Taq polymerase and then finally by standard PCR. Minus strand DNA is then made double stranded with Taq polymerase. Double-stranded DNA is then heat denatured to form single strands; plus and minus HCV specific primers are annealed to the complementary DNA templates, and the Taq polymerase, which is heat stable, synthesizes new plus and minus strand DNA from each respective primer–template pair. Initially, the sample tubes were opened after reverse transcription and RT inactivation to add additional primers and Taq polymerase for PCR. The separation of the RT and PCR steps was required because each enzyme operated under different buffer conditions, and because RT inhibited Taq polymerase

(Sellner, Coelen & Mackenzie, 1992). However, the opening of tubes halfway through the protocol resulted in crossover contamination of DNA from one sample to another. So some laboratories now use an enzyme called Tth in a one-step procedure, since the Tth enzyme has both RT and DNA polymerase activities (Young, Resnick & Myers, 1993). Other laboratories have worked out one-step RT/PCR protocols using both RT and Taq polymerase in the same tube without a major loss in sensitivity (Ahmad, Schiff & Baroudy, 1993). When this temperature-dependent cycling is repeated 30–40 times, one could theoretically amplify the original cDNA template to 2^n copies. As in most PCR protocols, the efficiency of PCR depends upon the primers used. The high genetic heterogeneity of HCV is a problem for its consistent detection in serum, but the highly conserved 5' UTR has turned out to be one of the best regions on which to base RT/PCR (Houghton et al., 1991) and detect the great majority of HCV infections in clinical samples.

In the early days, the resulting amplified product, or amplicon, was detected as a band of the expected size (defined as the distance on the template between the primers) by agarose gel electrophoresis and either ethidium bromide staining or by Southern blot hybridization. These original "home-brew" assays were not standardized, making comparison of sensitivity, specificity, reproducibility, and accuracy difficult among different laboratories (Zaaijer et al., 1993). Semiquantification has been achieved by adding known amounts of "spike" to each sample. This spike has sequences on either end that are identical to those of the amplicon, but it has an entirely different sequence (compared with the amplicon) between the primers. The ratio of spike to amplicon from the virus in the same tube following competitive amplification is the basis for semiquantification (Hagiwara et al., 1993; Zaaijer et al., 1993; Nakagawa et al., 1994). In an attempt to streamline the assay, and make it less labor intensive, the amplified products have been detected colorimetrically in 96-well plates (Shindo, Di Bisceglie & Silver, 1991). In these assays, visable color produced in each well is proportional to the amount of PCR product in the well and could be quickly measured by an ELISA reader. This assay format is relatively inexpensive and is the basis for the development of clinical kits (e.g., the Roche Amplicor) that can be used in hospital laboratories where the equipment may not be available for further automation of the PCR amplification and detection steps. This is especially important in countries within the developing world that have a high incidence of HCV and need to process many samples inexpensively. The development of these kits has also improved performance and comparability among laboratories, since all of the buffers used are the same and the controls are standardized (Damen et al., 1996).

The advent of "real-time PCR" (Oldach, 1999; Takeuchi et al., 1999) has reduced hands-on-time for these assays and has provided a means to measure

PCR and RT/PCR products accurately in the laboratory. Real-time PCR is based upon an increase in fluorescence that is directly proportional to the amount of amplified product. This results from cleavage of the HCV-specific probe during amplification and the loss of fluorescence quenching within the probe (Holland et al., 1991; Livak et al., 1995). The cycle number where fluorescence in a clinical sample exceeds a threshold level can be directly compared with that of a known internal control or spike (which is coamplified with the sample but gives off light at a different wavelength). Alternatively, fluorescence emitted by external controls of several known concentrations in different tubes could be used to provide a standard curve for the assay and to assess test sensitivity. With real-time PCR, the reduction in hands-on-time minimizes the chances of contamination and operator variability and reduces the sample turn-around-time from 1–2 or more days to several hours. The Roche COBAS AMPLICOR™ has combined thermocycler, automatic pipetter, incubator, washer, and reader in one automated instrument (Jungkind et al., 1996). This system presently offers both qualitative and quantitative (HCV MONITOR™) tests for HCV (Martell et al., 1999). It has recently been complemented by the COBAS AmpliPrep, which is a fully automated sample processor that saves more than 75% of hands-on-time for sample preparation compared with manual methods. The compatibility of the COBAS AmpliPrep with the HCV MONITOR™ and other similarly designed tests will facilitate the appearance of fully automated PCR within the next few years. Very recently, Roche has developed the TaqMan RT/PCR test for HCV RNA (Kleiber et al., 2000). This approach combines high sensitivity with a broad dynamic range, which is not only important in monitoring viral load during therapy but also in assessing virus clearance among acutely infected patients, in assessing viral reactivation, and in documenting a complete virological response to therapy (Dhumeaux, Doffoel & Galmiche, 1997; NIH, 1997). The sensitivity of the Taq-Man method is approximately 100 copies/ml viral RNA in a clinical sample, with a dynamic (linear) range of almost 5 logs and a turn-around-time of less than 3 hours. The increasing use of an international standard for HCV (Saldanha, Lelie & Heath, 1999) will permit realistic comparison of PCR-based assays among different laboratories, will permit comparative quantification between PCR and other detection methods, and will permit direct comparison of independently conducted antiviral trials.

Several other companies have developed alternative amplification technologies to detect HCV, although, with the exception of the bDNA assay, most of the others have not yet been widely used. For example, the transcription-mediated amplification system, developed by Gen-Probe, is an isothermal template amplification assay that can result in up to a billion-fold amplification within 30 minutes. The reaction depends upon addition of RNA polymerase (for DNA templates) plus RT (for RNA templates) to the nucleic acid. An acridinium ester-labeled HCV DNA probe is then used for hybridization to the amplified products, and the hybrids are detected by chemilluminescence. The assay appears to be more sensitive than RT/PCR and may be of some value in detecting complete virological end-of-treatment responders (Sarrazin et al., 2000b). While this assay could be done manually, Gen-Probe is developing a fully automated sytem (TIGRIS™) that will handle sample processing through detection steps. Another approach to HCV detection involves signal, and not template amplification, as exemplified by the bDNA assay. Bayer (formally Chiron) Diagnostics has recently developed the HCV RNA 3.0 Quantitative Assay, which has a dynamic range of more than 4 logs in an automated 96-well plate format. Although the bDNA shows good tolerance to sequence variability, has sensitivity approaching that of RT/PCR, and involves simple sample preparation, it is not yet approved for use as a clinical test in many countries. Organon Teknika Corporation (Boxtel, the Netherlands) has developed both qualitative and quantitative nucleic acid sequence-based amplification for the detection of HCV RNA (Sillekens, 1996). This assay can measure reproducibly down to about 10^4 copies/ml of viral RNA in blood, although its sensitivity is not equal with all HCV subtypes tested. The assay appears to be up to 10-fold more sensitive than the bDNA assay and of comparable sensitivity to the HCV MONI-TOR (Damen et al., 1999; Lunel et al., 1999). Finally, Abbott Laboratories (North Chicago, IL) has developed a procedure known as the asymmetric gap ligase chain reaction, which appears to be highly sensitive for the detection of HCV RNA but has not undergone further development or widespread application (Marshall et al., 1994). While it is likely that real-time RT/PCR will serve many of the needs for HCV RNA detection, other approaches of comparable specificity, sensitivity, and reproducibility may be less expensive and technically easier to conduct. Only time will determine the relative contribution of each approach to the detection of HCV.

20

Hepatitis C genotypes and quasispecies

The categorization of HCV isolates into genotypes occurred during the characterization of HCV clones in different laboratories by sequencing. This has led to the establishment of extensive phylogenetic trees, which are usually based upon comparative sequence analysis of subgenomic regions, such as those spanning core, E1, or NS5B (Bukh et al., 1995) (Section 3.2). Given the high sequence diversity of HCV, sequence analysis of these short regions has often provided enough information for definitive genotyping and, in many cases, subtyping as well (Bukh et al., 1993). Although sequencing is the "gold standard" for genotyping and subtyping, several faster methods have been designed to provide the same information. For example, RT/PCR products from different subgenomic regions of the viral genome have been generated using universal primers that presumably permit amplification of viral RNA from all genotypes and subtypes (Ch. 19). Following amplification using universal primers, one approach then uses genotype-specific primers for further (nested) amplification of only targets with the corresponding sequences (Kato et al., 1991; Okamoto et al., 1994, 1996). Genotype-specific core region primers could distinguish between 1a, 1b, 1c, 2a, 2b, and 3a sequences in the nested amplification step (Okamoto et al., 1992c, 1994). Alternatively, the RT/PCR products resulting from amplification using universal primers have been tested for hybridization to genotype-specific probes (Li et al., 1991, 1994; Takada et al., 1993) or have been digested with one or more restriction endonucleases to permit identification of digestion fragments that are genotype specific (Nakao et al., 1991; Murphy, Willems & Delage, 1994). Although all of these methods are useful, some clinical samples with divergent sequences in the regions of the primers do not amplify with universal primers. Samples may also fail to amplify further by nested PCR, hybridize to genotype-specific probes under stringent conditions, or cleave with the appropriate restriction endonuclease. Hence, these faster methods will only detect a limited number of existing genotypes and subtypes for which the tests were designed (Widell et al., 1994). This limits the utility of these and other assays, and DNA sequencing of RT/PCR amplified products still remains the most reliable method for both genotype and subtype determinations.

Characterization of quasispecies was originally carried out by RT/PCR amplification of the desired region (usually the HVR1), followed by cloning of the amplified products into bacteria, and standard DNA sequence analysis of multiple clones (Martell et al., 1992). Although highly informative, this approach is labor intensive and not adaptable to the high throughput that is needed to characterize many clones from multiple clinical samples. Instead, asymmetric PCR has been used to amplify one cDNA strand. The product(s) were then analyzed by non-denaturing gel electrophoresis, where the mobility of each single-stranded DNA was dependent upon its conformation, which, in turn, was sequence dependent (Enomoto et al., 1994). Most of the major quasispecies migrated to different positions on the gel and could be identified. In an alternative approach, called temperature-gradient gel electrophoresis, the products resulting from RT/PCR amplification were denatured, and one of the strands hybridized to a known HCV sequence. The products were then analyzed on a gel in which there was a temperature gradient. A perfect hybrid, or heteroduplex, was the most stable and had a higher melting temperature than heteroduplexes formed between a wild-type probe and a RT/PCR product that had one or more point mutations. The melting of the latter during the electrophoresis, and corresponding shift in mobility, signalled the presence of a mutation (a quasispecies) (Lu et al., 1995). In a variant of this approach, referred to as gel shift analysis, the mobility of the heteroduplex on a nondenaturing gel is dependent upon whether the hybrid is perfect or whether there is one or more regions in which there is no base pairing (quasispecies) (Wilson et al., 1995). In gel shift analysis, as in temperature gradient gel electrophoresis, the RT/PCR products are hybridized to a probe of known (wild-type HCV) sequence prior to analysis. Although each of these approaches are useful, they only detect the major quasispecies in a given serum sample. In addition, if a quasispecies sequence has little homology with the wild-type sequence used as probe, no heteroduplex will be formed and no quasispecies detected.

21

Replication of hepatitis C in tissue culture

The establishment of tissue culture systems that consistently support high levels of HCV replication is a priority not only for elucidating the replication cycle of the virus but also for screening of putative antiviral compounds. Although many groups have reported virus production in various tissue culture systems (Table 11.1), the low levels of virus produced over time has necessitated using RT/PCR for detection (Ch. 12). Given that HCV is closely related to flaviviruses (Miller & Purcell, 1990) (Table 2.1), it has been assumed that the replication cycle of HCV, like that of flaviviruses, would contain a minus strand intermediate (Chambers et al., 1990; Monath, 1990). The finding of HCV minus strand RNA in tissue culture cells (Table 11.1) and in liver samples (Fong et al., 1991b; Gerber et al., 1992; Negro et al., 1998) from infected patients is consistent with a role for minus strand in the replication cycle, although this has yet to be formally proven. From a technical perspective, detection of minus strand RNA is problematic at best, since it involves using strand-specific primers, which may also randomly prime on the viral plus strand (or on cellular mRNAs), resulting in false-positive results. In tissue culture systems that depend upon infection of susceptible cells with virus from an infectious serum, it is not always clear whether the RT/PCR results reflect de novo production of RNA and/or detection of RNA extracted from virus particles that simply adhered to the tissue culture cells. In addition, while the detection of virus proteins in various tissue culture systems is consistent with virus replication, it is not certain whether virus gene expression occurs in the absence of replication. Moreover, the demonstration that virus generated by several tissue culture systems is infectious in susceptible chimpanzees is highly suggestive of replication but has so far not permitted further development of the corresponding cell lines in which to learn more about replication and to screen compounds that may be effective against HCV. Independent approaches for minus strand RNA detection using RNase protection, for example, would help to solve the problem of amplifying misprimed templates, but these studies have not been reported. A convincing demonstration of minus strand in tissue culture cells would involve direct detection by Northern blotting. In addition, metabolic labeling with UTP would be a definitive way of showing de novo synthesis.

However, the systems currently available do not appear to produce enough virus for detection using these approaches. Hence, the question still remains as to what is the best way to prove HCV replication in tissue culture cells.

22

Enzyme activities of nonstructural protein 3

NS3 has protease, helicase and NTPase activities. NS3 protease assays have been developed using full-length NS3 or its serine protease domain (residues 1–181) (Section 2.4). Polypeptides made by in vitro translation (Bouffard et al., 1995; Hahm et al., 1995; Lin & Rice, 1995), and expressed in *E. coli* (Yamada et al., 1998), mammalian (Bartenschlager et al., 1993; Eckart et al., 1993; Grakoui et al., 1993b) or insect cells (Hirowatari et al., 1993; Overton et al., 1995) have been shown to be active. For the in vitro assays, translated NS3 was mixed with radiolabeled synthetic peptide containing the desired cleavage site, and the products assayed by sodium dodecyl sulfate polyacrylamide gel electrophoresis or reversed phase high pressure liquid chromatography. For some cleavage reactions, in vitro translated NS4A cofactor and commercially available microsomal membranes were added along with the synthetic substrate. Purified protease from *E. coli* has also been tested against radiolabeled substrates made by solid-phase peptide synthesis or by in vitro translation (Bianchi et al., 1996; Shimizu et al., 1996; Sudo et al., 1996). In some studies, recombinant NS3 contained a hexahistadine tag, which permitted easy purification by affinity chromatography using a nickel (Ni^{2+}) column that tightly bound the tag sequence (D'Souza et al., 1995; Kakiuchi et al., 1995). Interestingly, the use of a 4A/4B peptide substrate that contains an ester in place of an amide linkage at the cleavage site showed a more than 100-fold improvement in cleavage, permitting detection of NS3 activity with subnanomolar quantities of recombinant NS3 (Bianchi et al., 1996). The incorporation of an internally quenched depsipeptide fluorogenic substrate into the ester-containing substrate has permitted real-time measurement of NS3 protease activity, since the fluorescence that develops is directly proportional to substrate cleavage and loss of the quenching effect (Taliani et al., 1996). In an alternative approach, chimeric Sindbis or poliovirus was made with NCV NS3 so that the replication of these viruses depended upon the expression of NS3 protease activity. In both cases, NS3 cleavage sites were engineered into the chimeric viruses so that polypeptide maturation would be HCV NS3 specific (Hahm et al., 1996; Filocamo et al., 1997). Some of these approaches have provided simple assays for NS3 activity and have been formatted into high throughput for inhibitor screening.

In addition to protease activity, assays have also been developed to detect NS3-associated helicase and NTPase activities. Most of the helicase/NTPase assays use a NS3 fragment spanning the carboxy-terminal 400–631 residues, where both of these activities are located. Helicase activity has been reported in mammalian cells expressing NS3 (Hong et al., 1996), although most studies have been conducted with NS3 isolated from recombinant bacteria. Recombinant helicase/NTPase from *E. coli* has been purified as a hexahistidine-tagged molecule (Jin & Peterson, 1995; Kim et al., 1995; Gwack et al., 1996; Preugschat et al., 1996). Following the lysis of bacteria, recombinant NS3 was often insoluble within the inclusion body, and recovery required solubilization in 5 mol/l guanidine hydrochloride, followed by nickel-agarose affinity chromatography, and then renaturation following the removal of the guanidine (Jin & Peterson, 1995). The nickel affinity purified NS3 helicase has been further purified by Q-Sepharose (Gwack et al., 1996) or by poly(U)-Sepharose 4B chromatography (Tai et al., 1996). Renaturation has been monitored in an ATPase assay followed either by the loss of ATP, which is measured by a decrease in absorbance of the reaction mixture at 340 nm or by ADP production, monitored by high-pressure liquid chromatography as an increase in 260 nm absorbing material (Jin & Peterson, 1995). In independent work, recombinant NS3 helicase/NTPase was isolated from the soluble fraction of a bacterial lysate. NTPase activity was assayed by addition of $[\alpha\text{-}^{32}P]$-ATP and the hydrolysis products were analyzed by ascending thin-layer chromatography (Tai et al., 1996; Paolini et al., 2000a). Hence, NTPase activity has been used to monitor the functional integrity of NS3 following purification.

The importance of NTPase activity to the NS3-encoded helicase (Section 2.4) is highlighted by the finding that the helicase activity is energy dependent, with ATP as the preferred substrate for NS3 isolated from either bacteria (Suzich et al., 1993) or eucaryotic cells (Morgenstern et al., 1997). Divalent manganese and magnesium cations strongly stimulate both NTPase and helicase activities, with poly(U) and poly(dU) as preferred substrates (Suzich et al., 1993; Jin & Peterson, 1995; Preugschat et al., 1996). NS3 helicase (unwindase) activity depends upon the presence of a short single-stranded region at the end of the template, since fully double-stranded templates are resistant to unwinding (Jin & Peterson, 1995; Gwack et al., 1996; Tai et al., 1996). This observation is consistent with the flexibility in the secondary structure at the ends of the HCV RNA. In these helicase assays, one of the two strands in the substrate is radiolabeled so that the release of radiolabel from the double-stranded substrate becomes a measure of helicase (unwindase) activity. In practice, helicase activity is monitored over time by the relative amounts of radiolabeled double-stranded versus single-stranded RNA species, which migrate to different positions in native acrylamide gels following electrophoresis. Their ratio is then determined by PhosphorImager analysis (Kim et al., 1995; Tai et al., 1996; Paolini et al., 2000a). The substrates that are often used to assay helicase activity span the 5' UTR or 3' UTR sequences of HCV, which are also likely to be the natural substrates during infection. In these assays, the addition of excess poly(A) or poly(C) does not compete with poly(U) and poly(dU) as substrate for NS3 helicase. This is not surprising in light of the fact that the 3' UTR of the HCV genome contains a poly(U) stretch (Kolykhalov et al., 1996). This may be the natural site where unwinding is initiated, which then proceeds in a 3' to 5' direction during minus strand RNA synthesis (Hong et al., 1996). Although helicase activity is exquisitely sensitive to salt in vitro (Gwack et al., 1996; Tai et al., 1996), the association of NS3 with membrane-bound replication complexes in infected cells may effectively exclude intracellular salts. The development of these assays will contribute both to a better understanding of the mechanisms of these activities and to screening methods for new drug candidates against the virus.

The fact that NS3 helicase activity requires binding to HCV RNA has also been exploited in the development of RNA-binding assays. Three assay formats have been established. In the Northwestern assay for RNA binding, purified NS3 has been electrophoresed in sodium dodecylsulfate polyacrylamide gels, transferred to nitrocellulose, and the membranes extensively washed. To detect binding, the membranes were incubated with $[\alpha\text{-}^{32}P]$-labeled single-stranded RNA, washed, and exposed to X-ray film. In the filter binding assay, purified NS3 was added to a prewetted nitrocellulose filter. After washing, the filters containing NS3 were incubated with radiolabeled single-stranded RNA, washed again, and binding was assessed by scintillation counting. In the gel retardation assay, NS3 was incubated with a radiolabeled single-stranded RNA substrate, and the complexes analyzed by 20% polyacrylamide gel electrophoresis in Tris/borate/EDTA buffer in the absence of sodium dodecylsulfate. The results were again revealed by autoradiography (Gwack et al., 1996; Paolini et al., 2000a). In all of these assays, radiolabeled single-stranded RNA was made by in vitro transcription with a single $[\alpha\text{-}^{32}P]$-NTP. As with the NTPase activity, the RNA-binding assay has been used as a measure of NS3 function. Both of these activities, in addition to helicase (unwindase), are considered potential targets for antiviral drug development. Consequently, some groups have developed high throughput assays based upon these activities explicitly for antiviral drug screening (Hsu et al., 1998; Kwong & Risano, 1998; Kyono, Miyashiro & Taguchi, 1998).

23

Characterization of nonstructural protein 5B

Considerable information about the structural features of the HCV-encoded RdRp is now available from the crystal structure of the enzyme (Ago et al., 1999; Bressanelli et al., 1999; Lesburg et al., 1999) (Ch. 16). However, the lack of a highly productive tissue culture system that consistently supports virus replication (Ch. 11) has made it difficult to isolate replication complexes in order to study NS5B function in its appropriate context. For this reason, a number of laboratories have isolated recombinant HCV NS5B for functional studies as well as for drug screening (Behrens et al., 1996; Al et al., 1997, 1998; Lohmann et al., 1997; Yamashita et al., 1998; Hagehorn et al., 2000). Some of the initial attempts to isolate NS5B from recombinant insect cells or *E. coli* showed that a large percentage was insoluble. To solve this problem, NS5B was isolated under denaturing conditions and then refolded into active enzyme (Yuan et al., 1997), where it was shown to replicate HCV RNA as well as globin mRNA, poly(A), poly(C) and other templates in the absence of additional virus or host factors (Behrens et al., 1996; Al et al., 1997, 1998; Lohmann et al., 1997). Secondary structural analysis of HCV NS5B showed that it had a hydrophobic carboxy-terminus, which may explain its hydrophobicity and membrane association in HCV replication complexes. Removal of the hydrophobic 21 carboxy-terminal amino acid residues from NS5B facilitated purification and increased the yield of functional enzyme (Yamashita et al., 1998). For isolation of NS5B from baculovirus vectors and a SF9 insect expression system, cells were lysed in a nondenaturing solubilization buffer containing the nonionic detergent Triton X-100, the lysate clarified by centrifugation, and the supernatant subjected to sequential ion exchange (diethylaminoethyl cellulose), heparin, and poly(U)-Sepharose chromatography, followed by a high pressure liquid chromatography step (DeFrancesco et al., 1996b). Independent efforts using recombinant baculovirus vectors in insect cells made an NS5B molecule containing a hexahistidine tag on its carboxy-terminus, which allowed more rapid purification. Briefly, cell lysates were made in buffer containing no detergents. After clarification by centrifugation, the pellets were resuspended in buffer containing Triton X-100. Following centrifugation and resuspension of the pellets in buffer containing Triton X-100, the samples were sonicated, centrifuged again, and the supernatant subjected to nickel affinity chromatography (Lohmann et al., 1997). The last step positively selected for the hexahistidine-tagged NS5B, which specifically bound to the affinity column. One or more proteinase inhibitors were added to the buffers used for purification in order to inhibit NS5B degradation during purification. Similar protocols have been used to isolate enzymatically active untagged or hexahistadine-tagged NS5B from recombinant *E. coli* (Al et al., 1997, 1998; De Staercke et al., 1998; Yamashita et al., 1998). NS5B has also been expressed in mammalian cells, although the use of an inducible expression system resulted in more rapid identification of cells that express higher levels of NS5B (Heller et al., 1998). It will be of great interest to see whether mammalian cell systems can be developed to study the properties of NS5B in more detail. The establishment of a suitable reporter gene assay that could accurately measure NS5B activity would not only accelerate the isolation of cells making high levels of NS5B but would also allow its more ready characterization. Such characterization would include identification of viral and cellular proteins that regulate NS5B activity and inhibitors of that activity in the context of drug screening.

The properties of isolated NS5B have been studied by in vitro assays that are similar to each other and to those originally developed for the study of the RdRp from poliovirus (Wimmer, Hellen & Cao, 1993). In these assays, untagged or tagged NS5B has been added to a poly(A)-containing RNA template in a buffer containing oligo(T) or oligo(U) primers and one radiolabeled nucleoside tris-phosphate ($[^{32}P]$-NTP). After several hours of incubation, the radiolabeled RNA products were extracted and analyzed by polyacrylamide gels containing 7 mol/l urea (DeFrancesco et al., 1996b). Although RNA synthesis with synthetic templates was primer dependent, no primers were needed for RdRp activity when full-length HCV RNA was used as template (Tanaka et al., 1995). The latter is consistent with a copy-back mechanism for HCV replication (Section 2.5).

Part V

Some outstanding questions and emerging areas for investigation

24

Outstanding issues

The chapters of this book have provided a multi- and interdisciplinary outline of HCV. However, there is still so much more work that has to be done before the virus, its biology, and associated diseases are understood well enough to generate effective vaccines and new potent therapeutics. To this end, a sampling of outstanding questions in the field are presented below.

1. **What are some of the implications of the physical heterogeneity of hepatitis C?**

   Various studies have shown the density of HCV to vary from 1.03 to 1.20 g/ml (Bradley et al., 1991; Carrick et al., 1992; Miyamoto et al., 1992; Hijikata et al., 1993b; Thomssen et al., 1993; Kanto et al., 1994; Choo et al., 1995; Nakajima et al., 1996; Yoshikura et al., 1996). Although this may result from differences in the types or quantity of viral polypeptide that make up different virus particles, it seems more likely that this physical heterogeneity may be contributed by the association of virus particles with different types and amounts of host cell and serum components. The findings that LDLs and immunoglobulins are associated with HCV particles of different densities, and that virus from different densities also differ in infectivity, suggest that the host–virus relationship that develops after infection depends, in part, upon the physical composition of the virus particles. For example, complexing of virus particles with immunoglobulins may limit virus spread and infection of susceptible hepatocytes following a bout of hepatitis. In addition, the complexing of host proteins with the virus envelope may prevent or blunt immunological recognition of neutralizing determinants on the virus. Although genetic heterogeneity within the HVR1 sequences may also contribute to the escape of extracellular virus from neutralizing antibodies (Martell et al., 1992; Weiner et al., 1992; Shimizu et al., 1994), the development of weak or delayed immune responses to the virus may contribute importantly to virus persistence and the high rate of chronic infection seen worldwide (Battegay, 1996).

2. **What is the significance of genetic heterogeneity within the 5' untranslated region?**

   There are slight differences in the sequences of the 5' UTR among HCV genotypes and subtypes, although it is not possible at this time to assess accurately their roles in virus replication, gene expression, or pathogenesis. This is because of the lack of an appropriate tissue culture system in which to study replication and small animal models in which to study pathogenesis. Instead, published studies have presented the translational efficiency of a reporter gene cloned downstream from the IRES and 5' region of the HCV core gene. In one study, the results showed a twofold higher level of reporter gene expression when the IRES sequences in the expression vectors were from HCV genotypes 1 or 2 than when they were from genotype 3 (Buratti et al., 1997). In contrast, other independent observations showed that the IRES sequences from subtype 2b were slightly more active than those from 1b (Tsukiyama-Kohara et al., 1992). Further work showed that the sequences from HCV subtype 1a were about twofold more efficient in translation compared with those from 1b (Honda et al., 1996b). Other work showed that the IRES sequence in genotype 2 was more active than those from genotypes 1, 3, 4, 5, and 6 (Collier, Tang & Elliot, 1998). Although interesting, the differences in translational efficiency between most studies is small, and it is not known whether they reflect the situation in the intact HCV genome.

3. What is the tissue range for hepatitis C?

In addition to hepatocytes, evidence for HCV infection has been found in lymphoid cells isolated from bone marrow and lymph nodes (Gabrielli et al., 1994; Sugiyama et al., 1997). The detection of HCV markers in a variety of autoaggressive and autoimmune diseases (Table 7.1) (Cassani et al., 1992; Strassburg et al., 1996; Zignego & Brechot, 1999), combined with a higher than expected frequency of nonHodgkin's lymphoma in HCV-infected patients compared with the general population (La Civita et al., 1995; Ferri et al., 1997a; Zignego et al., 1997a), is also consistent with the hypothesis that lymphoid cells may support virus gene expression or replication. The transmission of HCV through saliva (Abe & Inchauspe, 1991) may indicate that it replicates in salivary glands. In this context, the development of sialadenitis in transgenic mice expressing the envelope proteins of HCV (Koike et al., 1997) shows that the salivary gland supports virus gene expression and may also be permissive for virus replication. However, it could also be the result of passive transmission of virus from the blood into the saliva. Likewise, the transmission of HCV through the conjunctiva (Sartori et al., 1993) may reflect either replication within the conjunctiva or passive transfer of virus though the conjunctiva into the bloodstream, or both.

4. What functions of nonstructural protein 5A are important for virus replication and hepatocarcinogenesis?

The significance of NS5A is not clearly understood. For example, it is not known whether there is a relationship between NS5A phosphorylation and *trans-*

activation, what the nature of the cellular kinase that phosphorylates NS5A is, or whether phosphorylation affects the ability of NS5A to interact with signal trans-duction molecules in the cytoplasm or transcription factors in the nucleus. It is not known whether NS5A *trans*-activation function brings about changes in host gene expression that favor host cell survival in the face of cytotoxic immune responses and/or whether it makes hepatocytes more "permissible" for virus replication. Moreover, the function of NS5A in the replication complexes of HCV is a mystery. Is NS5A always expressed in a viral replication complex or is some of it expressed free so that it could alter cellular pathways in the nucleus and cytoplasm? Is NS5A phosphorylation important for it to mediate IFN resis-tance? These are just some of the many concerns that need to be addressed in the future.

5. What determines the template specificity of hepatitis C encoded nonstructural protein 5B?

It may be impossible to explain fully the determinants of NS5B template specificity until a tissue culture system that consistently supports HCV replication at high levels becomes available. However, it seems likely that compartmentalization of NS5B and viral RNA within membrane-bound replication complexes is very important for replication to occur, since the scarcity of both in a newly infected cell would preclude them ever finding each other. The apparent requirement for a replication complex also appears to be important for insuring that NS5B replicates HCV RNA, and not heterologous cellular mRNA templates, as it does in vitro. In this context, the likely importance of compartmentalization is underscored by the realization that, if NS5B acted in the absence of a replication complex, virtually all of the activity would end up replicating cellular RNAs, which are abundant compared with viral RNAs, especially early after infection. The finding that soluble HCV NS5B does not bind HCV RNA in vitro (Lohmann et al., 1997) is consistent with the hypothesis that other HCV and/or host polypeptides in the replication complex are capable of direct binding, thereby acting as cofactors in viral replica-tion (Al et al., 1997, 1998), and/or that protein–protein interactions involving NS5B directs the latter to the viral RNA template in vivo. There is support for the latter mechanism in poliovirus replication (Andino, Rieckhof & Baltimore, 1990; Andino et al., 1993; Roehl et al., 1997). These protein–protein interactions may stabilize otherwise weak viral polymerase–RNA interactions, as in poliovirus (Richards & Ehrenfeld, 1998) and help to establish template specificity.

6. What happens when an asymptomatic individual is diagnosed as being infected by hepatitis C?

When a test result for HCV infection comes back positive, and this result is verified during follow-up, patients are counseled in order to minimize additional risks for the development of liver disease, reduce the risk of transmitting HCV, and to consider treatment options. To minimize additional risks for the development of liver disease, it is important for patients to stay away from alcohol, since alcohol exacerbates liver disease in chronically infected patients. Patients should also check with their doctor each time a new medication for an unrelated condition is considered, since some medicines may have adverse effects on an already damaged liver. In addition, immunization against HBV and HAV may be advised, since coinfection with these agents will make liver disease worse and successful treatment less likely.

To reduce the risk for HCV transmission, patients should not donate blood, blood fractions, organs, tissues, or semen. At home, they should not share razors, toothbrushes, or other personal items that may carry small amounts of contaminated blood. In addition, they should cover all cuts etc. to prevent the unintended spread of contaminated blood. Although sexual transmission of HCV to an uninfected spouse has been documented, the risk for sexual transmission is low. Hence, the CDC does not recommend any change in sexual practices, although the use of condoms and counseling of the uninfected spouse should be considered (CDC, 1998). For the infected woman, HCV is not a contraindication for pregnancy, although roughly 5% of children born to infected mothers become infected at the time of birth, and testing of newborns to HCV-positive mothers should be conducted. While no treatment exists that can prevent transmission to infants, the natural history of infection during childhood is mostly asymptomatic, although the long-term effects of neonatal infection still need to be studied. Finally, there is no indication that breast milk transmits HCV.

A positive HCV test should not adversely affect the everyday activities of most people. This is because HCV is not transmitted through the air, through food or water, by sharing glasses and eating utensils, or by casual contact. Therefore, it should not impact upon work, school, play, or child-care settings. However, infected persons should be assessed on a regular basis for biochemical evidence of liver disease, by checking blood ALT levels under the supervision of a specialist.

7. Should there be universal screening for hepatitis C RNA in all blood donors?

The risk for transmission of HCV after anti-HCV testing is now about 1 in 100 000 transfusions (van der Poel, 1999). This is probably a result of HCV virus concentrations in acute phase sera (prior to anti-HCV development) that may be as high as 10^8 virus genome equivalents/ml (Vrielink et al., 1995). In addition, if only one out of several thousand donor sera were contaminated with these levels of HCV, it is likely that infectious (and detectable) virus will be passed on to individuals at high risk for PTH even if these contaminated donor units are pooled with several thousand sera or blood fractions from HCV-free donors. Even though current inactivation methods for HCV reduce the viral load by approximately 6 logs (Prince et al., 2000), high-risk populations will still develop HCV infections. This transfer could be further reduced if donor sera were screened for HCV RNA, since this would pick up infectious sera from acute infections prior to the development of anti-HCV. It has been estimated that the risk for HCV infection with anti-HCV screening is 9.7 cases/million, while the risk for infection would fall to 2.7 cases/million if HCV RNA testing was implemented (Schreiber et al., 1996a,b). Although commercial assays for the detection of HCV RNA are available, they are quite expensive for routine use. In addition, the available virus inactivation methods are also quite expensive (Pereira, 1999), which, in part, is limiting their widespread application. The PCR technologies are technically demanding and expensive, so their universal application for HCV (and other pathogens) will come about only when standardized, automated, inexpensive, and simple amplification tests could be devised (Saldanha and Minor, 1996a,b). Even if all of these challenges were met, the implementation of routine screening would depend upon the results of retrospective and prospective studies, which would first have to demonstrate that such screening would further reduce the frequency of PTH in high-risk patients. Hence, it seems more probable that this technology would be first applied to screening blood and blood products destined for use in high-risk populations before it would be considered for more widespread screening.

8. What happens if there is a suspected exposure to hepatitis C through needlestick or some other source?

When an accidental exposure to HCV has been suspected, the time and nature of exposure should be reported as soon as possible to a physician. If the exposure is the result of a needle stick, or from a tube containing blood that may be from an infected person, then it would be helpful to have the needle or blood sample tested for HCV RNA by RT/PCR or some other sensitive amplification technique. According to published studies, the risk for getting HCV infection is not high, with two studies reporting 0/24 (Zuckerman et al., 1994) and 0/61 (Petrosillo, Puro & Ippolito, 1994) needlesticks resulting in infection, while another study showed 3/56 (5.4%) (Arai et al., 1996). Overall, the frequency of acquiring HCV from percutaneous exposure is up to 1 in 10 (Gerberding, 1995). Regardless of these numbers, it is important to seek medical attention as soon as possible, since it will be important to have serial blood samples taken and tested for the development of anti-HCV over the period of at least 12–18 months. Testing for the presence of HCV RNA would also be useful, if this assay is available. Unfortunately, there is no protective vaccine presently available to prevent infection, nor is there an effective hyperimmune gammaglobulin for protection against infection shortly after exposure.

9. Do different subtypes or quasispecies have different replicative abilities?

There are several areas where genetic heterogeneity in HCV could have an impact upon replicative ability. One has to do with the specificity of the NS3/NS4A protease (Section 2.4). This protease undergoes rapid *cis*-cleavage at Thr-1657 to yield mature NS3 and NS4A, which remain associated and act in *trans* to mediate processing of the other nonstructural proteins (Section 2.4). Using in vitro translation or transient expression into eucaryotic cells, NS3–NS4A cleavage was shown to be tolerant to substitutions of amino acids with small (Gly, Ala, Ser), large polar (Asn), or negatively charged (Asp) side chains. However, substitution of Thr-1657 with Arg, Phe, Tyr, or Ile, significantly decreased processing (Leinbach et al., 1994; Tanji et al., 1994b; Bartenschlager et al., 1995a). While these results suggest that polypeptide folding rather than primary sequence is important for processing (Bartenschlager et al., 1995a), it also suggests that different mutations at the NS3–NS4A processing site will result in different amounts of processing and different levels of virus replication (Section 2.5). In contrast, mutations at sites that NS3 cleaves in *trans* were susceptible to many different amino acid replacements, suggesting that the sequence context was important for specificity (Kolykhalov, Agapov & Rice, 1994; Bartenschlager et al., 1995a). Again, reduced cleavage efficiency may result in altered levels of virus gene expression and replication.

Variation within the IRES is another source of genetic heterogeneity that could have an impact upon virus gene expression and replication (Fig. 2.2). For example, one study showed that translation using the 5' UTR from genotype 3 was about half that of either 1b or 2a (Buratti et al., 1997). Independent work showed that the 5' UTR from subtype 2b was two- to fivefold more active in directing translation compared with the subtype 1b sequence, although the differences in the nucleotide sequences did not map to the IRES (Kamoshita et al., 1997). The high activity of subtype 2b IRES has been confirmed, while comparative analysis with the IRES from other subtypes showed that subtype 6a IRES had the lowest activity. Another study showed that the 5' UTR from subtype 1a was about twofold more efficient in directing translation than was the analogous sequence from subtype 1b; the sequence differences mapped to nucleotides upstream of the IRES in the 5' UTR (Honda et al., 1996b, 1999b). Collectively, these studies imply that mutations within the 5' UTR may affect the conformation of the IRES element and the efficiency of translation. However, IRES activity was determined by reporter gene assays using different sized fragments spanning the 5' UTR and sometimes part of the core region. This raises the question as to whether these differences would still occur when the IRES is in the natural context of the whole virus genome. Interestingly, mutations within domain IV of the IRES (Fig. 2.3), which contains the translation initiation codon for HCV, alter the efficiency of translation. This is because such mutations would affect the stability of the domain IV stem–loop, which needs to be melted in order to make room for 40S rRNA attachment (Honda et al., 1996a). Since neighboring secondary structure would also have an impact upon this "melting," up- or downstream mutations that alter the stability of the RNA secondary structure would also be predicted to alter translation efficiency. This is probably one of the reasons why the 5' region of the core gene is so highly conserved among different isolates of HCV.

10. What are some of the outstanding issues that remain to be addressed to understand the natural history of infection?

The outcome of chronic HCV infection is variable. It is not clear whether chronic hepatitis seen on liver biopsy invariably progresses to cirrhosis or whether there are markers that appear early on in chronic infection that predict the development of cirrhosis, although some risk factors have recently been identified (Table 4.1). This is important, since cirrhosis contributes importantly to morbidity and mortality (Ikeda et al., 1993; Niederau et al., 1998). Further, the silent (asymptomatic) nature of HCV infection in the transfusion setting (Alter et al., 1992) compared with the documentation of seriously ill people in tertiary care facilities (Kiyosawa et al., 1990; Tong et al., 1995) generates unintentional bias in the reporting and understanding of the full spectrum that constitutes the natural history of infection. To deal with this issue, long-term follow-up studies will need to be conducted, although following patients for 30 years will be a real challenge. The problem surrounding long-term follow-up is more than academic, since a more detailed understanding of natural history will be important in deciding who to treat, with what, and for how long. A more detailed understanding of natural history will also guide the development and evaluation of future therapeutics.

11. Why is it difficult to assess the prognostic significance of immune responses in hepatitis C infection?

The evolving quasispecies nature of HCV means that immune responses characterized from PBMC often do not match the major quasispecies existing in the infected individual at that time. This is true not only for antibodies but also for CTL responses, when strong CTL specificities may no longer target hepatocytes infected with different variants to those existing in the periphery. In addition, the immune responses that are relevant to pathogenesis at any time during infection are more likely to be found intrahepatically than in peripheral blood (Minutello et al., 1993). For example, intrahepatic Th cells seem to be enriched for reactivity to NS4 compared with Th cells in peripheral blood in that the intrahepatic cells provide the bulk of the help for NS4 antibody production (Minutello et al., 1993). Further, it is not clear whether the infiltration of lymphocytes and/or production of specific cytokines at any time during infection are the cause of the pathology or are triggered by other immune responses. In other words, it is difficult to establish cause and effect relationships between specific immune responses and different features of pathogenesis. If HCV is cytopathic, for example, then immune responses may simply be responding to damaged cells. The pathogenesis of infection may also be influenced by the immunogenetics of each person (McKiernan & Kelleher, 2000), which may contribute importantly to the timing and vigor of the immune responses that develop after acute infection. Finally, there does not seem to be a clear correlation between T cell responses to HCV proteins and the clinical outcome of chronic infection (Botarelli et al., 1993). These are just some of the reasons why it is difficult to assess the significance of immune responses to the pathogenesis of acute and chronic infection, although the development of an appropriate animal model would permit cause and effect experiments to be carried out that would clarify many of these issues.

12. Can cytotoxic T lymphocytes clear hepatitis C effectively from liver?

If 1–10% of hepatocytes in the human liver become infected (10^{9-10} cells), and there are at most 10^7 HCV CTL precursors (based on a 10^{-5} CTL precursor frequency from 10^{12} total lymphocytes in the body), then there would be one CTL for every 100–1000 infected hepatocytes. This suggests that antigen nonspecific lymphocytes are recruited and/or that noncytolytic cytokines partially control HCV.

13. Does hepatitis C play an important role in the pathogenesis of fulminant hepatitis?

HCV RNA has been found in 10–35% of patients with fulminant hepatitis (Inokuchi et al., 1996; Villamil et al., 1995), although it is not known whether the relationship is causal or coincidental.

14. What are the factors that lead to chronic infection?

Elucidating the factors leading to chronic HCV infection will be very important for understanding the natural history of infection and for the development of future therapeutics. Presently, it is likely that virus genetic variation (quasispecies) and inappropriate (quantitative and qualitative) immune responses following acute infection contribute importantly to the development and persistence of chronic infections. The development of viral quasispecies faster than they can be recognized and eliminated by neutralizing antibodies (against the envelope glycoproteins) helps to explain virus persistence (Houghton et al., 1991; Weiner et al., 1992). In addition, it can be envisaged that the development of cell-mediated immune responses against successive virus variants in immunodominant epitopes of the virus can result in the successive bouts of CLD characteristic of chronic

HCV infections (Koziel et al., 1993). The fact that diversity of quasispecies increases during chronic infection (Takaki et al., 2000) and that it decreases in tissue culture systems supporting HCV replication (Kato et al., 1995), are observations consistent with this hypothesis. The infection of extrahepatic sites, especially where immune responses do not eliminate virus-infected cells (i.e., where there is no immune-mediated pathology), represents reservoirs for virus replication and spread. Reseeding of the liver with virus variants from extrahepatic sites may also trigger new bouts of CLD. Another way HCV may contribute to chronicity involves the putative alteration of host signal transduction pathways by HCV core and/or truncated NS5A (if this exists) in infected cells. If this occurs in hepatocytes, it may result in their increased resistance to immune-mediated apoptosis, while if this occurs in infected lymphocytes, it may blunt the development of timely and appropriate immune responses aimed at virus elimination. This would especially be true if the core protein, for example, binds to TNF receptor family members and alters the transmission of apoptotic signals. While these possibilities are provocative, their rigorous testing will only come about when liver cell lines supporting sustained HCV replication, and animal models of HCV-associated CLDs, are successfully developed.

15. Does hepatitis C core antigen play a central role in hepatocarcinogenesis?

The results of some (Moriya et al., 1998) but not other transgenic mouse systems (Kawamura et al., 1997; Pasquinelli et al., 1997), suggest that core is directly involved with the development of HCC. However, if core is important, the question arises as to whether sustained, high levels of HCV core can be detected in the liver and/or tumors from chronically infected patients who develop HCV-associated HCC. To date, there are no data to suggest that core protein is detectable in the majority of HCC tissues examined, although antibody reagents differ among the various studies and may account for some of the differences. Given the centrality of HCV core to virus replication, and the finding of HCV replication in both tumor and nontumor cells (Gerber et al., 1992; Haruna et al., 1994), it seems likely that core is present in both compartments and can participate in the pathogenesis of HCC. However, the HCV core transgenic mice that develop HCC express core in the absence of virus replication. Additionally, since core is normally part of the virus replication complex, it is not clear how much "free" core is available to interact with cellular growth regulatory proteins and pathways relative to the fraction tied up as a structural protein in the nucleocapsid of the virus. Since many studies have documented the function(s) of HCV core in cell types other than hepatocytes, it is not clear whether these same interactions occur in infected hepatocytes or in liver-derived cell lines.

16. What are some of the putative steps whereby hepatitis C may transform hematopoietic cells?

The association of HCV infection with B cell lymphoproliferative disorders in patients, combined with the likely lymphotrophism of HCV (demonstrated both in vivo and in vitro), suggest that HCV alters the growth, survival, and function of B cells. For example, there is a report of one chronically infected patient with EMC who developed a chromosomal rearrangement involving the *bcl-2* locus during the benign phase of disease. This resulted in the accelerated development of lymphoma (Ellis et al., 1995). Since Bcl-2 is an important component of the antiapoptotic complement of the cell, its constitutive activation may contribute to lymphoproliferation. In this context, elevated Bcl-2 expression has been reported in HCV-infected patients with EMC (Monteverde, Ballare & Pileri, 1997). This is probably caused by a t(14:18) translocation, which places the *bcl-2* locus under control of the immunoglobulin heavy chain locus, resulting in Bcl-2 overexpression, which is a consistent and early event in the development of follicular lymphoma (Jaeger et al., 1994). Preliminary observations with many HCV-infected patients have reported a high frequency of this mutation (Zignego et al., 1997b). Finally, the finding that the HCV core stimulates *c-myc* expression (Ray et al., 1995, 1996a) (Section 5.4 and Ch. 6), and that *Myc* cooperates with Bcl-2 in tumor formation (Fanidi, Harrington & Evan, 1992), provides further evidence of a likely mechanism whereby HCV may contribute to the development of lymphoma.

17. What are the mechanism(s) of antiviral activities mediated by interferon?

IFN consists of a family of proteins (α, β, and γ) the production of which is often triggered by double-stranded viral RNA in infected cells or by viral antigens processed by virus-specific T lymphocytes. IFNs induce the synthesis of a PKR and 2',5'-oligoadenylate synthetase. The former inhibits the translation of virus proteins by phosphorylating and inactivating the translation initiation factor eIF2α, while the latter results in the enzymatic degradation of viral RNA into oligomers. IFN expression also results in upregulation of MHC class I and class II, enhances NK activity, and modulates antibody production by B cells. It is not clear whether the direct antiviral action or the immunomodulatory properties of the IFNs, or both, are operative in viral clearance and resolution of liver disease among treated patients.

18. Who is recommended for treatment?

Treatment is recommended for chronically infected patients at risk for the development of cirrhosis. These patients are persistently positive for HCV RNA and have elevated ALT. Upon liver biopsy, they demonstrate moderate liver inflammation, necrosis, and either portal or bridging fibrosis (NIH, 1997). It is not clear whether treatment should be initiated in patients with little or no fibrosis, mild inflammation, and minimal necrosis, since such patients are likely to progress very slowly to cirrhosis, if at all. In addition, it is not clear whether treatment should be initiated in patients with compensated cirrhosis (i.e., who lack jaundice, encephalopathy, variceal hemorrhage, or ascites). IFN treatment has not been approved for infected children less than 18 years of age or for adults greater than 60 years, which precludes their inclusion at the present time in IFN-based treatment protocols. Among the chronically infected patients who should not be treated are those with persistently normal transaminases, those with advanced cirrhosis who are at risk for decompensation, and infected alcoholics and intravenous drug users unless drinking and intravenous drug abuse are terminated. Treatment is also contraindicated in patients who are pregnant, in those with autoimmune diseases, with cytopenias, hyperthyroidism, and with clinical depression (NIH, 1997), since the last four conditions could be exacerbated by treatment.

19. Why do in vitro tissue culture systems fail to support high levels of hepatitis C replication?

It is not clear why high levels of HCV replication cannot be achieved in tissue culture systems, although it is likely that one or more host factors that support HCV infection to high levels in vivo are missing or are at suboptimal levels in the cells lines tested to date. Some of these cellular factors include eIF3 (Sizova et al., 1998), heterogeneous nuclear protein L (Hahm et al., 1998), PTB (Ali & Siddiqui, 1995), La antigen (Ali & Siddiqui, 1997), and other cellular proteins (Yen et al., 1995; Fukushi et al., 1997). Optimal levels of PTB, for example, may promote HCV RNA translation (Ali & Siddiqui, 1995), which is required for the formation of HCV replication complexes, although this remains to be shown. Of course, this does not provide a satisfactory explanation for the low levels of HCV replication observed upon infection of primary hepatocytes. A possible explanation for this may be that the conditions for infection or replication are not optimal in vitro. For example, it cannot be excluded that viral receptor(s) are either removed or their expression downregulated in the process of hepatocyte isolation. Alternatively, or in addition, it is possible that the culture conditions are not optimal for HCV replication. For example, MT-2C cells support HCV replication for a significantly longer period of time when grown at 32 °C than when grown at 37 °C (Mizutani et al., 1996a). In addition, it cannot be excluded that the primary site for HCV replication is in a cell type other than hepatocytes. For example, it is possible that HCV first replicates in Kupffer cells, in which HCV may acquire additional host-encoded proteins within the viral envelope that promote binding to and uptake by hepatocytes. The finding that bone marrow, lymph nodes, and many lymphoid cell lines are permissive for HCV is consistent with a role for Kupffer (macrophage-like) cells in the liver supporting HCV replication. Further, the relationship between HCV replication and cell cycle or state of cellular differentiation is not known. Clearly, tissue culture is characterized by considerable cellular growth during log phase, while HCV replication in the liver has to contend with mostly quiescent hepatocytes. The titer of virus in serum used to infect the cell lines may also contribute importantly to the amount of virus produced (Shimizu et al., 1993). Moreover, the diversity of quasispecies in different samples may limit their ability to infect and replicate in susceptible cells, since different quasispecies may have different replicative abilities. In this context, it would be expected that sera obtained from chronically infected patients and chimpanzees would have quasispecies with limited replicative capacity, since the quasispecies with higher replicative fitness would have been recognized and eliminated by the immune system earlier. The necessity to create a "consensus" sequence in order to get successful infection of chimpanzees is just one manifestation of how virus genetic heterogeneity may impact upon replicative fitness in vivo. Of course, the serum samples and individual molecular clones used for infection and transfection, respectively, of tissue culture cells are likely to reflect these same limitations, resulting in low levels of virus replication. The problem is that there is currently no way to select for quasispecies with high replicative fitness. While this list is not exhaustive, it highlights both the complexity of the problem and the challenges that lie ahead in order to attain the goal of a truly permissive cell culture system for HCV that sustains a high level of virus replication.

20. What are some of the problems that need to be addressed in the development of protective and/or therapeutic vaccines against hepatitis C?

A variety of approaches have been taken by different groups in attempts to develop HCV vaccines. For example, the induction of immune responses in mice immunized with polypeptide or recombinant DNA vaccines is an important first step in evaluating their immunogenicity, although at this time, it is not clear whether epitopes that are immunogenic in mice will also be immunogenic in chimpanzees or people. It is even less certain whether immunogenic epitopes actually play important roles in virus clearance, since mice are not naturally susceptible to HCV, and this question, therefore, could not be addressed in mice. There is also the potential problem that the therapeutic vaccination of chronically infected patients with liver disease will result in a life-threatening exacerbation of this disease instead of resolution. Given the variability in the pathogenesis and outcome of chronic infection, it may be difficult to design a single therapeutic vaccine that is effective in the majority of patients who need it. However, the finding that recovery from acute infection involves strong CD4[+] T cell responses to multiple virus antigens (Missale et al., 1996; Diepolder et al., 1997; Takaki et al., 2000), and that boosting HCV CTL responses may also improve responses to IFN therapy (Nelson et al., 1998), suggests that therapeutic vaccination may lead to an improved outcome. The finding of a limited distribution of quasispecies in patients who resolved acute infection, and evolution of quasispecies in patients who develop chronic infection (Farci et al., 2000), suggests a role for neutralization escape mutants in viral persistence and the possibility that immunization of acutely infected people may promote quasispecies evolution and the development of chronicity. In this regard, the development of antibodies against HCV envelope and core, as well as CTL against core, following DNA immunization of mice (Saito et al., 1997) represents an important first step in the development and evaluation of genetic vaccine candidates against this virus. The choice of HCV core for immunization stems from the fact that it is one of the most conserved proteins of the virus, and that the nucleocapsid of other viruses has been shown to trigger the generation of protective CTL responses. However, since both cellular and humoral immune responses have been documented for most of the other HCV antigens, the role of these responses, if any, to neutralization or resolution of infection remains an open question.

Given that the clearance of virus and resolution are likely to be dependent upon a strong polyspecific response to virus antigens, and that E1/E2 responses may not be completely neutralizing (Farci et al., 1992a), it is possible that protective and/or therapeutic vaccines will need to include other virus-encoded antigens. However, the inclusion of NS3 and/or core antigen may be problematic, since both of these proteins have been associated with hepatocellular transformation and the development of HCC in various systems (Sakamuro et al., 1995; Ray et al., 1995, 1996b, 1997, 1998a,b; Moriya et al., 1998). If further work shows that these antigens are important to the pathogenesis of chronic infection, or contribute to virus neutralization, it is possible that the appropriate immunodominant epitopes could be incorporated into DNA vaccines that would elicit the relevant immune responses but would not cause tumors. Then, if protective vaccines were not developed, it would be enough to vaccinate acutely infected people to prevent the onset of chronic infection and liver disease. It may be that, in the future, some sort of vaccination program may be used in conjunction with antiviral drugs in the management of HCV (Houghton, 2000).

21. What are the goals and prospects for the future treatment of hepatitis C?

The goal of HCV therapeutics is to bring about a sustained virological response that is accompanied by improved histopathology with a minimum of side effects from treatment. This outcome should reduce the risk for the development of cirrhosis and HCC. Future work should aim to optimize IFN/ribavirin combination therapy. If the experience with HIV therapeutics reveals anything, it is that blood-borne viruses are masters in maintaining chronic infections in the face of often strong, polyspecific immune responses. Since HIV and HCV rapidly mutate, combination therapy against critical proteins in the life cycle of each virus appears to be the best bet of controlling, and possibly eliminating, these viruses.

In the future design of therapeutics for HCV, complementary based therapies will probably be the most successful. The facts that acute, resolving hepatitis is associated with rapid, strong, and polyspecific immune responses and that most chronic infections lack these characteristics suggest that any immunotherapy directed against HCV should aim toward acute exacerbation of CLD, followed by resolution. A potential problem with this approach is that if the therapy targets the majority of the hepatocytes in the liver, this may result in severe hepatitis, liver failure, or worse. Another problem is being able to target all of the virus in chronically infected patients, since chronicity is often associated with increased quasispecies diversity. There has been discussion of targeting epitopes that are well conserved during infection, but it is not clear whether these well-conserved epitopes are those that are immunodominant and are important for the clearance of virus during infection. Hence, one consideration that may be important in the design of future therapeutics is to devise ways to limit quasispecies diversity during infection. One way that may be effective is to treat chronically infected patients with one or more antiviral compounds in order to reduce significantly virus titer within a week or two. This should reduce the virus load in both the serum and liver. Once virus load is reduced, it is anticipated that the appropriate immunotherapy would result in the appearance of rapid, strong, immune responses that have a much greater chance of eliminating the relatively small virus load from the blood and liver without causing more than an acute flare of hepatitis. Importantly, immunotherapy will establish memory responses that will keep the virus in check after the termination of antiviral therapy. Long-term antiviral therapy, especially in the absence of immunotherapy, would be expected to result in the development of drug-resistant virus mutants with variable pathogenic potential. The challenge for both the basic scientist and the clinician today is how to formulate meaningful therapies that highlight the strengths of the immune system as well as attack the weaknesses of the virus.

25

Prospects

The "silent" epidemic of hepatitis C is no longer silent, thanks to the discovery and molecular cloning of the virus, coupled with the development and deployment of assays that specifically detect anti-HCV and HCV RNA in infected patients. These combined approaches have reduced the risk of acquiring HCV from contaminated blood to almost zero. On the clinical level, the challenge is to try to stem the magnitude of the epidemic in the foreseeable future by intensifying community outreach and education programs designed to avoid infection: making the public aware of the remaining major risk factors, including IV drug abuse and the problems of transmission associated with multiple sexual partners. For those already infected, the need for counseling has never been greater, not only for the prevention of transmission but also in making important therapeutic decisions that patients can live with. Fortunately, the use of IFN and ribavirin combination therapy has provided a great deal of hope for chronically infected patients, who otherwise have a very high risk for the development of end-stage liver disease. There is still a long way to go before all patients with chronic HCV infection can be effectively and safely treated. The combination of high throughput screening assays (using individual virus gene products produced by recombinant DNA technology), and the willingness of physicians to introduce some of the best candidates into clinical trials, will invariably lead to an improvement in the therapeutic tools available and the outcome of infection. Still, at the basic science level, this process would be accelerated by the development of a fully permissive tissue culture system that supports HCV replication and of a small animal model that not only replicates the virus but also develops HCV-associated CLD. This is especially true because drugs that are active against one virus gene product need to be evaluated against the whole virus, and because it is of central importance to know whether these putative compounds are effective against both virus and associated liver diseases in a preclinical setting. A successful tissue culture system and small animal model would also provide unprecedented opportunities to understand the replication cycle of HCV, the nature of virus–host cell interactions at the molecular level, the pathogenesis of chronic infection, and the development of HCC. Perhaps one of the biggest challenges to stem the spread of HCV in the future is the development of a safe and effective protective vaccine, and, lacking that, a therapeutic vaccine. The variability in the natural history and pathogenesis of chronic infection, combined with the genetic heterogeneity of HCV, poses difficult challenges in any proposed immunotherapy, since it is not known what combination of immune responses (including their timing and strength) is responsible for virus clearance in the small percentage of acutely infected patients who resolve infection. Given all of these variables, it seems probable that broadly effective treatments against HCV will have to target multiple virus activities and also modulate immune responses, building upon the lessons learned from combination therapies developed for HIV. It is hoped that this book, and others like it, will stimulate the broad-based inter- and multidisciplinary approach that will accelerate both basic research and clinical application. As a result, HCV infection may be reduced to a treatable, curable virus infection within our lifetimes and those of our patients.

References

Aach, R. D., Stevens, C. E., Hollinger, F. B. et al. (1991) Hepatitis C virus infection in post-transfusion hepatitis (analysis with first- and second-generation assays). *New England Journal of Medicine*, **325**, 1325–9.

Abbas, A. K., Murphy, K. M. & Sher, A. (1996) Functional diversity of helper T lymphocytes. *Nature*, **383**, 787–93.

Abdelaal, M., Rowbottom, D., Zawawi, T., Scott, T. & Gilpin, C. (1994) Epidemiology of hepatitis C virus: a study of male blood donors in Saudi Arabia. *Transfusion*, **34**, 135–7.

Abe, K. & Inchauspe, G. (1991) Transmission of hepatitis C by saliva. *Lancet*, **337**, 248.

Abe, K., Inchauspe, G., Shikata, T. & Prince, A. M. (1991) Three different patterns of hepatitis C virus infection in chimpanzees. *Hepatology*, **15**, 690–95.

Abe, K., Kurata, T., Teramoto, Y., Shiga, J. & Shikata, T. (1993) Lack of susceptibility of various primates and woodchucks to hepatitis C virus. *Journal of Medical Primatology*, **22**, 433–4.

Abou-Elella, A., Gramlich, T., Fritsch, C. & Gansler, T. (1996) c-*myc* amplication in hepatocellular carcinoma predicts unfavorable prognosis. *Modern Pathology*, **9**, 95–8.

Abuaf, N., Lunel, F., Giral, P. et al. (1993) Non-organ specific auto-antibodies associated with chronic hepatitis C virus hepatitis. *Journal of Hepatology*, **18**, 359–64.

Agnello, V., Abel, G., Elfahal, M., Knight, G. B. & Zhang, Q. X. (1999) Hepatitis C virus and other Flaviviridae viruses enter cells via low density lipoprotein receptor. *Proceedings of the National Academy of Sciences of the USA*, **96**, 12766–71.

Ago, H., Adachi, T., Yoshida, A. et al. (1999) Crystal structure of the RNA-dependent RNA polymerase of hepatitis C virus. *Structure with Folding and Design*, **7**, 1417–26.

Ahmad, N., Schiff, G. M. & Baroudy, B. M. (1993) Detection of viremia by a one step polymerase chain reaction method in hepatitis C virus infection. *Virus Research*, **30**, 303–15.

Ahmed, M. M., Shaw, J. C., Elias, E. & Mutimer, D. J. (1995) Isolation and culture of biliary epithelial cells (BEC) from explanted hepatitis C virus (HCV) infected liver. *Journal of Hepatology*, **23**, 97A.

Aizaki, H., Saito, A., Kusakawa, I. et al. (1996) Mother-to-child transmission of a hepatitis C virus variant with an insertional mutation in its hypervariable region. *Journal of Hepatology*, **25**, 608–13.

Al, R. H., Xie, Y., Wang, Y., De Staercke, C., van Beers, E. H. & Hagedorn, C. H. (1997) Expression of recombinant hepatitis C virus NS5B. *Nucleic Acids Symposium Series*, **36**, 197–9.

Al, R. H., Xie, Y., Wang, Y. & Hagedorn, C. H. (1998) Expression of recombinant hepatitis C virus NS5B in *Escherichia coli. Virus Research,* **53**, 141–9.

Alberti, A., Morsica, G., Chemello, L. et al. (1992) Hepatitis C viremia and liver disease in symptom-free individuals with anti-HCV. *Lancet,* **340**, 697–8.

Ali, N. & Siddiqui, A. (1995) Interaction of polypyrimidine tract binding protein with the 5' noncoding region of the hepatitis C virus RNA genome and its functional requirement in internal initiation of translation. *Journal of Virology,* **69**, 6367–75.

Ali, N. & Siddiqui, A. (1997) The La antigen binds 5' noncoding region of the hepatitis C virus RNA in the context of the initiator AUG codon and stimulates internal ribosome entry site mediated translation. *Proceedings of the National Academy of Sciences of the USA,* **94**, 2249–54.

Alimzhanov, M. B., Kuprash, D. V., Kosco-Vibois, M. H. et al. (1997) Abnormal development of secondary lymphoid tissues in lymptoxin β-deficient mice. *Proceedings of the National Academy of Sciences of the USA,* **94**, 9302–7.

Allain, J. P. (2000) Genomic screening for blood-borne viruses in transfusion settings. *Clinical and Laboratory Haematology,* **22**, 1–10.

Allander, T., Medin, C., Jacobson, S. H., Grillner, L. & Persson, M. A. (1994) Hepatitis C transmission in a hemodialysis unit: molecular evidence for spread of virus among patients not sharing equipment. *Journal of Medical Virology,* **43**, 415–19.

Alt, M., Renz, R., Hofschneider, P. H. & Caselmann, W. H. (1997) Core specific antisense phosphorothioate oligodeoxynucleotides as potent and specific inhibitors of hepatitis C viral translation. *Archives of Virology,* **142**, 589–99.

Alt, M., Eisenhardt, S., Serwe, M., Renz, R. Engels, J. W. & Caselmann, W. H. (1999) Comparative inhibitory potential of differently modified antisense oligodeoxynucleotides on hepatitis C virus translation. *European Journal of Clinical Investigation,* **29**, 868–76.

Alter, H. J. (1988) Transfusion-associated non-A, non-B hepatitis: the first decade. In *Viral Hepatitis and Liver Disease,* ed. A. J. Zuckerman, pp. 537–42. New York: Alan R Liss.

Alter, H. J. & Bradley, D. W. (1995) Non-A, non-B hepatitis unrelated to the hepatitis C virus. *Seminars in Liver Disease,* **15**, 110–20.

Alter, H. J., Holland, P. V., Purcell, R. H. et al. (1972) Posttransfusion hepatitis after exclusion of commercial and hepatitis B antigen positive donors. *Annals of Internal Medicine,* **77**, 691–9.

Alter, H. J., Holland, P. V., Morrow, A. G., Purcell, R. H. Feinstone, S. M. & Moritsugu, Y. (1975) Clinical and serological analysis of transfusion-associated hepatitis. *Lancet,* **ii**, 838–41.

Alter, H. J., Purcell, R., Holland, P. & Popper, H. (1978) Transmissible agent in non-A, non-B hepatitis. *Lancet,* **i**, 459–63.

Alter, H. J., Purcell, R. H., Holland, P. V., Alling, D. W. & Koziol, D. E. (1981) Donor transaminase and recipient hepatitis: impact on blood transfusion services. *Journal of the American Medical Association,* **246**, 630–4.

Alter, H. J., Purcell, R. H., Shih, J. W. et al. (1989a) Detection of antibody to hepatitis C virus in prospectively followed transfusion recipients with acute and chronic non-A, non-B hepatitis. *New England Journal of Medicine,* **321**, 1495–1500.

Alter, H. J., Jett, B. W., Polito, A. J. et al. (1991) Analysis of the role of hepatitis C virus in transfusion-associated hepatitis. In *Viral Hepatitis and Liver Disease,* eds. R. B. Hollinger, S. M. Lemon & H. S. Margolis, pp. 396–402. Baltimore, MD: Williams & Wilkins.

Alter, H. J., Sanchez-Pescador, R., Urdea, M. S. et al. (1995) Evaluation of branched DNA signal amplification for the detection of hepatitis C virus RNA. *Journal of Viral Hepatitis*, **2**, 121–32.

Alter, M. J. (1990) Epidemiology of community-acquired hepatitis C. In *Viral Hepatitis and Liver Disease*, eds. F. B. Hollinger, S. M. Lemon & H. Margolis, pp. 410–13, Baltimore, MD: Williams & Wilkins.

Alter, M. J. (1993a) Epidemiology of hepatitis C in the West. *Seminars in Liver Disease*, **15**, 5–14.

Alter, M. J. (1993b) The detection, transmission, and outcome of hepatitis C virus infection. *Infectious Agents and Disease*, **2**, 155–66.

Alter, M. J. (1997) Epidemiology of hepatitis C. *Hepatology*, **26**(Suppl.), 62–5.

Alter, M. J., Gerety, R. J., Smallwood, L. A. et al. (1982) Sporadic non-A, non-B hepatitis: frequency and epidemiology in an urban US population. *Journal of Infectious Diseases*, **145**, 886–93.

Alter, M. J., Coleman, P. J., Alexander, W. J. et al. (1989b) Importance of heterosexual activity in the transmission of hepatitis B and non-A, non-B hepatitis. *Journal of the American Medical Association*, **262**, 1201–5.

Alter, M. J., Hadler, S. C., Judson, F. N. et al. (1990) Risk factors for acute non-A, non-B hepatitis in the United States and association with hepatitis C virus infection. *Journal of the American Medical Association*, **264**, 2231–5.

Alter, M. J., Margolis, H. S., Krawczynski, K. et al. (1992) The natural history of community-acquired hepatitis C in the United States. *New England Journal of Medicine*, **327**, 1899–1905.

Andino, R., Rieckhof, G. E. & Baltimore, D. (1990) A functional ribonucleoprotein complex forms around the 5' end of poliovirus RNA. *Cell*, **63**, 369–80.

Andino, R., Rieckhof, G. E., Achacoso, P. L. & Baltimore, D. (1993) Poliovirus RNA synthesis utilizes an RNP complex formed around the 5'-end of the viral RNA. *EMBO Journal*, **12**, 3587–98.

Ando, K., Moriyama, T., Guidotti, L. G. et al. (1993) Mechanism of class I restricted immunopathology: a transgenic mouse model of fulminant hepatitis. *Journal of Experimental Medicine*, **178**, 1541–54.

Antonelli, G., Currenti, M., Turriziani, E. & Dianzani, F. (1992) Relative frequency of nonneutralizing antibodies to interferon (IFN) in hepatitis patients treated with different IFN-α preparations. *Journal of Infectious Diseases*, **165**, 593–4.

Arai, Y., Noda, K., Enomoto, N. et al. (1996) A prospective study of hepatitis C virus infection after needlestick accidents. *Liver*, **16**, 331–4.

Araki, K., Miyazaki, J., Hino, O. et al. (1989) Expression and replication of hepatitis B virus genome in transgenic mice. *Proceedings of the National Academy of Sciences of the USA*, **86**, 207–11.

Arankalle, V. A., Tungatkar, S. P. & Banerjee, K. (1996) Anti-HCV positivity among blood donor population from Puna, India (1981–1994). *Vox Sanguinis*, **69**, 75.

Arbuthnot, P., Bralet, M. P., Thomassin, H., Danan, J. L., Brechot, C. & Ferry, N. (1995) Hepatoma cell specific expression of a retrovirally transferred gene is achieved by a α-fetoprotein but not insulin-like growth factor II regulatory sequences. *Hepatology*, **22**, 1788–96.

Arichi, T., Saito, T., Major, M. E. et al. (2000) Prophylactic DNA vaccine for hepatitis C virus (HCV) infection: HCV specific cytotoxic T lymphocyte induction and protection from HCV recombinant vaccinia infection in an HLA-A2.1 transgenic mouse model. *Proceedings of the National Academy of Sciences of the USA,* **97**, 297–302.

Asabe, S. I., Tanji, Y., Satoh, S., Kaneko, T., Kimura, K. & Shimotohno, K. (1997) The N-terminal region of hepatitis C virus-encoded NS5A is important for NS5A-dependent phosphorylation. *Journal of Virology,* **71**, 790–6.

Ashwell, A. & Morrell, A. G. (1974) The role of surface carbohydrates in the hepatic recognition and transport of circulating glycoproteins. *Advances in Enzymology Related to Areas of Molecular Biology,* **41**, 99–128.

Attwood, M. R., Bennett, J. M., Campbell, A. D. et al. (1999) The design and synthesis of potent inhibitors of hepatitis C virus NS3-4A proteinase. *Antiviral Chemistry and Chemotherapy,* **10**, 259–73.

Autschbach, F., Meuer, S. C., Moebius, U. et al. (1991) Hepatocellular expression of lymphocyte function-associated antigen 3 in chronic hepatitis. *Hepatology,* **14**, 223–30.

Babinet, C., Farza, H., Morello, D., Hadchouel, M. & Pourcel, C. (1985) Specific expression of hepatitis B surface antigen (HBsAg) in transgenic mice. *Science,* **230**, 1160–3.

Baginski, S. G., Pevear, D. C., Seipel, M. et al. (2000) Mechanism of action of a pestivirus antiviral compound. *Proceedings of the National Academy of Sciences of the USA,* **97**, 7981–6.

Balachandran, S., Kim, C. N., Yeh, W. C., Mak, T. W., Bhalla, K. & Barber, G. N. (1998) Activation of the dsRNA-dependent protein kinase, PKR, induces apoptosis through FADD-mediated death signaling. *EMBO Journal,* **17**, 6888–02.

Ballardini, G., Groff, P., Giostra, F. et al. (1995a) Hepatocellular codistribution of c100, c33, c22, and NS5 hepatitis C virus antigens detected by using immunopurified polyclonal spontaneous human antibodies. *Hepatology,* **21**, 730–4.

Ballardini, G., Groff, P., Pontisso, P. et al. (1995b) Hepatitis C virus (HCV) genotype: tissue HCV antigens, hepatocellular expression of HLA-A, B, C and intercellular adhesion-1 molecules. *Journal of Clinical Investigation,* **95**, 2067–75.

Baltimore, D. (1988) Intracellular immunization. *Nature,* **335**, 395–6.

Barba, G., Harper, F., Harada, T. et al. (1997) Hepatitis C virus core protein shows a cytoplasmic localization and associates to cellular lipid storage droplets. *Proceedings of the National Academy of Sciences of the USA,* **94**, 1200–5.

Barnaba, V., Franco, A., Alberti, A., Benvenuto, R. & Balsano, F. (1990) Selective killing of hepatitis B envelope antigen-specific B cells by class I restricted, exogenous antigen specific T lymphocytes. *Nature,* **345**, 258–60.

Barrera, J. M., Bruguera, M., Guadalue-Ercilla, M. et al. (1995a) Persistent hepatitis C viremia after acute self-limiting posttransfusion hepatitis C. *Hepatology,* **21**, 639–44.

Barrera, J. M., Francis, B., Ercilla, G. et al. (1995b) Improved detection of anti-HCV in post-transfusion hepatitis by a third generation ELISA. *Vox Sanguinis,* **68**, 15–18.

Bartenschlager, R., Ahlborn-Laake, L., Mous, J. & Jacobsen, H. (1993) Nonstructural protein 3 of the hepatitis C virus encodes a serine-type proteinase required for cleavage at the NS3/4 and NS4/5 junctions. *Journal of Virology,* **67**, 3835–44.

Bartenschlager, R., Ahlborn-Laake, L., Mous, J. & Jacobsen, H. (1994) Kinetic and structural analyses of hepatitis C virus polyprotein processing. *Journal of Virology,* **68**, 5045–55.

Bartenschlager, P., Ahlborn-Laake, L., Yasargil, K., Mous, J. & Jacobsen, H. (1995a) Substrate determinants for cleavage in *cis* and in *trans* by the hepatitis C virus NS3 proteinase. *Journal of Virology,* **69**, 198–205.

Bartenschlager, R., Lohmann, V., Wilkinson, T. & Koch, J.O. (1995b) Complex formation between the NS3 serine type proteinase of the hepatitis C virus and NS4A and its importance for polyprotein maturation. *Journal of Virology,* **69**, 7519–28.

Baru, M., Axelrod, J.H. & Nur, I. (1995) Liposome-encapsulated DNA-mediated gene transfer and synthesis of human factor IX in mice. *Gene,* **161**, 143–50.

Battegay, M. (1996) Immunity to hepatitis C virus. A further piece of the puzzle. *Hepatology,* **24**, 961–3.

Battegay, M., Fikes, J., Di Bisceglie, A. M. et al. (1995) Patients with chronic hepatitis C have circulating cytotoxic T cells which recognize hepatitis C virus encoded peptides binding to HLA-A2.1 molecules. *Journal of Virology,* **49**, 2462–70.

Baur, M., Hay, U., Novacek, G., Dittrich, C. & Ferenci, P. (1992) Prevalence of antibodies to hepatitis C virus in patients with hepatocellular carcinoma in Austria. *Archives of Virology,* **4**, 76–80.

Bazan, J.F. & Fletterick, R.J. (1989) Detection of a trypsin-like serine protease domain in flaviviruses and pestiviruses. *Virology,* **171**, 637–9.

Beeson, P.B. (1943) Jaundice occurring one to four months after transfusion of blood or plasma: Report of seven cases. *Journal of the American Medical Association,* **121**, 1332–4.

Behrens, J. (2000) Control of beta-catenin signaling in tumor development. *Annals of the New York Academy of Sciences,* **910**, 21–33.

Behrens, S. E., Tomei, L., DeFrancesco, R. (1996) Identification and properties of the RNA-dependent RNA polymerase of hepatitis C virus. *EMBO Journal,* **15**, 12–22.

Bell, H., Hellum, K., Harthug, S. et al. (1997) Genotype, viral load and age as independent predictors of treatment outcome of interferon-alpha 2a treatment in patients with chronic hepatitis C. *Scandinavian Journal of Infectious Diseases,* **29**, 17–22.

Bellobuono, A., Mondazzi, L., Tempini, S., Silini, E., Vicari, F. & Ideo, G. (1997) Ribavirin and interferon alpha combination therapy vs. interferon alpha alone in the retreatment of chronic hepatitis C: a randomized clinical trial. *Journal of Viral Hepatitis,* **4**, 185–91.

Bendelac, A., Lantz, O., Quimby, M. E., Yewdell, J. W., Bennink, J. R. & Brutkiewicz, R. R. (1995) CD1 recognition by mouse NK1+ T lymphocytes. *Science,* **268**, 863–5.

Benvegnu, L. & Alberti, A. (1996) Risk factors and prevention of hepatocellular carcinoma in HCV infection. *Digestive Diseases and Sciences,* **41**(Suppl.), 49–55.

Benvegnu, L., Fattovich, G., Noventa, F. et al. (1994) Concurrent hepatitis B and C infection and risk of hepatocellular carcinoma. *Cancer,* **27**, 2442–8.

Benvegnu, L., Pontisso, P., Cavalletto, D., Noventa, F., Chemello, L. & Alberti, A. (1997) Lack of correlation between hepatitis C virus genotypes and clinical course of hepatitis C virus related cirrhosis. *Hepatology,* **25**, 211–5.

Bertoletti, A. & Maini, M. K. (2000) Protection or damage: a dual role for the virus-specific cytotoxic T lymphocyte response in hepatitis B and C infection. *Current Opinion in Immunology,* **12**, 403–8.

Bertoletti, A., D'Elios, M. M., Boni, C. et al. (1997) Different cyokine profiles of intrahepatic T cells in chronic hepatitis B and hepatitis C virus infections. *Gastroenterology,* **112**, 193–9.

Bertolini, L., Lacovacci, C. & Carloni, G. (1993) The human bone marrow derived B cell line CE, susceptible to hepatitis C virus infection. *Research in Virology*, **144**, 281–5.

Bhattacherjee, V., Prescott, L. E., Pike, I. et al. (1995) Use of NS-4 peptides to identify type-specific antibody to hepatitis C virus genotypes 1, 2, 3, 4, 5 and 6. *Journal of General Virology*, **76**, 1737–48.

Bianchi, E., Steinkuhler, C., Taliani, M., Urbani, A., DeFrancesco, R. & Pessi, A. (1996) Synthetic depsipeptide substrates for the assay of human hepatitis C virus protease. *Analytical Biochemistry*, **237**, 239–44.

Bianchi, L., Desmet, V. J., Popper, H., Scheuer, P. J., Aledort, L. M. & Berk, P. D. (1987) Histologic patterns of liver disease in hemophiliacs, with special reference to morphologic characteristics of non-A, non-B hepatitis. *Seminars in Liver Disease*, **7**, 203–9.

Bjorkander, J., Cunningham-Rudles, C., Lundin, P., Olsson, R., Soderstrom, F. & Hanson, L. A. (1988) Intravenous immunoglobulin prophylaxis causing liver damage in 16 of 77 patients with hypogammaglobulinaemia or IgG subclass deficiency. *American Journal of Medicine*, **84**, 107–11.

Blajchman, M. A., Bull, S. B. & Feinman, S. V. (1995) Post-transfusion hepatitis: impact of non-A, non-B hepatitis surrogate tests. Canadian post-transfusion hepatitis prevention study group. *Lancet*, **345**, 21–5.

Blendis, L., Wong, F. & Sherman, M. (2000) Interferon therapy prevents hepatocellular carcinoma in some patients with chronic HCV: the role of fibrosis. *Gastroenterology*, **118**, 446–8.

Blight, K. & Gowans, E. (1995) *In situ* hybridization and immunohistochemical staining of hepatitis C virus products. *Viral Hepatitis Reviews*, **1**, 143–55.

Blight, K. J., Kolykhalov, A. A. & Rice, C. M. (2000) Efficient initiation of HCV RNA replication in cell culture. *Science*, **290**, 1972–4.

Blight, K., Lesniewski, R. R., LaBrooy, J. T. & Gowans, E. J. (1994) Detection and distribution of hepatitis C specific antigens in naturally infected liver. *Hepatology*, **20**, 553–7.

Blumberg, A., Zehnder, C. & Burckhardt, J. J. (1995) Prevention of hepatitis C infection in haemodialysis units. A prospective study. *Nephrology, Dialysis and Transplantation*, **10**, 230–3.

Blumberg, B. S., Alter, H. J. & Visnich, S. (1965). A 'new' antigen in leukemia sera. *Journal of the American Medical Association*, **191**, 541–6.

Boige, V., Laurent-Puig, P., Fouchet, P. et al. (1997) Concerted nonsyntenic allelic losses in hyperploid hepatocellular carcinoma as determined by a high-resolution alleotype. *Cancer Research*, **57**, 1986–90.

Booth, J. C., Kumar, U., Webster, D., Monjardino, J. & Thomas, H. C. (1998) Comparison of the rate of sequence variation in the hypervariable region of E2/NS1 region of hepatitis C virus in normal and hypogammaglobulinemic patients. *Hepatology*, **27**, 223–7.

Borowski, P., Ochlmann, K., Heiland, M. & Laufs, R. (1997) Nonstructural protein 3 of hepatitis C virus blocks the distribution of free catalytic subunit of cyclic AMP-dependent protein kinase. *Journal of Virology*, **71**, 2838–43.

Bortolotti, F., Giachino, R., Vajro, P. et al. (1995) Recombinant interferon-alfa therapy in children with chronic hepatitis C. *Hepatology*, **22**, 1623–7.

Bosma, G., Custer, R. & Bosma, M. (1983) A severe combined immunodeficiency mutation in the mouse. *Nature,* **301,** 527–30.

Botarelli, P., Brunetto, M. R., Minutello, M. A. et al. (1993) T lymphocyte response to hepatitis C virus in different clinical courses of infection. *Gastroenterology,* **104,** 580–7.

Boudot-Thoraval, F., Pawlotsky, J. M., Thiers, V. et al. (1993) Lack of mother-to-infant transmission of hepatitis C virus in human immunodeficiency virus seronegative woman: a prospective study with hepatitis C virus RNA testing. *Hepatology,* **17,** 772–7.

Bouffard, P., Bartenschlager, R., Ahlborn-Laake, L. et al. (1995) An *in vitro* assay for hepatitis C virus NS3 proteinase. *Virology,* **209,** 52–9.

Bradley, D. W. (2000) Studies of non-A, non-B hepatitis and characterization of the hepatitis C virus in chimpanzees. *Current Topics in Microbiology and Immunology,* **242,** 1–23.

Bradley, D. W., Cook, E. H., Maynard, J. E. et al. (1979) Experimental infection of chimpanzees with antihemophilic (factor VIII) materials: recovery of virus-like particles associated with non-A, non-B hepatitis. *Journal of Medical Virology,* **3,** 253–69.

Bradley, D. W., Maynard, J. E., Cook, E. H. et al. (1980) Non-A/non-B hepatitis in experimentally infected chimpanzees: cross-challenge and electron microscopic studies. *Journal of Medical Virology,* **6,** 185–201.

Bradley, D. W., Maynard, J. E., Popper, H. et al. (1981) Persistent non-A, non-B hepatitis in experimentally infected chimpanzees. *Journal of Infectious Diseases,* **143,** 210–18.

Bradley, D. W., Maynard, J. E., Krawczynski, K. Z. et al. (1982) Non-A, non-B hepatitis in chimpanzees infected with Factor VIII agent: evidence of persistent hepatic disease. In *Viral Hepatitis: 1981 International Symposium,* eds. W. Szmuness, H. J. Alter, & J. E. Maynard, pp. 319–29 New York: Franklin Institute Press.

Bradley, D. W., Maynard, J. E., Popper, H. et al. (1983) Posttransfusion non-A, non-B hepatitis: Physiochemical properties of two distinct agents. *Journal of Infectious Diseases,* **148,** 254–65.

Bradley, D., McCaustland, K., Cook., E. H., Ebert, J. W. & Maynard, J. E. (1984a) Non-A, non-B hepatitis in chimpanzees: effects of immunosuppression on course of disease and recovery of tubule-forming agent from infected liver. In *Viral Hepatitis and Liver Disease,* pp. 451–8. New York: Grune & Stratton.

Bradley, D. W., Schable, C. A., McCaustland, K. A. et al. (1984b) Hepatitis A virus: growth characteristics of *in vivo* and *in vitro* propagated wild and attenuated virus strains. *Journal of Medical Virology,* **14,** 373–86.

Bradley, D. W., McCaustland, K. A., Cook., E. H., Schable, C. A., Ebert, J. W. & Maynard, J. E. (1985) Posttransfusion non-A, non-B hepatitis in chimpanzees: Physiochemical evidence that the tubule forming agent is a small enveloped virus. *Gastroenterology,* **88,** 773–9.

Bradley, D., McCaustland, K., Krawczynski, K., Spelbring, J., Humphrey, C. & Cook, E. H. (1991) Hepatitis C virus: buoyant density of the factor VIII-derived isolate in sucrose. *Journal of Medical Virology,* **34,** 206–8.

Brechot, C. (1994) Hepatitis C virus genetic variability: clinical implications. *American Journal of Gastroenterology,* **89**(Suppl.), 41–7.

Brechot, C., Hadchouel, M., Scotto, J. et al. (1981) State of hepatitis B virus DNA in hepatocytes of patients with hepatitis B surface antigen positive and negative liver disease. *Proceedings of the National Academy of Sciences of the USA,* **78,** 3906–10.

Bressanelli, S., Tomei, L., Roussel, A. et al. (1999) Crystal structure of the RNA-dependent RNA polymerase of hepatitis C virus. *Proceedings of the National Academy of Sciences of the USA*, **96**, 13034–9.

Bresters, D., Mauser-Bunschuten, E. P., Reesink, H. W. et al. (1993) Sexual transmission of hepatitis C virus. *Lancet*, **342**, 210–11.

Bronkhorst, C. M. & ten Kate, F. J. (1998) Liver histology in hepatitis C. *Current Studies in Hematology and Blood Transfusion*, **62**, 119–34.

Brown, E. A., Zhang, H., Ping, L. H. & Lemon, S. M. (1992) Secondary structure of the 5' nontranslated regions of hepatitis C virus and pestivirus genomic RNAs. *Nucleic Acids Research*, **20**, 5041–5.

Brown, J. J., Parashar, B., Moshage, H. et al. (2000) A long-term hepatitis B viremia model generated by transplanting nontumorigenic immortalized human hepatocytes in Rag-2 deficient mice. *Hepatology*, **31**, 173–81.

Brown-Driver, V., Eto, T., Lesnik, E., Anderson, K. P. & Hanecak, R. C. (1999) Inhibition of translation of hepatitis C virus RNA by 2-modified antisense oligonucleotides. *Antisense and Nucleic Acid Drug Development*, **9**, 145–54.

Bruno, S., Silini, E., Crosignani, A. et al. (1997) Hepatitis C virus genotypes and risk of hepatocellular carcinoma in cirrhosis: a prospective study. *Hepatology*, **25**, 754–8.

Bruix, J., Barrera, J. M., Calvet, X. et al. (1989) Prevalence of antibodies to hepatitis C virus in Spanish patients with hepatocellular carcinoma and hepatic cirrhosis. *Lancet*, **ii**, 1004–6.

Buck, K. W. (1996) Comparison of the replication of positive-stranded RNA viruses of plants and animals. *Advances in Virus Research*, **47**, 159–251.

Buendia, M. A. (2000) Genetics of hepatocellular carcinoma. *Seminars in Cancer Biology*, **10**, 185–200.

Bui, L. A., Butterfield, L. H., Kim, J. Y. et al. (1997) *In vivo* therapy of hepatocellular carcinoma with a tumor-specific adenoviral vector expressing interleukin 2. *Human Gene Therapy*, **8**, 2173–82.

Bukh, J., Purcell, R. H. & Miller, R. H. (1992) Sequence analysis of the 5' noncoding region of hepatitis C virus. *Proceedings of the National Academy of Sciences of the USA*, **89**, 4942–6.

Bukh, J., Purcell, R. H. & Miller, R. H. (1993) At least 12 genotypes of hepatitis C virus predicted by sequence analysis of the putative E1 gene of isolates collected worldwide. *Proceedings of the National Academy of Sciences of the USA*, **90**, 8234–8.

Bukh, J., Purcell, R. H. & Miller, R. H. (1994) Sequence analysis of the core gene of 14 hepatitis C virus genotypes. *Proceedings of the National Academy of Sciences of the USA*, **91**, 8239–43.

Bukh, J., Miller, R. H. & Purcell, R. H. (1995) Genetic heterogeneity of hepatitis C virus: quasispecies and genotypes. *Seminars in Liver Disease*, **15**, 41–63.

Bukh, J., Emerson & Purcell, R. H. (1997) Genetic heterogeneity of hepatitis C virus and related viruses. In *Viral Hepatitis and Liver Disease*, eds. M. Rizzetto, R. H. Purcell, J. L. Gerin & G. Verme, pp. 167–75, Torino: Edizioni Minerva Medica.

Buratti, E., Gerotto, M., Pontisso, P., Alberti, A., Tisminetzky, S. G. & Baralle, F. E. (1997) *In vivo* translational efficiency of different hepatitis C virus 5' UTRs. *FEBS Letters*, **411**, 275–80.

Buratti, E., Tisminetzky, S. G., Zotti, M. & Baralle, F. E. (1998) Functional analysis of the interaction between HCV 5' UTR and putative subunits of eucaryotic translation initiation factor IF3. *Nucleic Acids Research*, **26**, 3179–87.

Burk, R. D., DeLoia, J. A., ElAwady, M. K. & Gearhart, J. D. (1988) Tissue preferential expression of the hepatitis B virus (HBV) surface antigen gene in two lines of HBV transgenic mice. *Journal of Virology*, **62**, 649–54.

Burman, P., Karlsson, F. A., Oberg, K. & Alm. G. (1985) Autoimmune thyroid disease in interferon-treated patients. *Lancet*, **ii**, 100–1.

Busch, M. P., Korelitz, J. J., Kleinman, S. H., Lee, S. R., AuBuchon, J. P. & Schreiber, G. B. (1995) Declining value of alanine aminotransferase in screening of blood donors to prevent post-transfusion hepatitis B and C virus infection. The retrovirus epidemiology donor study. *Transfusion*, **35**, 903–10.

Busch, M. P., Wilber, J. C., Johnson, P., Tobler, L. & Evans, C. S. (1992) Impact of specimen handling and storage on detection of hepatitis C virus RNA. *Transfusion*, **32**, 420–5.

Busch, M. P., Tobler, L., Quan, S. et al. (1993) A pattern of 5-1-1 and c100-3 only on hepatitis C virus (HCV) recombinant immunoblot assays does not reflect HCV infection in blood donors. *Transfusion*, **33**, 84–8.

Byrne, J. A. & Oldstone, M. B. A. (1984) Biology of cloned cytotoxic T lymphocytes specific for lymphocytic choriomeningitis virus: clearance of virus *in vivo*. *Journal of Virology*, **51**, 682–6.

Cabot, B., Esteban, J. L., Martell, M. et al. (1997) Structure of replicating hepatitis C virus (HCV) quasispecies in the liver may not be reflected by analysis of circulating HCV virions. *Journal of Virology*, **71**, 1732–4.

Cacciarelli, T. V., Martinez, O. M., Gish, R. G., Villanueva, J. C. & Krams, S. M. (1996) Immunoregulatory cytokines in chronic hepatitis C virus infection: pre- and posttreatment with interferon alpha. *Hepatology*, **24**, 6–9.

Cacoub, P., Fabiani, F. L., Messel, L. et al. (1994) Mixed cryoglobulinemia and hepatitis C virus. *American Journal of Medicine*, **96**, 124–32.

Cai, Z. & Sprent, J. (1996) Influence of antigen dose and costimulation on the primary response of CD8 T cells *in vitro*. *Journal of Experimental Medicine*, **183**, 2247–57.

Camma, C., Almasio, P. & Craxi, A. (1996) Interferon as treatment for acute hepatitis C: a meta-analysis. *Digestive Diseases and Sciences*, **41**, 1248–55.

Canese, M. G., Rizzetto, M., Novara, R., London, W. T. & Purcell, R. H. (1984) Experimental infection of chimpanzees with the HBsAg associated delta virus: an ultrastructural study. *Journal of Medical Virology*, **13**, 63–72.

Cao, G., Kuriyama, S., Du, P. et al. (1997) Complete regression of established murine hepatocellular carcinoma by *in vivo* tumor necrosis factor α gene transfer. *Gastroenterology*, **112**, 501–10.

Carloni, G., Iacovacci, S., Sargiacomo, M. et al. (1993) Susceptibility of human liver cell cultures to hepatitis C virus infection. *Archives of Virology*, **8**, 31–9.

Carman, W. F., Zanetti, A. R., Karayiannis, P. et al. (1990) Vaccine-induced escape mutant of hepatitis B virus. *Lancet*, **336**, 325–9.

Carrick, R. J., Schlauder, G. G., Peterson, D. A. & Mushahwar, I. K. (1992) Examination of the buoyant density of hepatitis C virus by the polymerase chain reaction. *Journal of Virological Methods*, **39**, 279–89.

Carucci, P., Gane, E. J., Riordan, S. et al. (1997) Hepatitis C virus-specific T helper cell responses in recurrent hepatitis C after liver transplanation. *Journal of Hepatology*, **26**, A145.

Caselmann, W. H., Eisenhardt, S. & Alt, M. (1997) Synthetic antisense oligodeoxynucleotides as potential drugs against hepatitis C. *Intervirology*, **40**, 394–9.

Cassani, F., Muratori, L., Manotti, P. et al. (1992) Serum autoantibodies and the diagnosis of type-1 autoimmune hepatitis in Italy: a reappraisal in the light of hepatitis C virus infection. *Gut*, **33**, 1260–3.

CDC (Centers for Disease Control and Prevention) (1998) Recommendations for prevention and control of hepatitis C virus (HCV) infection and HCV-related chronic disease. *Morbidity and Mortality Weekly Reports*, **47** (RR-19), 1–39.

Cerny, A. & Chisari, F. V. (1999) Pathogenesis of chronic hepatitis C: immunological features of hepatic injury and viral persistence. *Hepatology*, **30**, 595–01.

Cerny, A., McHutchinson, J. G., Pasquinelli, C. et al. (1995) Cytotoxic T lymphocyte response to hepatitis C virus-derived peptides containing the HLA A2.1 binding motif. *Journal of Clinical Investigation*, **95**, 521–30.

Chambers, T. J., Hahn, C. S., Galler, R. & Rice, C. M. (1990) Flavivirus genome organization, expression, and replication. *Annual Review of Microbiology*, **44**, 649–88.

Chan, S.-W., McOmish, F., Holmes, E. C. et al. (1992) Analysis of a new hepatitis C virus type and its phylogenetic relationship to existing variants. *Journal of General Virology*, **73**, 1131–41.

Chang, J., Yang, S. H., Cho, Y. G., Hwang, S. B., Hahn, Y. S. & Sung, Y. C. (1998) Hepatitis C virus core from two different genotypes has an oncogenic potential but is not sufficient for transforming primary rat embryo fibroblasts in cooperation with the H-*ras* oncogene. *Journal of Virology*, **72**, 3060–5.

Chang, K. M., Rehermann, B. & Chisari, F. V. (1997a) Immunopathology of hepatitis C. *Springer Seminars in Immunopathology*, **19**, 57–68.

Chang, K. M., Rehermann, B., McHutchison, J. G. et al. (1997b). Immunological significance of cytotoxic T lymphocyte epitope variants in patients chronically infected by the hepatitis C virus. *Journal of Clinical Investigation*, **100**, 2376–85.

Chang, K. M., Gruener, N. H., Southwood, S. et al. (1999) Identification of HLA-A3 and -B7 restricted CTL response to hepatitis C virus in patients with acute and chronic hepatitis C. *Journal of Immunology*, **162**, 1156–64.

Chauveau, P., Courouce, A. M., Naret, C., Poignet, J. L., Ramdame, M. & Delons, S. (1992) Prevalence of antibodies to hepatitis C virus (HCV) by second generation test in hemodialyzed patients. *Journal of the American Society of Nephrology*, **3**, 398.

Chayama, K., Tsubota, A., Arase, Y. et al. (1995) Genotype, slow decrease in virus titer during interferon treatment and high degree of sequence variability of hypervariable region are indicative of poor response to interferon treatment in patients with chronic hepatitis type C. *Journal of Hepatology*, **23**, 648–53.

Chayama, K., Tsubota, A., Kobayashi, M. et al. (1997) Pretreatment virus load and multiple amino acid substitutions in the interferon sensitivity-determining region predict the outcome of interferon treatment in patients with chronic genotype 1b hepatitis C virus infection. *Hepatology*, **25**, 745–9.

Chazouilleres, O., Kim, M., Combs, C. et al. (1994) Quantification of hepatitis C virus RNA in liver transplant recipients. *Gastroenterology*, **106**, 994–9.

Chemello, L., Bonetti, P., Cavalletto, L. et al. and the TriVeneto Viral Hepatitis Group (1995a)

Randomized trial comparing three different regimens of alpha-2a interferon in chronic hepatitis C. *Hepatology,* **22**, 700–6.

Chemello, L., Cavalletto, L., Bernardinello, E., Guido, M., Pontisso, P. & Alberti, A. (1995b) The effect of interferon alfa and ribavirin combination therapy in naive patients with chronic hepatitis C. *Journal of Hepatology,* **23**(Suppl. 1), 8–12.

Chen, C. H., Sheu, J. C., Wang, J. T. et al. (1994) Genotypes of hepatitis C virus in chronic liver disease in Taiwan. *Journal of Medical Virology,* **44**, 234–6.

Chen, C. M., You, L. R., Hwang, L. H. & Lee, Y. H. W. (1997) Direct interaction of hepatitis C virus core protein with the cellular lymphotoxin-β receptor modulates the signal pathway of the lymphotoxin-β receptor. *Journal of Virology,* **71**, 9417–26.

Chen, M., Yun, Z. B., Sallberg, M. et al. (1995) Detection of hepatitis C virus RNA in the cell fraction of saliva before and after oral surgery. *Journal of Medical Virology,* **45**, 223–6.

Chen, M., Sallberg, M., Sonnerborg, A. et al. (1999) Limited humoral immunity in hepatitis C virus infections. *Gastroenterology,* **116**, 135–43.

Chien, D. Y., Xhoo, Q. L., Tabrizi, A. et al. (1992) Diagnosis of hepatitis C virus (HCV) infection using an immunodominant chronic polypeptide to capture circulating antibodies. Revaluation of the role of HCV in liver disease. *Proceedings of the National Academy of Sciences of the USA,* **89**, 10011–15.

Chien, D. Y., Choo, Q. L., Ralston, R. et al. (1993) Persistence of HCV despite antibodies to both putative envelope glycoproteins. *Lancet,* **342**, 933.

Chisari, F. V. (1997) Cytotoxic T cells and viral hepatitis. *Journal of Clinical Investigation,* **99**, 1472–7.

Chisari, F. V., Pinkert, C. A., Milich, D. R. et al. (1985) A transgenic mouse model of the chronic hepatitis B surface antigen carrier state. *Science,* **230**, 1157–60.

Cho, H. S., Ha, N. C., Kang, L. W. et al. (1998) Crystal structure of RNA helicase from genotype 1b hepatitis C virus. A feasible mechanism of unwinding duplex RNA. *Journal of Biological Chemistry,* **273**, 15045–52.

Cho, S. H., Yoon, J. I., Chang, J. E., Ahn, B. M., Lee, C. H. & Lee, Y. I. (1993) Genomic typing of hepatitis C viruses from Korean patients: implications of genome variation in the E2/NS1 region. *Biochemical and Biophysical Research Communications,* **196**, 780–8.

Choo, K. B., Liew, L. N., Chong, K. Y., Lu, R. H. & Cheng, W. T. (1991a) Transgenome transcription and replication in the liver and extrahepatic tissues of a human hepatitis B virus transgenic mouse. *Virology,* **182**, 785–92.

Choo, Q. L., Kuo, G., Weiner, A. J., Overby, L. R., Bradley, D. W. & Houghton, M. (1989) Isolation of a cDNA clone derived from a blood-borne non-A, non-B viral hepatitis genome. *Science,* **244**, 359–62.

Choo, Q. L., Berger, K., Kuo, G. & Houghton, M. (1990) Detection and mapping of immunologic epitopes expressed by bacterial cDNA clones of the hepatitis C virus. In *Viral Hepatitis and Liver Disease,* eds. F. B. Hollinger, S. M. Lemon & H. S. Margolis, pp. 345–6, Philadelphia: PA: Williams & Wilkins.

Choo, Q. L., Richman, K. H., Han, J. H. et al. (1991b) Genetic organization and diversity of the hepatitis C virus. *Proceedings of the National Academy of Sciences of the USA,* **88**, 2451–5.

Choo, Q. L., Kuo, G., Ralston, R. et al. (1994) Vaccination of chimpanzees against infection by the hepatitis C virus. *Proceedings of the National Academy of Sciences of the USA*, **91**, 1294–8.

Choo, S., So, H., Cho, J. M. & Ryu, W. (1995) Association of hepatitis C virus particles with immunoglobulin: a mechanism for persistent infection. *Journal of General Virology*, **76**, 2337–41.

Chouaib, S., Asselin-Paturel, C., Mami-Chouaib, F., Caignard, A. & Blay, J. Y. (1997) The host–tumor immune conflict: from immunosuppression to resistance and destruction. *Immunology Today*, **18**, 493–7.

Chu, M., Mierzwa, R. & Truumees, I. (1996) Structure of sch 68631: a new hepatitis C virus proteinase inhibitor from *Streptomyces* sp. *Tetrahedron Letters*, **37**, 7229–32.

Chu, M., Mierzwa, R., He, L. et al. (1999) Isolation and structure of SCH 351633: a novel hepatitis C virus (HCV) NS3 protease inhibitor from the fungus *Penicillium griseofulvum*. *Bioorganic and Medicinal Chemistry Letters*, **9**, 1949–52.

Chung, K. M., Song, O. K. & Jang, S. K. (1997) Hepatitis C virus nonstructural protein 5A contains potential transcriptional activator domains. *Molecular Cellular Biology*, **7**, 661–7.

Clemens, M. J. & Elia, A. (1997) The double-stranded RNA-dependent protein kinase PKR: structure and function. *Journal of Interferon and Cytokine Research*, **17**, 503–24.

Cocquerel, L., Duvet, S., Meunier, J. C. et al. (1999) The transmembrane domain of hepatitis C virus glycoprotein E1 is a signal for static retention in the endoplasmic reticulum. *Journal of Virology*, **73**, 2641–9.

Collier, A. J., Tang, S. & Elliot, R. M. (1998) Translational efficiencies of the 5′ untranslated region from representatives of the six major genotypes of hepatitis C virus using a novel bicistronic reporter assay system. *Journal of General Virology*, **79**, 2359–66.

Collier, J. & Heathcote, J. (1998) Hepatitis C viral infection in the immunosuppressed patient. *Hepatology*, **27**, 2–6.

Colombo, M., Kuo, G., Choo, Q. L. et al. (1989) Prevalence of antibodies to hepatitis C virus in Italian patient with hepatocellular carcinoma. *Lancet*, **ii**, 1006–8.

Colombo, M. (1992) Hepatocellular carcinoma. *Journal of Hepatology*, **15**, 225–36.

Congia, M., Clemente, M. G., Dessi, C. et al. (1996) HLA class II gene in chronic hepatitis C virus-infection and associated immunological disorders. *Hepatology*, **24**, 1338–41.

Conry-Cantilena, C., Van Raden, M., Gibble, J. et al. (1996) Routes of infection, viremia, and liver disease in blood donors found to have hepatitis C virus infection. *New England Journal of Medicine*, **334**, 1691–6.

Contreras, M., Barbara, J. A. J., Anderson, C. C. et al. (1991) Low incidence of non-A, non-B post-transfusion hepatitis in London confirmed by hepatitis C virus serology. *Lancet*, **337**, 753–7.

Cooper, S., Erickson, A., Adams, E. et al. (1999) Analysis of a successful immune response against hepatitis C virus. *Immunity*, **10**, 439–49.

Corrao, G. & Arico, S. (1998) Independent and combined action of hepatitis C virus infection and alcohol consumption on the risk of symptomatic liver cirrhosis. *Hepatology*, **17**, 914–9.

Craig, J. R., Klatt, E. C. & Yu, M. (1991) Role of cirrhosis and the development of HCC: evidence from histologic studies and large population studies. In *Etiology, Pathology and Treatment of Hepatocellular Carcinoma in North America*, eds. E. Tabor, A. M. Di Bisceglie & R. H. Purcell, pp. 177–90. The Woodlands: Portfolio Publishing.

Cramp, M. E., Carucci, P., Underhill, J., Naoumov, N. V., Williams, R. & Donaldson, P. T. (1998) Association between HL-A class II genotype and spontaneous clearance of hepatitis C viraemia. *Journal of Hepatology*, **29**, 207–13.

Cramp, M. E., Carucci, P., Rossol, S. et al. (1999) Hepatitis C virus (HCV) specific immune responses in anti-HCV positive patients with hepatitis C viraemia. *Gut*, **44**, 424–9.

Craske, J. & Spooner, R. (1978) Evidence for existence of two types of factor VIII-associated non-B transfusion hepatitis. *Lancet*, **ii**, 1051–52.

Cribier, B., Schmitt, C., Bingen, A., Kirn, A. & Keller, F. (1995) *In vitro* infection of peripheral blood mononuclear cells by hepatitis C virus. *Journal of General Virology*, **76**, 2485–91.

Crowe, J., Doyle, C., Fielding, J. F. et al. (1995) Presentation of hepatitis C in a unique uniform cohort 17 years from inoculation. *Gastroenterology*, **108**, 1054A.

Cui, J., Shin, T., Kawano, T. et al. (1997) Requirement for Valpha14 NKT cells in IL-12 mediated rejection of tumors. *Science*, **278**, 1623–6.

Cuypers, H. T. M., Bresters, D., Winkel, I. N. et al. (1992) Storage conditions of blood samples and primer selection affect the yield of cDNA polymerase chain reaction products of hepatitis C virus. *Journal of Clinical Microbiology*, **30**, 3220–24.

Czaja, A. J., Carpenter, H. A., Santrach, P. J. & Moore, S. B. (1995) D-related human leukocyte antigens and disease severity in chronic hepatitis C. *Hepatology*, **22**(Suppl.), 339A.

Dales, S., Eggers, H. J., Tamm, I. & Palade, G. E. (1965) Electron microscopic study of the formation of poliovirus. *Virology*, **26**, 379–89.

Damen, M. & Bresters, D. (1998) Hepatitis C treatment. In *Hepatitis C Virus*, ed. H. W. Reesink, pp. 181–207. Basel: Karger.

Damen, M., Cuypers, H. T. M., Zaaijer, H. L. et al. (1996) International collaborative study on the second EUROHEP HCV-RNA reference panel. *Journal of Virological Methods*, **58**, 175–85.

Damen, M., Sillekens, P., Cuypers, H. T., Frantzen, I. & Melsert, R. (1999) Characterization of the quantitative HCV NASBA assay. *Journal of Virological Methods*, **82**, 45–54.

Darke, P. L., Jacobs, A. R., Waxman, L. & Kuo, L. C. (1999) Inhibition of hepatitis C virus NS2/3 processing by NS4A peptides–implications for control of viral processing. *Journal of Biological Chemistry*, **274**, 34511–14.

Dash, S., Halim, A. B., Tsuji, H., Hiramatsu, N. & Gerber, M. A. (1997) Transfection of HepG2 cells with infectious hepatitis C virus genome. *American Journal of Pathology*, **151**, 363–73.

Davis, A. R. & Kowalik, A. M. (1996) Hepatitis C virus transmission to heterosexual partners: Bedroom or bathroom hazard? *Medical Journal of Australia*, **164**, 126.

Davis, G. L. (1992) Chronic hepatitis. In *Liver and Biliary Diseases*, ed. N. Kaplowitz, pp. 289–299. Baltimore, MD: Williams & Wilkins.

Davis, G. L. (2000) Current therapy for chronic hepatitis C. *Gastroenterology*, **118**(Suppl.), 104–14.

Davis, G. L. & Lau, J. Y. N. (1997) Factors predictive of a beneficial response to therapy of hepatitis C. *Hepatology*, **26**(Suppl.), 122–7.

Davis, G. L., Lau, J. Y. N., Urdea, M. S. et al. (1994) Quantitative detection of hepatitis C virus RNA with a solid-phase amplification method: definition of optimal conditions for specimen collection and clinical application in interferon-treated patients. *Hepatology*, **19**, 1337–41.

Dawson, G. J., Lesneiwski, R. R., Steward, I. L. et al. (1991) Detection of antibodies to hepatitis C virus in US blood donors. *Journal of Clinical Microbiology*, **29**, 551–6.

De Alava, E., Camps, J., Pardo-Mindan, J. et al. (1993) Histological outcome of chronic hepatitis C treated with a 12-month course of lymphoblastoid alfa interferon. *Liver*, **13**, 73–9.

Debure, A., Degos, F., Pol, S. et al. (1988) Liver diseases and hepatic complications in renal transplant patients. *Advances in Nephrology*, **17**, 375–400.

DeFrancesco, R., Urbani, A., Nardi, M. C., Tomei, L., Steinkuhler, C. & Tramontano, A. (1996a) A zinc binding site in viral serine proteinases. *Biochemistry*, **35**, 13282–7.

DeFrancesco, R., Behrens, S. E., Tomei, L., Altamura, S. & Jiricny, J. (1996b) RNA-dependent RNA polymerase of hepatitis C virus. In *Methods in Enzymology: Viral polymerases and related proteins*, eds. L. C. Kuo, D. B. Olsen & S. S. Carroll, pp. 58–67. San Diego, CA: Academic Press.

de Lamballerie, X., Olmer, M., Bouchouareb, D., Zandotti, C. & De Micco, P. (1996) Nosocomial transmission of hepatitis C virus in haemodialysis patients. *Journal of Medical Virology*, **49**, 296–302.

Deleersnyder, V., Pillez, A., Wychowski, C. et al. (1997) Formation of native hepatitis C virus glycoprotein complexes. *Journal of Virology*, **71**, 697–704.

Delwaide, J. & Gerard, C. (2000) Evidence-based medicine treatment of chronic hepatitis C. Liege Study Group on Viral Hepatitis. *Revue Medicale de Liege*, **55**, 337–40.

Deng, R. & Brock, K. V. (1993) 5' and 3' untranslated regions of pestivirus genome: primary and secondary structure analyses. *Nucleic Acids Research*, **21**, 1949–57.

Depraetere, V. & Golstein, P. (1997) Fas and other cell death signaling pathways. *Seminars in Immunology*, **9**, 93–107.

Deriabin, P. G., Isaeva, E. I., Viazov, S. O., Samokhvalov, E. K. & Cossart, Y. E. (1997) Chronic infection of swine embryonal kidney cells PS caused by hepatitis C virus. *Voprosy Virusologii*, **42**, 259–63.

Desmet, V. J., Gerber, M., Hoofnagle, J. H., Manns, M. & Scheuer, P. J. (1994) Classification of chronic hepatitis: diagnosis, grading and staging. *Hepatology*, **19**, 1513–20.

De Staercke, C., Al, R. H., Xie, Y. & Hagedorn, C. H. (1998) Expression of hepatitis C virus NS5B polymerase in *E. coli* and characterization. *Fifth International Meeting on Hepatitis C Virus and Related Viruses: Molecular Virology and Pathogenesis*, Venice, Italy, June 1998.

Dhumeaux, D., Doffoel, M. & Galmiche, J. P. (1997) A French consensus conference on hepatitis C: screening and treatment. *Journal of Hepatology*, **27**, 941–4.

Diamantis, I. D., McGandy, C. E., Chen, T. J., Liaw, Y. F., Gudat, F. & Bianchi, L. (1992) Hepatitis B X gene expression in hepatocellular carcinoma. *Journal of Hepatology*, **15**, 400–3.

Di Bisceglie, A. M. (1995) Hepatitis C and hepatocellular carcinoma. *Seminars in Liver Disease*, **15**, 64–9.

Di Bisceglie, A. M. (1997) Hepatitis C and hepatocellular carcinoma. *Hepatology*, **26**(Suppl.), 34S–8S.

Di Bisceglie, A. M., Martin, P., Kassianides, C. et al. (1989) Recombinant interferon alpha therapy for chronic hepatitis C: a randomized, double-blind, placebo-controlled trial. *New England Journal of Medicine*, **321**, 1506–10.

Di Bisceglie, A. M., Goodman, Z. D., Ishak, K. G., Hoofnagle, J. H., Melpolder, J. J. & Alter, H. J. (1991) Long term clinical and histopathological follow up of chronic posttransfusion hepatitis. *Hepatology*, **14**, 969–74.

Di Bisceglie, A. M., Conjeevaram, H. S., Fried, M. W. et al. (1995) Ribavirin as therapy for chronic hepatitis C: a randomized, double blind, placebo-controlled trial. *Annals of Internal Medicine*, **123**, 897–903.

Dickson, R. C., Mizokami, M., Orito, E., Qian, K. P. & Lau, J. Y. (1999) Quantification of serum HCV core antigen by fluorescent enzyme immunoassay in liver transplant recipients with recurrent hepatitis C: clinical and virologic implications. *Transplantation*, **68**, 1512–16.

Diehl, A. M., Chacon, M. & Wagner, P. (1988) The effect of chronic ethanol feeding on ornithine decarboxylase activity and liver regeneration. *Hepatology*, **8**, 237–42.

Dienes, H., Feinstone, S. & Popper, H. (1980) Non-A, non-B and GB-hepatitis in marmosets. *Gastroenterology*, **79**, 1072.

Dienes, H., Popper, H., Arnold, W. & Lobeck, H. (1982) Histologic observations in human hepatitis non-A, non-B. *Hepatology*, **2**, 552–71.

Dienstag, J. L. (1983) Non-A, non-B hepatitis. I. Recognition, epidemiology and clinical features. *Gastroenterology*, **85**, 439–62.

Diepolder, H. M., Zachoval, R., Hoffmann, R. M. et al. (1995) Possible mechanism involving T lymphocyte response to nonstructural protein 3 in viral clearance in acute hepatitis C virus infection. *Lancet*, **346**, 1006–7.

Diepolder, H. M., Gerlach, J. T., Zachoval, R. et al. (1997) Immunodominant CD4+ T cell epitope within nonstructural protein 3 in acute hepatitis C virus infection. *Journal of Virology*, **71**, 6011–19.

Diepolder, H. M., Hoffmann, R. M., Gerlach, J. T., Zachoval, R., Jung, M. C. & Pape, G. R. (1998) Immunopathogenesis of HCV infection. *Current Studies in Hematology and Blood Transfusion*, **62**, 135–51.

Di Marco, S., Rizzi, M., Volpari, C. et al. (2000) Inhibition of the hepatitis C virus NS3/4A protease. The crystal structures of two protease-inhibitor complexes. *Journal of Biological Chemistry*, **275**, 7152–7.

Dimasi, N., Martin, E., Volpari, C. et al. (1997) Characterization of engineered hepatitis C virus NS3 protease inhibitors affinity selected from human pancreatic secretory trypsin inhibitor and minibody repertoires. *Journal of Virology*, **71**, 7461–9.

Dittmann, S., Roggendorf, M., Durkop, J., Wiese, M., Lorbeer, B. & Deinhardt, F. (1991) Long-term persistence of hepatitis C virus antibodies in a single source outbreak. *Journal of Hepatology*, **13**, 323–7.

Dodd, R. Y. (1992) Hepatitis C virus, antibodies and infectivity: paradox, pragmatism and policy. *American Journal of Clinical Pathology*, **97**, 4–6.

Doherty, P. C., Allan, W. & Eichelberger, M. (1992) Roles of ab and gd T cell subsets in viral immunity. *Annual Review of Immunology*, **10**, 123–51.

Doi, H., Yoon, S., Homma, M. & Hotta, H. (1994) Identification of hepatitis C virus subtype 3b (HCV-3b) among Japanese patients with liver diseases using highly efficient primers for reverse transcription-polymerase chain reaction. *Microbiology and Immunology*, **38**, 159–63.

Domingo, E. & Holland, J. J. (1994) Mutations rates and rapid evolution of RNA viruses. In *Evolutionary Biology of Viruses*, ed. S. S. Morse, pp. 161–84. New York: Raven Press.

Domingo, E., Escarmis, C., Sevilla, N. et al. (1996) Basic concepts in RNA virus evolution.

Federation of American Societies for Experimental Biology Journal, 10, 859–64.

Donahue, F. G., Munoz, A., Ness, P. M. et al. (1992) The declining risk of post-transfusion hepatitis C virus infection. *New England Journal of Medicine,* 327, 369–73.

D'Souza, E. D., Grace, K., Sangar, D. V., Rowlands, D. J. & Clarke, B. E. (1995) *In vitro* cleavage of hepatitis C virus polyprotein substrates by purified recombinant NS3 protease. *Journal of General Virology,* 76, 1729–36.

Dufour, M. C. (1994) Chronic liver disease and cirrhosis. In *Digestive Diseases in the United States: Epidemiology and Impact,* ed. J. E. Everhart US Department of Health and Human Services, Public Health Service, National Institutes of Health, National Institute of Diabetes and Digestive and Kidney Diseases, NIH Publication No. 94–1447, pp. 615–45, Washington, DC: US Government Printing Office.

Dusheiko, G., Weiss, H. S., Brown, D. et al. (1994) Hepatitis C virus genotypes: an investigation of type specific differences in geographic origin and disease. *Hepatology,* 19, 13–18.

Dusheiko, G., Main, J., Thomas, H. et al. (1996) Ribavirin treatment for patients with chronic hepatitis C: results of a placebo-controlled study. *Journal of Hepatology,* 25, 591–8.

Duvet, S., Dubuisson, J., Ermonval, M., Cacan, R. & Verbert, A. (1999) Retention and degradation of *N*-glycoproteins in the rough endoplasmic reticulum. *Bioscience Reports,* 19, 491–8.

Ebeling, F., Naukkarinen, R. & Leikola, J. (1990) Recombinant immunoblot assay for hepatitis C virus antibody as a predictor of infectivity. *Lancet,* 335, 982–3.

Eckart, M. R., Selby, M., Masiarz, F. et al. (1993) The hepatitis C virus encodes a serine protease involved in processing of the putative nonstructural proteins from the viral polyprotein precursor. *Biochemical and Biophysical Research Communications,* 192, 399–406.

Ehrenfeld, E. & Semler, B. L. (1995) Anatomy of the poliovirus internal ribosome entry site. *Current Topics in Microbiology and Immunology,* 203, 65–83.

Ellis, M., Rathaus, M., Amiel, A., Manor, Y., Klein, A. & Lishner, M. (1995) Monoclonal lymphocyte proliferation and *bcl-2* rearrangement in essential mixed cryoglobulinemia. *European Journal of Clinical Investigation,* 25, 833–7.

Encke, J., zu Putlitz, J., Geissler, M. & Wands, J. R. (1998) Genetic immunization generates cellular and humoral immune responses against the nonstructural proteins of the hepatitis C virus in a murine model. *Journal of Immunology,* 161, 4917–23.

Enomoto, N., Takada, A., Nakao, T. & Date, T. (1990) There are two major types of hepatitis C virus in Japan. *Biochemical and Biophysical Research Communications,* 170, 1021–5.

Enomoto, N., Kurosaki, M., Marumo, F. & Sato, C. (1994) Fluctuation of hepatitis C virus quasispecies in persistent infection and interferon treatment revealed by single-strand conformation polymorphism analysis. *Journal of General Virology,* 75, 1361–9.

Enomoto, N., Sakuma, I., Asahina, Y. et al. (1995) Comparison of full-length sequences of interferon-sensitive and resistant hepatitis C virus 1b. *Journal of Clinical Investigation,* 96, 224–30.

Enomoto, N., Sakuma, I., Asahina, Y. et al. (1996) Mutations in the nonstructural protein 5A gene and response to interferon in patients with chronic hepatitis C virus 1b infection. *New England Journal of Medicine,* 334, 77–81.

Erickson, A. L., Houghton, M., Choo, Q. L. et al. (1993) Hepatitis C virus specific CTL responses in the liver of chimpanzees with acute and chronic hepatitis C. *Journal of Immunology*, **151**, 4189–99.

Esteban, J. I., Esteban, R., Viladomiu, L. et al. (1989) Hepatitis C virus antibodies among risk groups in Spain. *Lancet*, **ii**, 294–7.

Esteban, J. I., Lopez-Talavera, J. C., Genesca, J. et al. (1991) High rate of infectivity and liver disease in blood donors with antibodies to hepatitis C virus. *Annals of Internal Medicine*, **115**, 443–9.

Esteban, J. I., Gomez, J., Martell, M. et al. (1996) Transmission of hepatitis C virus by a cardiac surgeon. *New England Journal of Medicine*, **334**, 555–60.

Esteban, J. K., Gonzalez, A., Hernandez, J. M. et al. (1990) Evaluation of antibodies to hepatitis C virus in a study of transfusion-associated hepatitis. *New England Journal of Medicine*, **323**, 1107–12.

Eyster, M. E., Diamondstone, L. S., Lien, J. M., Ehmann, W. C., Quan, S. & Goedert, J. J. (1993) Natural history of hepatitis C virus infection in multi-transfused hemophiliacs: effect of co-infection with human immunodeficiency virus. *Journal of Acquired Immune Deficiency Syndrome and Human Retrovirology*, **6**, 602–10.

Failla, C., Tomei, L. & DeFrancesco, R. (1995) An amino-terminal domain of the hepatitis C virus NS3 proteinase is essential for interaction with NS4A. *Journal of Virology*, **69**, 1769–77.

Fanidi, A., Harrington, E. A. & Evan, G. I. (1992) Cooperative interaction between *c-myc* and *bcl-2* proto-oncogenes. *Nature*, **359**, 554–6.

Farci, P., Alter, H. J., Wang, D. et al. (1991) A long-term study of hepatitis C virus replication in non-A, non-B hepatitis. *New England Journal of Medicine*, **325**, 98–104.

Farci, P., Alter, H. J., Govindarajan, S. et al. (1992a) Lack of protective immunity against reinfection with hepatitis C virus. *Science*, **258**, 135–40.

Farci, P., London, W. T., Wong, D. C. et al. (1992b) The natural history of infection with hepatitis C virus (HCV) in chimpanzees: comparison of serologic responses measured with first- and second-generation assays and relationship to HCV viremia. *Journal of Infectious Diseases*, **165**, 1006–11.

Farci, P., Alter, H. J., Wong, D. C. et al. (1994) Prevention of hepatitis C virus infection in chimpanzees after antibody-mediated *in vitro* neutralization. *Proceedings of the National Academy of Sciences of the USA*, **91**, 7792–6.

Farci, P., Melpolder, J. C., Shimoda, A. et al. (1996a) Studies of HCV quasispecies in patients with acute resolving hepatitis compared to those who progress to chronic hepatitis. *Hepatology*, **24**, 350A.

Farci, P., Shimoda, A., Wong, D. et al. (1996b) Prevention of hepatitis C virus infection in chimpanzees by hyperimmune serum against the hypervariable region of the envelope protein. *Proceedings of the National Academy of Sciences of the USA*, **93**, 15394–99.

Farci, P., Shimoda, A., Colana, A. et al. (2000) The outcome of acute hepatitis C predicted by the evolution of the viral quasispecies. *Science*, **288**, 339–44.

Farza, H., Hadchouel, M., Scotto, J., Tiollais, P., Babinet, C. & Pourcel, C. (1988) Replication and gene expression of hepatitis B virus in a transgenic mouse that contains the complete viral genome. *Journal of Virology*, **62**, 4144–52.

Fattovich, G., Betterle, C., Brollo, L. et al. (1991) Autoantibodies during α-interferon therapy for chronic hepatitis B. *Journal of Medical Virology*, **34**, 132–5.

Fattovich, G., Giustina, G., Degos, F. et al. (1997) Morbidity and mortality in compensated cirrhosis type C: a retrospective follow-up study of 384 patients. *Gastroenterology*, **112**, 463–72.

Favero, M. S. & Alter, M. J. (1996) The reemergence of hepatitis B virus infection in hemodialysis centers. *Seminars in Dialysis*, **9**, 373–4.

Feinstone, S. M., Kapilian, A. Z. & Purcell, R. H. (1973) Hepatitis A: detection by immune electron microscopy of a virus-like antigen associated with acute illness. *Science*, **182**, 1026–8.

Feinstone, S. M., Kapilian, A. Z., Purcell, R. H., Alter, H. J. & Holland, P. V. (1975) Transfusion-associated hepatitis not due to viral hepatitis type A or B. *New England Journal of Medicine*, **292**, 767–70.

Feinstone, S. M., Alter, H. J., Dienes, H. P. et al. (1981) Non-A, non-B hepatitis in chimpanzees and marmosets. *Journal of Infectious Diseases*, **144**, 588–98.

Feinstone, S. M., Mihalik, K. B., Kamimura, T., Alter, H. J., London, W. T. & Purcell, R. H. (1983) Inactivation of hepatitis B virus and non-A, non-B hepatitis by chloroform. *Infection and Immunity*, **41**, 816–21.

Feitelson, M. A. (1996) Hepatocellular injury in hepatitis B and C virus infections. In *Clinics in Laboratory Medicine. Hepatitis and Chronic Liver Disease*, eds. M. A. Feitelson & M. A. Zern, pp. 307–24, Philadelphia, PA: Saunders.

Feitelson, M. A., and Duan, L. X. (1997) Hepatitis B virus X antigen in the pathogenesis of chronic infections and the development of hepatocellular carcinoma. *American Journal of Pathology*, **150**, 1141–57.

Feitelson, M. A., Lega, L., Guo, J. et al. (1994) Pathogenesis of post-transfusion viral hepatitis in children with β-thalassemia. *Hepatology*, **19**, 558–68.

Feitelson, M. A., Duan, L.-X., Guo, J. et al. (1995) X region deletion variants of hepatitis B virus in surface antigen negative and non-A, non-B hepatitis virus infections. *Journal of Infectious Diseases*, **172**, 713–22.

Feray, C., Gigou, M., Samuel, D. et al. (1994) The course of hepatitis C virus infection after liver transplantation: clinical and virological features. *Hepatology*, **20**, 1137–43.

Feray, C., Gigou, M., Samuel, D. et al. (1995) Influence of the genotypes of hepatitis C virus on the severity of recurrent liver disease after liver transplantation. *Gastroenterology*, **108**, 1088–96.

Fernadez, I., Castellano, G., Domingo, M. J. et al. (1997) Influence of viral genotype and the level of viremia on the severity of liver injury and the response to interferon therapy. *Scandinavian Journal of Gastroenterology*, **32**, 70–6.

Ferrari, C., Valli, A., Galati, L. et al. (1994) T cell response to structural and nonstructural hepatitis C virus antigens in persistent and self-limited hepatitis C virus infections. *Hepatology*, **19**, 286–95.

Ferri, C., Monti, M., La Civita, L. et al. (1993) Infection of peripheral blood mononuclear cells by hepatitis C virus in mixed cryoglobulinemia. *Blood*, **82**, 3701–4.

Ferri, C., La Civita, L., Caracciolo, F., Bellesi, G. & Zignego, A. L. (1997a) Hepatitis C virus infection and lymphoproliferative disorders. *Blood*, **88**, 4730.

Ferri, C., La Civita, L., Fazzi, P. et al. (1997b) Interstitial lung fibrosis and rheumatic disorders in patients with hepatitis C virus infection. *British Journal of Rheumatology*, **36**, 360–5.

Filocamo, G., Pacini, L. & Migliaccio, G. (1997) Sindbis viruses dependent on the NS3 protease of hepatitis C virus. *Journal of Virology*, **71**, 1417–27.

Fiore, R. J., Potenza, D., Monno, L. et al. (1995) Detection of HCV RNA in serum and seminal fluid from HIV-1 coinfected intravenous drug addicts. *Journal of Medical Virology*, **46**, 364–7.

Fischler, B., Lindh, G., Lindgren, S. et al. (1996) Vertical transmission of hepatitis C virus infection. *Scandinavian Journal of Infectious Diseases*, **28**, 353–6.

Fong, T. L., Di Bisceglie, A. M., Waggoner, J. G., Banks, S. M. & Hoofnagle, J. H. (1991a) The significance of antibody to hepatitis C virus in patients with chronic hepatitis B. *Hepatology*, **14**, 64–7.

Fong, T. L., Shindo, M., Feinstone, S. M., Hoofnagle, J. H. & Di Bisceglie, A. (1991b) Detection of replicative intermediates of hepatitis C viral RNA in liver and serum of patients with chronic hepatitis C. *Journal of Clinical Investigation*, **88**, 1058–60.

Fong, T. L., Charboneau, F., Valinluck, B. & Govindarajan, S. (1993) The stability of serum hepatitis C viral RNA in various handling and storage conditions. *Archives of Pathology and Laboratory Medicine*, **117**, 150–1.

Fournier, C., Sureau, C., Coste, J. et al. (1998) *In vitro* infection of adult normal human hepatocytes in primary culture by hepatitis C virus. *Journal of General Virology*, **79**, 2367–74.

Francki, R. I. B., Fauquet, C. M., Knudson, D. L. & Brown, F. (1991) Classification and nomenclature of viruses: Fifth Report of the International Committee on Taxonomy of Viruses. *Archives of Virology*, **2**(Suppl.), 223.

Frank, C., Mohamed, M. K., Strickland, G. T. et al. (2000) The role of parenteral antischistosomal therapy in the spread of hepatitis C virus in Egypt. *Lancet*, **355**, 887–91.

Fujita, T., Ishido, S., Muramatsu, S., Itoh, M. & Hotta H. (1996) Suppression of actinomycin D-induced apoptosis by the NS3 protein of hepatitis C virus. *Biochemical and Biophysical Research Communications*, **229**, 825–31.

Fukuda, K., Vishnuvardhan, D., Sekiya, S. et al. (2000) Isolation and characterization of RNA aptamers specific for the hepatitis C virus nonstructural protein 3 protease. *European Journal of Biochemistry*, **267**, 3685–94.

Fukuda, R., Ishimura, N., Nguyen, X. T. et al. (1995) Gene expression of perforin and granzyme A in the liver of chronic hepatitis C: comparison with peripheral blood mononuclear cells. *Microbiology and Immunology*, **39**, 873–7.

Fukuma, T., Enomoto, N., Marumo, F. & Sato, C. (1998) Mutations in the interferon-sensitivity determining region of hepatitis C virus and transcriptional activity of the nonstructural region 5A protein. *Hepatology*, **28**, 1147–53.

Fukumoto, T., Berg, T., Ju, Y. et al. (1996) Viral dynamics of hepatitis C early after orthotopic liver transplantation: evidence for rapid turnover of serum virions. *Hepatology*, **24**, 1351–4.

Fukushi, S., Katayama, K., Kurihara, C. et al. (1994) Complete 5′ noncoding region is necessary for the efficient internal initiation of hepatitis C virus RNA. *Biochemical and Biophysical Research Communications*, **199**, 425–32.

Fukushi, S., Kurihara, C., Ishiyama, N., Hoshino, F. B., Oya, A. & Katayama, K. (1997) The sequence element of the internal ribosome entry site and a 25-kilodalton cellular protein contribute to efficient internal initiation of translation of hepatitis C virus RNA. *Journal of*

Virology, **71**, 1662–6.

Fuller-Pace, F. V. (1994) RNA helicases: modulator of RNA structure. *Trends in Cell Biology*, **4**, 271–4.

Fusconi, M., Lenzi, M., Maraldini, G. & Bianchi, F. (1990) Anti-HCV testing in autoimmune hepatitis and primary biliary cirrhosis. *Lancet*, **336**, 822–3.

Gabrielli, A., Manzin, A., Candela, M. et al. (1994) Active hepatitis C virus infection in bone marrow and peripheral blood mononuclear cells from patients with mixed cryoglobulinemia. *Clinical Experimental Immunology*, **97**, 87–93.

Gale, M. Jr, Korth, M. J., Tang, N. M. et al. (1997) Evidence that hepatitis C virus resistance to interferon is mediated through repression of the PKR protein kinase by the nonstructural 5A protein. *Virology*, **230**, 217–27.

Gale, M. Jr, Blakely, C. M., Kwieciszewski, B. et al. (1998a) Control of PKR protein kinase by hepatitis C virus nonstructural 5A protein: molecular mechanisms of kinase regulation. *Molecular and Cellular Biology*, **18**, 5208–12.

Gale, M. Jr, Korth, M. J. & Katze, M. G. (1998b) Repression of the PKR protein kinase by hepatitis C virus: a potential mechanism for interferon resistance. *Clinical Diagnostic Virology*, **10**, 157–62.

Galun, E., Burakova, T., Ketzinel, M. et al. (1995) Hepatitis C virus viremia in SCID–BNX mouse chimera. *Journal of Infectious Diseases*, **172**, 25–30.

Garcia-Bengoechea, M., Emparanza, H., Sarriugarte, A. et al. (1995) Antibodies to hepatitis C virus: a cross-sectional study in patients attending a trauma unit or admitted to hospital for elective surgery. *European Journal of Gastroenterology and Hepatology*, **7**, 237–41.

Garcia-Monzon, C., Jara, P., Fernandez-Berjemo, M. et al. (1998) Chronic hepatitis C in children: a clinical and immuno-histological comparative study with adult patients. *Hepatology*, **98**, 1696–1701.

Garfein, R. S., Doherty, M. C., Monterroso, E. R., Thomas, D. L., Nelson, K. E. & Vishov, D. (1998) Prevalence and incidence of hepatitis C virus infection among young adult injection drug users. *Journal of Acquired Immune Deficiency Syndrome and Human Retrovirology*, **18**(Suppl. 1), 11–19.

Garoff, H. & Li, K. J. (1998) Recent advances in gene expression using alphavirus vectors. *Current Opinion in Biotechnology*, **9**, 464–9.

Garson, J. A., Ring, C., Tuke, P. & Tedder, R. S. (1990) Enhanced detection by PCR of hepatitis C virus RNA. *Lancet*, **336**, 878–9.

Garson, J. A., Clewley, J. P., Simmonds, P. et al. (1992) Hepatitis C viremia in United Kingdom blood donors. *Vox Sanguinis*, **62**, 218–23.

Gerber, M. A., Shieh, Y. S. C., Shim, K. S. et al. (1992) Detection of replicative hepatitis C virus sequences in hepatocellular carcinoma. *American Journal of Pathology*, **141**, 1271–7.

Gerberding, J. L. (1995) Management of occupational exposures to blood-borne viruses. *New England Journal of Medicine*, **332**, 444–51.

Gerken, G., Teuber, G., Goergen, B. & Meyer zum Buschenfelde, K. H. (1995) Interferon-alpha retreatment in chronic hepatitis C. *Journal of Hepatology*, **22**(Suppl. 1), 118–21.

Gerlach, J. T., Diepolder, H. M., Jung, M. C. et al. (1999) Recurrence of hepatitis C virus after loss of virus specific CD4[+] T cell response in acute hepatitis C. *Gastroenterology*, **117**, 933–41.

Gerotto, M., Sullivan, D. G., Polyak, S. J. et al. (1999) Effect of retreatment with interferon alone or interferon plus ribavirin on hepatitis C virus quasispecies diversification in nonresponder patients with chronic hepatitis C. *Journal of Virology,* **73,** 7241–7.

Ghosh, A. K., Stelle, R., Meyer, K., Fay, R. & Ray, R. B. (1999) Hepatitis C virus NS5A protein modulates cell cycle regulatory genes and promotes cell growth. *Journal of General Virology,* **80,** 1179–83.

Gilli, P., Soffritti, S., de Paoli-Vitali, E. & Bedani, P. L. (1995) Prevention of hepatitis C virus in dialysis units. *Nephron,* **70,** 301–6.

Giuggio, V. M., Bonkovsky, H. L., Smith, J. & Rothman, A. L. (1998) Inefficient recognition of autologous viral sequences by intrahepatic hepatitis C virus specific cytotoxic T lymphocytes in chronically infected subjects. *Virology,* **251,** 132–40.

Glue, P., Rouzier-Panis, R., Raffanel, C. et al. (2000) A dose-ranging study of pegylated interferon alfa-2b and ribavirin in chronic hepatitis C. The Hepatitis C Intervention Therapy Group. *Hepatology,* **32,** 647–53.

Gomez, J., Martell, M., Quer, J., Cabot, B. & Esteban, J. I. (1999) Hepatitis C viral quasispecies. *Journal of Viral Hepatitis,* **6,** 3–16.

Gonzalez-Peralta, R. P., Liu, W. Z., Davis, G. L., Qian, K. P. & Lau, J. Y. (1997) Modulation of hepatitis C virus quasispecies heterogeneity by interferon-alpha and ribavirin therapy. *Journal of Viral Hepatitis,* **4,** 99–106.

Gonzalez-Peralta, R. P., Davis, G. L. & Lau, J. Y. (1994a) Pathogenetic mechanisms of hepatocellular damage in chronic hepatitis C virus infection. *Journal of Hepatology,* **21,** 255–9.

Gonzalez-Peralta, R. P., Fang, J. W., Davis, G. L. et al. (1994b) Optimization for the detection of hepatitis C virus antigens in the liver. *Journal of Hepatology,* **20,** 143–7.

Goodman, Z. D. & Ishak, K. G. (1995) Histopathology of hepatitis C virus infection. *Seminars in Liver Disease,* **15,** 70–81.

Gorbalenya, A. E. & Koonin, E. V. (1993) Helicases: amino acid sequence comparison and structure-function relationship. *Current Opinion in Structural Biology,* **3,** 419–29.

Gorbalenya, A. E. & Snijder, E. J. (1996) Viral cysteine proteinases. *Perspectives in Drug Discovery and Design,* **6,** 64–86.

Gorbalenya, A. E., Donchenko, A. P., Koonin, E. V., Blinov, V. M. (1989) N-terminal domains of putative helicases of flavi- and pestiviruses may be serine proteases. *Nucleic Acids Research,* **17,** 3889–97.

Gordon, S. C., Patel, A. H., Kulesza, G. W., Barnes, R. E. & Silverman, A. L. (1992) Lack of evidence for the heterosexual transmission of hepatitis C. *American Journal of Gastroenterology,* **87,** 1849–51.

Grakoui, A., McCourt, D. W., Wychowski, C., Feinstone, S. M. & Rice, C. M. (1993a) A second hepatitis C virus encoded proteinase. *Proceedings of the National Academy of Sciences of the USA,* **90,** 10583–7.

Grakoui, A., McCourt, D. W., Wychowski, C., Feinstone, S. M. & Rice, C. M. (1993b) Characterization of the hepatitis C virus encoded serine proteinase: determination of proteinase-dependent polyprotein cleavage sites. *Journal of Virology,* **67,** 2832–43.

Greenblatt, M. S., Feitelson, M. A., Zhu, M. et al. (1997) Integrity of p53 in hepatitis B X antigen positive and negative hepatocellular carcinomas. *Cancer Research,* **57,** 426–32.

Gretch, D. R., Bacchi, C. E., Corey, L. et al. (1995a) Persistent hepatitis C virus infection after liver transplantation. *Hepatology*, **22**, 1–9.

Gretch, D. R., de la Rosa, C., Carithers, R. L., Wilson, R. A., Williams, B. & Corey, L. (1995b) Assessment of hepatitis C viremia using molecular amplification technologies: correlations and clinical implications. *Annals of Internal Medicine*, **123**, 321–9.

Gretch, D. R., Polyak, S. J., Willson, R. A. & Carithers, R. L., Jr (1996) Treatment of chronic hepatitis C virus infection: a clinical and virological perspective. *Advances in Experimental Medicine and Biology*, **394**, 207–24.

Grossman, M. & Wilson, J. M. (1993) Retroviruses: delivery vehicle to the liver. *Current Opinion in Genetics and Development*, **3**, 110–14.

Gumperz, J. E., Roy, C., Makowska, A. et al. (2000) Murine CD1d-restricted T cell recognition of cellular lipids. *Immunity*, **12**, 211–21.

Gumucio, J. J. & Berkowitz, C. M. (1992) Structural organization of the liver and function of the hepatic acinus. In *Liver and Biliary Diseases*, ed. N. Kaplowitz, pp. 2–17. Baltimore, MD: Williams & Wilkins.

Gunji, T., Kato, N., Hijikata, M., Hayashi, K., Saitoh, S. & Shimotohno, K. (1994) Specific detection of positive and negative stranded hepatitis C viral RNA using chemical RNA modification. *Archives of Virology*, **134**, 293–302.

Gupta, S. (2000) Hepatic polyploidy and liver growth control. *Seminars in Cancer Biology*, **10**, 161–71.

Gwack, T., Kim, D. W., Hang, J. H. & Choe, J. (1996) Characterization of RNA binding activity and RNA helicase activity of the hepatitis C virus NS3 protein. *Biochemical and Biophysical Research Communications*, **225**, 654–9.

Haber, M. M., West, A. B., Haber, A. D. & Reuben, A. (1995) Relationship of aminotransferases to liver histological status in chronic hepatitis C. *American Journal of Gastroenterology*, **90**, 1250–7.

Haddad, J., Deny, P., Munz-Gotheil, C. et al. (1992) Lymphocytic sialadenitis of Sjögren's syndrome associated with chronic hepatitis C virus liver disease. *Lancet*, **339**, 321–3.

Hadiwandowo, S., Tsuda, F., Okamoto, H. et al. (1994) Hepatitis B virus subtypes and hepatitis C virus genotypes in patients with chronic liver disease or on maintenance hemodialysis in Indonesia. *Journal of Medical Virology*, **43**, 182–6.

Hadziyannis, S. J., Giannoulis, G., Hadiziyannis, E. et al. (1993) Hepatitis C virus infection in Greece and its role in chronic liver disease and hepatocellular carcinoma. *Journal of Hepatology*. **17**, S72–7.

Hagehorn, C. H., van Beers, E. H. & De Staercke, C. (2000) Hepatitis C virus RNA-dependent RNA polymerase (NS5B polymerase). *Curent Topics in Microbiology and Immunology*, **242**, 225–60.

Hagiwara, H., Hayashi, N., Mita, E. et al. (1993) Quantitative analysis of hepatitis C virus RNA in serum during interferon alfa therapy. *Gastroenterology*, **104**, 877–83.

Hahm, B., Back, S. H., Lee, T. G., Wimmer, E. & Jang, S. K. (1996) Generation of a novel poliovirus with a requirement of hepatitis C virus protease NS3 activity. *Virology*, **226**, 318–26.

Hahm, B., Kim, Y, K., Kim, J. H., Kim, T. Y. & Jang, S. K. (1998) Heterogeneous nuclear ribonuclear protein L interacts with the 3' border of the internal ribosomal entry site of hepatitis C virus. *Journal of Virology*, **72**, 8782–8.

Hahm, S., Han, D. S., Back, S. H. et al. (1995) NS3-4A of hepatitis C virus is a chymotrypsin-like protease. *Journal of Virology*, **69**, 2534–9.

Halfon, P., Khiri, H., Gerolami, V. et al. (1996) Impact of virus handling and storage conditions on quantitative detection of hepatitis C virus RNA. *Journal of Hepatology*, **25**, 307–11.

Han, C. J., Lee, H. S., Kim, H. S., Choe, J. H. & Kim, C. Y. (1997) Hepatitis C virus genotypes in Korea and their relationship to clinical outcome in type C chronic liver diseases. *Korean Journal of Internal Medicine*, **12**, 21–7.

Han, D. S., Hahm, B., Rho, H. M. & Jang, S. K. (1995) Identification of the serine proteinase domain in NS3 of the hepatitis C virus. *Journal of General Virology*, **76**, 985–93.

Han, J. H., Shyamala, V., Richman, K. H. et al. (1991) Characterization of the terminal regions of hepatitis C viral RNA: identification of conserved sequences in the 5' untranslated region and poly(A) tails at the 3' end. *Proceedings of the National Academy of Sciences of the USA*, **88**, 1711–5.

Han, W., Hu, Z. L., Jiang, X. J. & Decicco, C. P. (2000) Alpha-ketoamides, alpha-ketoesters and alpha-diketones as HCV NS3 protease inhibitors. *Bioorganic and Medicinal Chemistry Letters*, **10**, 711–13.

Hanecak, R., Brown-Driver, V., Fox, M. C. et al. (1996) Antisense oligonucleotide inhibition of hepatitis C virus expression in transformed hepatocytes. *Journal of Virology*, **70**, 5203–12.

Hanson, J. L., Long, A. M. & Schultz, S. C. (1997) Structure of the RNA-dependent RNA polymerase of poliovirus. *Structure*, **5**, 1109–22.

Hanson, M. R. & Polesky, H. F. (1987) Evaluation of routine anti-HBc screening of volunteer blood donors: a questionable surrogate test for non-A, non-B hepatitis. *Transfusion*, **27**, 107–8.

Hantz, O., Vitvitski, L. & Trepo, C. (1980) Identification of hepatitis B-like virus particles in serum and liver. *Journal of Medical Virology*, **5**, 73–86.

Harada, S., Watanabe, Y., Takeuchi, K. et al. (1991) Expression of processed core protein of hepatitis C virus in mammalian cells. *Journal of Virology*, **65**, 3015–21.

Harrison, A. K., Murphy, F. A. & Gardner, J. J. (1982) Visceral target organs in systemic St Louis encephalitis virus infections in hamsters. *Experimental Molecular Pathology*, **37**, 292–304.

Haruna, Y., Hayashi, N., Kamada, T., Hytiroglou, P., Thung, S. N. & Gerber, M. A. (1994) Expression of hepatitis C virus in hepatocellular carcinoma. *Cancer*, **73**, 2253–8.

Hasan, F., Jeffers, L. J., DeMedina, M. et al. (1990) Hepatitis C-associated hepatocellular carcinoma. *Hepatology*, **12**, 589–91.

Hatzakis, A., Katsoulidou, A., Kaklamani, E. et al. (1996) Hepatitic C virus 1b is the dominant genotype in HCV-related carcinogenesis: a case control study. *International Journal of Cancer*, **68**, 51–3.

Hayashi, J., Kishihara, Y., Yamaji, K. et al. (1997) Hepatitis C viral quasispecies and liver damage in patients with chronic hepatitis C virus infection. *Hepatology*, **25**, 697–701.

Hayashi, J., Aoki, H., Kajino, K., Moriyama, M., Arakawa, Y. & Hino, O. (2000) Hepatitis C virus core protein activates the MAPK/ERK cascade synergistically with tumor promoter TPA, but not with epidermal growth factor or transforming growth factor α. *Hepatology,* **32,** 958–61.

He, L. F., Alling, D., Popkin, T., Shapiro, M., Alter, H. J. & Purcell, R. H. (1987) Determining the size of non-A, non-B hepatitis by filtration. *Journal of Infectious Diseases,* **156,** 636–40.

Healey, C. J., Chapman, R. W. G. & Fleming, K. A. (1995) Liver histology in hepatitis C infection: a comparison between patients with persistently normal or abnormal transaminases. *Gut,* **37,** 274–8.

Heathcote, E. J., Shiffman, M. L., Cooksley, G. E. et al. (2000) Peginterferon alfa-2a in patients with chronic hepatitis C and cirrhosis. *New England Journal of Medicine,* **343,** 1673–80.

Heilek, G. M. & Peterson, M. G. (1997) A point mutation abolishes the helicase but not the nucleoside triphosphatase activity of hepatitis C virus NS3 protein. *Journal of Virology,* **71,** 6264–6.

Heim, M. H., Moradpour, D. & Blum, H. E. (1998) Expression of hepatitis C virus proteins inhibits signal transduction through the Jak-Stat pathway. *Hepatology,* **28,** 321A.

Heintges, T., zu Putlitz, J. & Wands, J. R. (1999) Characterization and binding of intracellular antibody fragments to the hepatitis C virus core protein. *Biochemical and Biophysical Research Communications,* **263,** 410–18.

Heller, A., Windheim, M., Berger, N. & Pfaff, E. (1998) Characterization of constitutive and inducible cell lines expressing hepatitis C virus NS5B. *Fifth International Meeting on Hepatitis C Virus and Related Viruses: Molecular Virology and Pathogenesis.* Venice, Italy, June 1998.

Hellings, J. A., van der Veen-Du Prie, J., Snelting-van Densen, R. & Stute, R. (1985) Preliminary results of transmission experiments of non-A, non-B hepatitis by mononuclear leucocytes from a chronic patient. *Journal of Virological Methods,* **10,** 321–6.

Herion, D. W., Malayaman, N., Hoofnagle, J. H. & Liang, T. J. (1998) Interaction of hepatitis C virus (HCV) NS5A with a cellular signaling protein involved in receptor tyrosine kinase mitogenic pathway. *Fifth International Meeting on Hepatitis C Virus and Related Viruses,* Venice, Italy, June, 1998.

Hetland, G., Skaug, K., Larsen, J., Maland, A., Stromme, J. H. & Storvold, G. (1990) Prevalence of anti-HCV in Norwegian blood donors with anti-HBc or increased ALT levels. *Transfusion,* **30,** 776–9.

Higashi, Y., Kakumu, S., Yoshioka, K. et al. (1993) Dynamics of genome change in the E2/NS1 region of hepatitis C virus *in vivo. Virology,* **197,** 659–68.

Higashitsuji, H., Itoh, K., Nagao, T. et al. (2000) Reduced stability of retinoblastoma protein by gankyrin, an oncogenic ankyrin-repeat protein overexpressed in hepatomas. *Nature Medicine,* **6,** 96–9.

Hijikata, M., Kato, N., Ootsuyama, Y., Nakagawa, M. & Shimotohno, K. (1991) Gene mapping of the putative structural region of the hepatitis C virus genome by *in vitro* processing analysis. *Proceedings of the National Academy of Sciences of the USA,* **88,** 5547–51.

Hijikata, M., Mizushima, H., Akagi, T. et al. (1993a) Two distinct proteinase activities required for the processing of a putative nonstructural precursor protein of hepatitis C virus. *Journal of Virology,* **67,** 4665–75.

Hijikata, M., Mizushima, H., Tanji, HY. et al. (1993b) Proteolytic processing and membrane association of putative nonstructural proteins of hepatitis C virus. *Proceedings of the National Academy of Sciences of the USA*, **90**, 10773–7.

Hijikata, M., Shimizu, Y. K., Kato, H. et al. (1993c) Equilibrium centrifugation studies of hepatitis C virus: evidence for circulating immune complexes. *Journal of Virology*, **67**, 1953–8.

Hiramatsu, N., Hayashi, N., Haruna, Y. et al. (1992) Immunohistochemical detection of hepatitis C virus-infected hepatocytes in chronic liver disease with monoclonal antibodies to core, envelope, and NS3 regions of the hepatitis C virus. *Hepatology*, **16**, 306–11.

Hiramatsu, N., Hayashi, N., Katayama, K. et al. (1994) Immunohistochemical detection of Fas antigen in liver tissue of patients with chronic hepatitis C. *Hepatology*, **19**, 1354–9.

Hiramatsu, N., Hayashi, N., Kasahara, A. et al. (1995) Improvement of liver fibrosis in chronic hepatitis C patients treated with natural interferon alpha. *Journal of Hepatology*, **22**, 135–42.

Hiramatsu, N., Dash, S. & Gerber, M. A. (1997) HCV cDNA transfection to HepG2 cells. *Journal of Viral Hepatitis*, **4**(Suppl. 1), 61–7.

Hiranuma, K., Tamaki, S., Nishimura, Y. et al. (1999) Helper T cell determinant peptide contributes to induction of cellular immune responses by peptide vaccines against hepatitis C virus. *Journal of General Virology*, **80**, 187–93.

Hirohashi, S. (1998) Inactivation of the E-cadherin mediated cell adhesion system in human cancers. *American Journal of Pathology*, **153**, 333–9.

Hirowatari, Y., Hijikata, M., Tanji, Y. et al. (1993) Two proteinase activities in HCV polypeptide expressed in insect cells using baculovirus vector. *Archives of Virology*, **133**, 349–56.

Hirowatari, Y., Hijikata, M. & Shimotohno, K. (1995) A novel method for analysis of viral proteinase activity encoded by hepatitis C virus in cultured cells. *Analytical Biochemistry*, **225**, 113–20.

Hodgson, P. D., Grant, M. D. & Michalak, T. I. (1999) Perforin and Fas/Fas ligand-mediated cytotoxicity in acute and chronic woodchuck viral hepatitis. *Clinical and Experimental Immunology*, **118**, 63–70.

Hodinka, R. L. (1998) The clinical utility of viral quantitation using molecular methods. *Clinical and Diagnostic Virology*, **10**, 25–47.

Hofgartner, W. T., Polyak, S. J., Sullivan, D., Carithers, R. L., Jr & Gretch, D. R. (1997) Mutations in the NS5A gene of hepatitis C virus in North American patients infected with HCV genotype 1a or 1b. *Journal of Medical Virology*, **53**, 118–26.

Hohne, M., Schaefer, S., Seifer, M., Feitelson, M. A., Paul, D. & Gerlich, W. H. (1990) Malignant transformation of immortalized transgenic hepatocytes after transfection with hepatitis B virus DNA. *EMBO Journal*, **9**, 1137–45.

Holland, J. J., de la Torre, J. C. & Steinhauer, D. A. (1992) RNA virus populations as quasi-species. *Current Topics in Microbiology and Immunology*, **176**, 1–20.

Holland, P. M., Abramson, R. D., Watson, R. & Gelfand, D. H. (1991) Detection of specific polymerase chain reaction product by utilizing the 5'–3' exonuclease activity of *Thermus aquaticus*. *Proceedings of the National Academy of Sciences of the USA*, **88**, 7276–80.

Hollinger, F. B., Gitnick, G., Aach, R. D. et al. (1978) Non-A, non-B hepatitis transmission in chimpanzees: a project of the transfusion-transmitted viruses study group. *Intervirology*, **10**, 60–8.

Honda, A., Arai, Y., Hirota, N. et al. (1999a) Hepatitis C virus structural proteins induce liver cell injury in transgenic mice. *Journal of Medical Virology*, **59**, 281–9.

Honda, M., Kaneko, S., Sakai, A., Unoura, M., Murakami, S. & Kobayashi, K. (1994) Degree of diversity of hepatitis C quasispecies and progression of liver disease. *Hepatology*, **20**, 1144–51.

Honda, M., Brown, E. A. & Lemon, S. M. (1996a) Stability of a stem–loop involving the initiator AUG controls the efficiency of internal initiation of translation on hepatitis C virus RNA. *RNA*, **2**, 955–68.

Honda, M., Rijnbrand, R., Abell, G., Kim, D. & Lemon, S. M. (1999b) Natural variation in translation activities of the 5' nontranslated RNAs of genotypes 1a and 1b hepatitis C virus: evidence for a long range RNA-RNA interaction outside of the internal ribosomal entry site. *Journal of Virology*, **73**, 4941–51.

Honda, M., Ping, L. H., Rijnbrand, R. C. A. et al. (1996b) Structural requirements for initiation of translation by internal ribosome entry within genome-length hepatitis C virus RNA. *Virology*, **222**, 31–42.

Hong, Z., Ferrari, E., Wright-Minogue, J. et al. (1996) Enzymatic characterization of hepatitis C virus NS3/4A complexes expressed in mammalian cells by using the herpes simplex virus amplicon system. *Journal of Virology*, **70**, 4261–8.

Hong, Z., Beaudet-Miller, M., Lanford, R. E. et al. (1999) Generation of transmissible hepatitis C virions from a molecular clone in chimpanzees. *Virology*, **256**, 36–44.

Hoofnagle, J. H. (1991) Thrombocytopenia during interferon-alpha therapy. *Journal of the American Medical Association*, **266**, 849.

Hoofnagle, J. H. (1997) Hepatitis C: the clinical spectrum of disease. *Hepatology*, **26**(Suppl. 1), 15–20.

Hoofnagle, J. H., Gerety, R. J., Ni, L. Y. & Barker, L. F. (1973) Antibody to hepatitis B virus core in man. *Lancet*, **ii**, 869–73.

Hoofnagle, J. H., Seeff, L. B., Bales, Z. B. & Zimmerman, H. J. (1978) Type B hepatitis after transfusion with blood containing antibody to hepatitis B core antigen. *New England Journal of Medicine*, **298**, 1379–83.

Hoofnagle, J. H., Mullen, K. D., Jones, D. B. et al. (1986) Treatment of chronic non-A, non-B hepatitis with recombinant human alpha interferon: a preliminary report. *New England Journal of Medicine*, **315**, 1575–8.

Hoofnagle, J. H., Shafritz, D. A. & Popper, H. (1987) Chronic type B hepatitis and the "healthy" HBsAg carrier state. *Hepatology*, **7**, 758–63.

Hopf, U., Moller, B., Kuther, D. et al. (1990) Long-term follow-up of posttransfusion and sporadic chronic hepatitis non-A, non-B and frequency of circulating antibodies to hepatitis C virus (HCV). *Journal of Hepatology*, **10**, 69–76.

Hopf, U., Berg, T., Konig, V., Kuther, S., Heuft, H. G. & Lobeck, H. (1996) Treatment of chronic hepatitis C with interferon alpha: long term follow-up and prognostic relevance of HCV genotypes. *Journal of Hepatology*, **24**(Suppl. 2), 67–73.

Horiike, N., Nonaka, T., Kumamoto, J., Kajino, K., Onji, M. & Ohta, Y. (1993) Hepatitis C virus plus and minus strand RNA in hepatocellular carcinoma and adjoining nontumourous liver. *Journal of Medical Virology*, **41**, 312–15.

Hotta, H., Doi, H., Hayashi, T. et al. (1994) Analysis of the core and E1 envelope region sequences of a novel variant of hepatitis C virus obtained in Indonesia. *Archives of Virology*, **136**, 53–62.

Houghton, M. C. (1996) Hepatitis C viruses. In *Fields Virology* 3rd edn, eds. B. N. Fields, D. M. Knipe & P. M. Howley, pp. 1035–58, Philadelphia, PA: Lippincott-Raven.

Houghton, M. C. (2000) Strategies and propects for vaccination against the hepatitis C virus. *Current Topics in Microbiology and Immunology*, **242**, 327–39.

Houghton, M., Weiner, A., Han, J., Kuo, G. & Choo, Q. L. (1991) Molecular biology of the hepatitis C viruses: implications for diagnosis, development and control of viral disease. *Hepatology*, **14**, 381–8.

Howard, C. R., Gray, L., D'Mello, F., Christopher, J. & Craske, J. (1998) Nucleic acid vaccines for hepatitis viruses. *Developments in Biological Standardization*, **92**, 157–62.

Hoyos, M., Sarion, J. V., Perex-Castellanos Prieto, M., Marty, M. L., Garrigues, V. & Berenguer, J. (1989) Prospective assessment of donor blood screening for antibody to hepatitis B core antigen as a means of preventing posttransfusion non-A, non-B hepatitis. *Hepatology*, **9**, 449–51.

Hruby, M. A. & Schauf, V. (1978) Transfusion-related short-incubation hepatitis in hemophilic patients. *Journal of the American Medical Association*, **240**, 1355–7.

Hsieh, T. Y., Matsumoto, M., Chou, H. C. et al. (1998) Hepatitis C virus core protein interacts with heterogeneous nuclear ribonuclearprotein K. *Journal of Biological Chemistry*, **273**, 17651–9.

Hsu, C. C., Hwant, L. H., Huang, Y. W., Chi, W. K., Chu, Y. D. & Chen, D. S. (1998) An ELISA for RNA helicase activity application as an assay of the NS3 helicase of hepatitis C virus. *Biochemical and Biophysical Research Communications*, **253**, 594–9.

Hsu, H. C., Jeng, Y. M., Mao, T. L., Chu, J. S., Lai, P. L. & Peng, S. Y. (2000) Beta-catenin mutations are associated with a subset of low-stage hepatocellular carcinoma negative for hepatitis B virus and with favorable prognosis. *American Journal of Pathology*, **157**, 763–70.

Hu, G. J., Wang, R. Y., Han, D. S., Alter, H. J. & Shih, J. W. (1999) Characterization of the humoral and cellular immune responses against hepatitis C virus core induced by DNA based immunization. *Vaccine*, **17**, 3160–70.

Huang, H., Fujii, H., Sankila, A. et al. (1999) β-Catenin mutations are frequent in human hepatocellular carcinomas associated with hepatitis C virus infection. *American Journal of Pathology*, **155**, 1795–1801.

Hussy, P., Langen H., Mous, J. & Jacobsen, H. (1996) Hepatitis C virus core protein: carboxy-terminal boundaries of two processed species suggest cleavage by a signal peptide peptidase. *Virology*, **224**, 93–104.

Hwang, S. B., Lo, S. Y., Ou, J. H. & Lai, M. M. C. (1995) Detection of cellular proteins and viral core protein interacting with the 5' untranslated region of hepatitis C virus RNA. *Journal of Biomedical Science*, **2**, 227–36.

Hwang, S. B., Park, K. J., Kim, Y. S., Sung, Y. C. & Lai, M. M. (1997) Hepatitis C virus NS5B protein is a membrane-associated phosphoprotein with a predominantly perinuclear localization. *Virology*, **227**, 439–46.

Iacovacci, S., Sargiacomo, M., Parolini, I., Ponzetto, A., Peschle, C. & Carloni, G. (1993)

Replication and multiplication of hepatitis C virus genome in human fetal liver cells. *Research in Virology*, **144**, 275–9.

Ichimura, H., Tamura, I., Kurimura, O. et al. (1994) Hepatitis C virus genotypes, reactivity to recombinant immunoblot assay 2 antigens and liver disease. *Journal of Medical Virology*, **43**, 212–5.

Ide, Y., Zhang, L., Chen, M. et al. (1996) Characterization of the nuclear localization signal and subcellular distribution of hepatitis C virus nonstructural protein NS5A. *Gene*, **182**, 203–11.

Ide, Y., Tanimoto, A., Sasaguri, Y. & Padmanabhan, R. (1997) Hepatitis C virus NS5A protein is phosphorylated *in vitro* by a stably bound protein kinase from HeLa cells and by cAMP-dependent protein kinase A-α catalytic subunit. *Gene*, **201**, 151–8.

Iio, S., Hayashi, N., Mita, E. et al. (1998) Serum levels of soluble Fas antigen in chronic hepatitis C patients. *Journal of Hepatology*, **29**, 517–23.

Iizuka, N., Najita, L., Franzusoff, A. & Sarnow, P. (1994) Cap dependent and cap independent translation by internal initiation of mRNA in cell extracts prepared from *Saccharomyces cervise*. *Molecular and Cellular Biology*, **14**, 7322–30.

Ikeda, K., Saitoh, S., Koida, I. et al. (1993) A multivariate analysis of risk factors for hepatocellular carcinogenesis: a prospective observation in 795 patients with viral and alcoholic cirrhosis. *Hepatology*, **18**, 47–53.

Ikeda, K., Saitoh, S., Arase, Y. et al. (1999) Effect of interferon therapy on hepatocellular carcinogenesis in patients with chronic hepatitis type C: a long-term observation study of 1643 patients using statistical bias correction with proportional hazard analysis. *Hepatology*, **29**, 1124–30.

Ikeda, M., Sugiyama, K., Mizutani, T. et al. (1998) Human hepatocyte clonal cell lines that support persistent replication of hepatitis C virus. *Virus Research*, **56**, 157–67.

Ilan, E., Burakova, T., Dagan, S. et al. (1999) The hepatitis B virus–*Trimera* mouse: a model for human HBV infection and evaluation of anti-HBV therapeutic agents. *Hepatology*, **29**, 553–62.

Inchauspe, G. (1997) Gene vaccination for hepatitis C. *Springer Seminars in Immunopathology*, **19**, 211–21.

Inchauspe, G., Vitvitski, L., Major, M. E. et al. (1997a) Plasmid DNA expressing a secreted or a nonsecreted form of hepatitis C virus nucleocapsid: comparative studies of antibody and T-helper responses following gene immunization. *DNA and Cell Biology*, **16**, 185–95.

Inchauspe, G., Major, M. E., Nakano, I., Vitvitski, L. & Trepo, C. (1997b) DNA vaccination for the induction of immune responses against hepatitis C virus proteins. *Vaccine*, **15**, 853–6.

Ingallinella, P., Altamura, S., Bianchi, E. et al. (1998) Potent peptide inhibitors of human hepatitis C virus NS3 protease are obtained by optimizing the cleavage products. *Biochemistry*, **37**, 8906–14.

Inokuchi, K., Nakata, K., Hamasaki, K. et al. (1996) Prevalence of hepatitis B or C virus infection in patients with fulminant viral hepatitis. An analysis using polymerase chain reaction. *Journal of Hepatology*, **24**, 258–64.

Inoue,Y., Miyazaki, M., Ohashi, R. et al. (1998) Ubiquitous presence of cellular proteins that specifically bind to the 3' terminal region of hepatitis C virus. *Biochemical and Biophysical Research Communications*, **245**, 198–203.

Iorio, R., Pensati, P., Porzio, S., Fariello, L., Guida, S. & Vegnente, A. (1996) Lymphoblastoid interferon alfa treatment in chronic hepatitis C. *Archives of Diseases of Children,* **74,** 152–6.

Irving, W. L., Day, S. & Johnston, I. D. (1993) Idiopathic pulmonary fibrosis and hepatitis C virus infection. *American Review of Respiratory Diseases,* **148,** 1683–4.

Ishido, S. & Hotta H. (1998) Complex formation of the nonstructural protein 3 of hepatitis C virus with the p53 tumor suppressor. *FEBS Letters,* **438,** 258–62.

Ishido, S., Fujita, T. & Hotta, H. (1998) Complex formation of NS5B with NS3 and NS4A proteins of hepatitis C virus. *Biochemical and Biophysical Research Communications,* **244,** 35–40.

Ishii, K., Rosa, D., Watanabe, Y. et al. (1998) High titers of antibodies inhibiting the binding of envelope to human cells correlate with natural resolution of chronic hepatitis C. *Hepatology,* **28,** 1117–20.

Ito, T., Tahara, S. M. & Lai, M. M. C. (1998) The 3' untranslated region of hepatitis C virus RNA enhances translation from an internal ribosomal entry site. *Journal of Virology,* **72,** 8789–96.

Ito, J., Mukaigawa, J., Zuo, J., Hirabayashi, Y., Mitamura, K. & Yasui, K. (1996) Cultivation of hepatitis C virus in primary hepatocyte culture from patients with chronic hepatitis C results in release of high titre infectious virus. *Journal of General Virology,* **77,** 1043–54.

Itoh, Y., Iwakiri, S., Kitayima, K. et al. (1986) Lack of detectable reverse transcriptase activity in human and chimpanzee sera with a high infectivity for non-A, non-B hepatitis. *Journal of General Virology,* **67,** 777–9.

Iwarson, S., Schaff, Z., Seto, B., Norkrans, G. & Gerety, R. J. (1985) Retrovirus-like particles in hepatocytes of patients with transfusion-acquired non-A, non-B hepatitis. *Journal of Medical Virology,* **16,** 37–45.

Jacob, J. R., Burk, K. H., Eichberg, J. W., Dreesman, G. R. & Lanford, R. E. (1990) Expression of infectious viral particles by primary chimpanzee hepatocytes isolated during the acute phase of non-A, non-B hepatitis. *Journal of Infectious Diseases,* **161,** 1121–7.

Jaeger, U., Karth, G. D., Knapp, S., Friedl, J., Laczika, K. & Kusec, R. (1994) Molecular mechanism of the t(14:18)–a model for lymphoid-specific chromosomal translocations. *Leukemia and Lymphoma,* **14,** 197–202.

Jang, S. K., Krausslich, M. J. H., Nicklin, G. M., Duke, A. C., Palmenberg, A. C. & Wimmer, E. (1988) A segment of the 5' nontranslated region of encephalomyocarditis virus RNA directs internal entry of ribosomes during *in vitro* translation. *Journal of Virology,* **62,** 2636–43.

Janot, C., Courouce, A. M. & Maniez, M. (1989) Antibodies to hepatitis C virus in French blood donors. *Lancet,* **ii,** 796–7.

Jarvis, B. & Faulds, D. (1999) Lamivudine. A review of its therapeutic potential in chronic hepatitis B. *Drugs,* **58,** 101–41.

Jeng, J.-E. & Tsai, J. F. (1991) Hepatitis C virus antibody in hepatocellular carcinoma in Taiwan. *Journal of Medical Virology,* **34,** 74–7.

Jiang, W. & Bond, J. S. (1992) Families of metalloendopeptidases and their relationships. *FEBS Letters,* **312,** 110–14.

Jin, D. Y., Wang, H. L., Zhou, Y. et al. (2000) Hepatitis C virus core protein-induced loss of LZIP function correlates with cellular transformation. *EMBO Journal,* **19,** 729–40.

Jin, L. & Peterson, D. L. (1995) Expression, isolation and characterization of the hepatitis C virus ATPase/RNA helicase. *Archives of Biochemistry and Biophysics*, **323**, 47–53.

Jin, Y., Fuller, L., Carreno, M. et al. (1997) The immune reactivity role of HCV induced liver infiltrating lymphocytes in hepatocellular damage. *Journal of Clinical Immunology*, **17**, 140–53.

Jungkind, D. L., DiRenzo, S., Beavis, K. G. & Silverman, N. S. (1996) Evaluation of an automated COBAS AMPLICOR™ PCR system for detection of several infectious agents and the impact on laboratory management. *Journal of Clinical Microbiology*, **34**, 2778–83.

Kabiri, M., Tabor, E. & Gerety, R. J. (1979) Antigen-antibody system associated with non-A, non-B hepatitis detected by indirect immunofluorescence. *Lancet*, **ii**, 221–4.

Kafri, T., Blomer, U., Peterson, D. A., Gage, F. H. & Verma, I. (1997) Sustained expression of genes delivered directly into liver and muscle by lentiviral vectors. *Nature Genetics*, **17**, 314–17.

Kahn, N. C. & Hollinger, F. B. (1986) Non-A, non-B hepatitis agent. *Lancet*, **i**, 41.

Kaito, M., Watanabe, S., Tsukiyama-Kohara, K. et al. (1994) Hepatitis C virus particle detected by immunoelectron microscopic study. *Journal of General Virology*, **75**, 1755–60.

Kakimi, K., Guidotti, L. G., Koezuka, Y., and Chisari, F. V. (2000) Natural killer T cell activation inhibits hepatitis B virus replication *in vivo*. *Journal of Experimental Medicine*, **192**, 921–30.

Kakiuchi, N., Hijikata, M., Komoda, Y., Tanji, Y., Hirowatari, Y. & Shimotohno, K. (1995) Bacterial expression and analysis of cleavage activity of HCV serine proteinase using recombinant and synthetic substrate. *Biochemical and Biophysical Research Communications*, **210**, 1059–65.

Kaldor, J. M., Archer, G. T., Buring, M. L. et al. (1992) Risk factors for hepatitis C virus infection in blood donors: a case-control study. *Medical Journal of Australia*, **157**, 227–30.

Kamei, A., Tamaki, S., Taniyama, H. et al. (2000) Induction of hepatitis C virus-specific cytotoxic T lymphocytes in mice by an intrahepatic inoculation with an expression plasmid. *Virology*, **273**, 120–6.

Kamer, G. & Argos, P. (1984) Primary structural comparison of RNA-dependent polymerases from plant, animal and bacterial viruses. *Nucleic Acids Research*, **12**, 7269–82.

Kamoshita, N., Tsukiyama-Kohara, K., Kohara, M. & Nomoto, A. (1997) Genetic analysis of internal ribosomal entry site on hepatitis C virus RNA: implication for involvement of the high ordered structure and cell type specific transacting factors. *Virology*, **233**, 9–18.

Kanai, K., Kako, M. & Okamoto, H. (1992) HCV genotypes in chronic hepatitis C and response to interferon. *Lancet*, **339**, 1543.

Kanai, Y., Ushijima, S., Hui, A. M. et al. (1997) The E-cadherin gene is silenced by CpG methylation in human hepatocellular carcinomas. *International Journal of Cancer*, **71**, 355–9.

Kanazawa, Y., Hayashi, N., Mita, E. et al. (1994) Influence of viral quasispecies on effectiveness of interferon therapy in chronic hepatitis C patients. *Hepatology*, **20**, 1121–30.

Kaneko, T., Tanji, Y., Satoh, S. et al. (1994) Production of two phosphoproteins from the NS5A region of the hepatitis C viral genome. *Biochemical and Biophysical Research Communications*, **205**, 320–6.

Kaneko, T., Moriyama, T., Udaka, K. et al. (1997) Impaired induction of cytotoxic T lymphocytes by antagonism of a weak agonist borne by a variant hepatitis C virus epitope. *European Journal of Immunology,* **27**, 1782–7.

Kaneko, Y. B., Harada, M., Kawano, T. et al. (2000) Augmentation of Vα14 NKT cell-mediated cytotoxicity by interleukin-4 in an autocrine mechanism resulting in the development of concanavalin A-induced hepatitis. *Journal of Experimental Medicine,* **191**, 105–14.

Kanto, T., Hayashi, N., Takehara, T. et al. (1994) Buoyant density of hepatitis C virus recovered from infected hosts: two different features in sucrose equilibrium density gradient centrifugation related to degree of inflammation. *Hepatology,* **19**, 296–302.

Kao, J. H., Lai, M. Y., Chen, P. J., Hwang, L. H. & Chen, D. S. (1996) Serum hepatitis C virus titers in the progression of type C chronic liver disease with special emphasis on patients with type 1b infection. *Journal of Clinical Gastroenterology,* **23**, 280–3.

Katayama, T., Kikuchi, S., Tanaka, Y. et al. (1990) Blood screening for non-A, non-B hepatitis by hepatitis C virus antibody assay. *Transfusion,* **30**, 374–6.

Kato, N., Hijikata, M., Ootsuyama, Y. et al. (1990) Molecular cloning of the human hepatitis C virus genome from Japanese patients with non-A, non-B hepatitis. *Proceedings of the National Academy of Sciences of the USA,* **87**, 9524–8.

Kato, N., Ootsuyama, Y., Ohkoshi, S. et al. (1991) Distribution of plural HCV types in Japan. *Biochemical and Biophysical Research Communications,* **181**, 279–85.

Kato, N., Ootsuyama, Y., Sekiya, H. et al. (1994) Genetic drift in hypervariable region 1 of the viral genome in persistent hepatitis C virus infection. *Journal of Virology,* **68**, 4776–84.

Kato, N., Nakazawa, T., Mizutani, T. & Shimotohno, K. (1995) Susceptibility of human T-lymphotropic virus type 1 infected cell line MT-2 to hepatitis C virus infection. *Biochemical and Biophysical Research Communications,* **206**, 863–9.

Kato, N., Ikeda, M., Mizutani, T. et al. (1996) Replication of hepatitis C virus in cultured non-neoplastic human hepatocytes. *Japanese Journal of Cancer Research,* **87**, 787–92.

Kato, N., Lan, K. H., Ono-Nita, S. K., Shiratori, Y. & Omata, M. (1997) Hepatitis C virus nonstructural region 5A protein is a potent transcriptional activator. *Journal of Virology,* **71**, 8856–9.

Kawamura, T., Furusaka, A., Koziel, M. et al. (1997) Transgenic expression of hepatitis C virus structural proteins in the mouse. *Hepatology,* **25**, 1014–21.

Kawamura, T., Takeda, K., Mediratta, S. K. et al. (1998) Critical role of NK1[e] T cells in IL-12 induced immune responses *in vivo. Journal of Immunology,* **160**, 16–9.

Kawata, A., Une, Y., Hosokawa, M., Uchino, J. & Kobayashi, H. (1992) Tumor infiltrating lymphocytes and prognosis of hepatocellular carcinoma. *Japanese Journal of Clinical Oncology,* **22**, 256–63.

Kay, M. A., Baley, P., Rothenberg, S. et al. (1992) Expression of human α_1-antitrypsin in dogs after autologous transplantation of retroviral transduced hepatocytes. *Proceedings of the National Academy of Sciences of the USA,* **89**, 89–93.

Kennedy, J., Vicari, A. P., Saylir, V. et al. (2000) A molecular analysis of NKT cells: identification of a class-I restricted T cell-associated molecule (CRTAM). *Journal of Leukocyte Biology,* **67**, 725–34.

Kerkhoff, E., Hoeben, R., Loffler, S., Troppmair, J., Lee, J. E. & Rapp, U. R.(1998) Regulation of c-*myc* expression by Ras/Raf signalling. *Oncogene,* **16**, 211–16.

Kew, M. C., Houghton, M., Choo, Q. L. & Kuo, G. (1990) Hepatitis C virus antibodies in southern African blacks with hepatocellular carcinoma. *Lancet*, **335**, 873–4.

Kim, C. M., Koike, K., Saito, I., Miyamura, T. & Jay, G. (1991) HBX gene of hepatitis B virus induces liver cancer in transgenic mice. *Nature*, **351**, 317–20.

Kim, D. W., Gwack, Y., Han, J. H. & Choe, J. (1995) C-terminal domain of the hepatitis C virus NS3 protein contains an RNA helicase activity. *Biochemical and Biophysical Research Communications*, **215**, 160–6.

Kim, J. L., Morgenstern, K. A., Lin, C. et al. (1996) Crystal structure of the hepatitis virus NS3 proteinase domain complexed with a synthetic NS4A cofactor peptide. *Cell*, **87**, 343–55.

Kim, J. L., Morgenstern, K. Al., Griffith, J. P. et al. (1998) Hepatitis C virus NS3 RNA helicase domain with a bound oligonucleotide: the crystal structure provides insights into the mode of unwinding. *Structure*, **6**, 89–100.

Kimura, O., Yamaguchi, Y., Gunning, K. B., Teeter, L. D., Husain, F. & Kuo, M. T. (1994) Retroviral delivery of DNA into the livers of transgenic mice bearing premalignant and malignant hepatocellular carcinomas. *Human Gene Therapy*, **5**, 845–52.

Kirchhoff, S., Koromilas, A. E., Schaper, F., Grashof, M., Sonenberg, N. & Hauser, H. (1995) IRF-1 induced cell growth inhibition and interferon induction requires the activity of the protein kinase PKR. *Oncogene*, **11**, 439–45.

Kirkwood, T. B. & Bangham, C. R. (1994) Cycles, chaos, and evolution in virus cultures: a model of defective interfering particles. *Proceedings of the National Academy of Sciences of the USA*, **91**, 8685–9.

Kitchen, A. D., Wallis, P. A. & Gorman, A. M. (1996) Donor-to-donor and donor-to-patient transmission of hepatitis C virus. *Vox Sanguinis*, **70**, 112–13.

Kiyosawa, K., Akahane, Y., Nagata, A., Koike, Y. & Furuta, S. (1982) The significance of blood transfusion in non-A, non-B chronic liver disease in Japan. *Vox Sanguinis*, **43**, 45–52.

Kiyosawa, K., Akahane, Y., Nagata, A. & Furuta, S. (1984) Hepatocellular carcinoma after non-A, non-B posttransfusion hepatitis. *American Journal of Gastroenterology*, **79**, 777–81.

Kiyosawa, K., Sodeyama, T., Tanaka, E. et al. (1990) Interrelationship of blood transfusion, non-A, non-B hepatitis and hepatocellular carcinoma: analysis by detection of antibody to hepatitis C. *Hepatology*, **12**, 671–5.

Kleiber, J., Walter, T., Haberhausen, G., Tsang, S., Babiel, R. & Rosenstraus, M. (2000) Performance characteristics of a quantitative, homogeneous TaqMan RT/PCR test for HCV RNA. *Journal of Molecular Diagnostics*, **2**, 158–66.

Klinck, R., Westhof, E., Walker, S., Afshar, M., Collier, A. & Aboul-Ela, F. (2000) A potential RNA drug target in the hepatitis C virus internal ribosomal entry site. *RNA-A Publication of the RNA Society*, **6**, 1423–31.

Kline, W. E., Bowman, R. J., Ennis McCurdy, K. K., O'Malley, J. P. & Sandler, S. G. (1987) Hepatitis B core antibody (anti-HBc) in blood donors in the United States: Implications for surrogate testing programs. *Transfusion*, **27**, 99–102.

Knodell, R. G., Conrad, M. E. & Dienstag, J. L. (1975) Etiological spectrum of post-transfusion hepatitis. *Gastroenterology*, **69**, 1278–85.

Knowles, B. B., Howe, C. C. & Aden, D. P. (1980) Human hepatocellular carcinoma cell lines secrete the major plasma proteins and hepatitis B surface antigen. *Science*, **209**, 497–9.

Kodama, T., Tamaki, T., Katabami, S. et al. (1993) Histological findings in asymptomatic hepatitis C virus carriers. *Journal of Gastroenterology and Hepatology*, **8**, 403–5.

Koeberl, D. D., Alexander, I. E., Halbert, C. L., Russel, D. W. & Miller A. D. (1997) Persistent expression of human clotting factor IX from mouse liver after intravenous injection of adeno-associated virus vectors. *Proceedings of the National Academy of Sciences of the USA*, **94**, 1426–31.

Koff, R. S. (1997) Therapy in chronic hepatitis C: say goodbye to the 6-month interferon regimen. *American Journal of Gastroenterology*, **91**, 2072–4.

Koff, R. S. & Dienstag, J. L. (1995) Extrahepatic manifestations of hepatitis C and the association with alcoholic liver disease. *Seminars in Liver Disease*, **15**, 101–9.

Koike, K., Moriya, K., Ishibashi, K. et al. (1995) Expression of hepatitis C virus envelope proteins in transgenic mice. *Journal of General Virology*, **76**, 3031–8.

Koike, K., Moriya, K., Ishibashi, K. et al. (1997) Sialadenitis histologically resembling Sjögren syndrome in mice transgenic for hepatitis C virus envelope genes. *Proceedings of the National Academy of Sciences of the USA*, **94**, 233–6.

Koizumi, K., Enomoto, N., Kurosaki, M. et al. (1995) Diversity of quasispecies in various disease stages of chronic hepatitis C virus infection and its significance in interferon treatment. *Hepatology*, **22**, 30–5.

Kolho, E. K. & Krusius, T. (1992) Risk factors for hepatitis C virus antibody positivity in blood donors in a low risk country. *Vox Sanguinis*, **63**, 192–7.

Kolykhalov, A. A., Agapov, E. V. & Rice, C. M. (1994) Specificity of the hepatitis C virus NS3 serine proteinase: effects of substitutions at the 3/4A, 4A/4B, 4B/5A, and 5A/5B cleavage sites on polyprotein processing. *Journal of Virology*, **68**, 7525–33.

Kolykhalov, A. A., Feinstone, S. M. & Rice, C. M. (1996) Identification of a highly conserved sequence element at the 3' terminus of hepatitis C virus genome RNA. *Journal of Virology*, **70**, 3363–71.

Kolykhalov, A. A., Agapov, E. V., Blight, K .L., Mihalik, K., Feinstone, S. M. & Rice, C. M. (1997) Transmission of hepatitis C by intrahepatic inoculation with transcribed RNA. *Science*, **277**, 570–4.

Kondo, R., Feitelson, M. A. & Strayer, D. S. (1998) Use of SV40 to immunize against hepatitis B surface antigen: implications for the use of SV40 as a gene transduction vehicle and for its application as an immunizing agent. *Gene Therapy*, **5**, 575–82.

Kondo, T., Suda, T., Fukuyama, H., Adachi, M. & Nagata, S. (1997) Essential roles of the Fas ligand in the development of hepatitis. *Nature Medicine*, **3**, 409–13.

Koonin, E. V. (1991) The phylogeny of RNA-dependent RNA polymerases of positive-strand RNA viruses. *Journal of General Virology*, **72**, 2197–06.

Koretz, R. L., Suffin, S. C. & Gitnick, G. L. (1976) Post-transfusion chronic liver disease. *Gastroenterology*, **71**, 797–803.

Koretz, R. L., Abbey, H., Coleman, E. & Gitnick, G. (1993a) Non-A, non-B post-transfusion hepatitis: looking back in the second decade. *Annuals of Internal Medicine*, **119**, 110–15.

Koretz, R. L., Brezina, M., Polito, A. J. et al. (1993b) Non-A, non-B posttransfusion hepatitis: comparing C and non-C hepatitis. *Hepatology*, **17**, 361–5.

Korolev, S., Yao, N., Lohman, T. M., Weber, P. C. & Waksman, G. (1998) Comparisons between the structures of HCV and Rep helicases reveal structural similarities between SF1 and SF2 superfamilies of helicases. *Protein Science*, **7**, 1–6.

Korth, M. J. & Katze, M. G. (2000) Evading the interferon response: hepatitis C virus and the interferon-induced protein kinase, PKR. *Current Topics in Microbiology and Immunology*, **242**, 197–224.

Kozak, M. (1989) The scanning model for translation: an update. *Journal of Cell Biology*, **108**, 229–41.

Kozarsky, K. F. & Wilson, J. M. (1993) Gene therapy: adenovirus vectors. *Current Opinion in Genetics and Development*, **3**, 499–503.

Koziel, M. J. (1997) The role of immune responses in the pathogenesis of hepatitis C virus infection. *Journal of Viral Hepatitis*, **4**(Suppl. 2), 31–41.

Koziel, M. J. & Walker, B. D. (1997) Characteristics of the intrahepatic cytotoxic T lymphocyte response in chronic hepatitis C virus infection. *Springer Seminars in Immunopathology*, **19**, 69–83.

Koziel, M. J., Dudley, D., Wong, J. T. et al. (1992) Intrahepatic cytotoxic T lymphocytes specific for hepatitis C virus in persons with chronic hepatitis. *Journal of Immunology*, **149**, 3339–44.

Koziel, M. J., Dudley, D., Afdhal, N. et al. (1993) Hepatitis C virus (HCV)-specific cytotoxic T lymphocytes recognize epitopes in the core and envelope proteins of HCV. *Journal of Virology*, **67**, 7522–32.

Koziel, M. J., Dudley, D., Afdhal, N. et al. (1995) HLA class I restricted cytotoxic T lymphocytes specific for hepatitis C virus. Identification of multiple epitopes and characterization of patterns of cytokine release. *Journal of Clinical Investigation*, **96**, 2311–21.

Koziol, D. E., Holland, P. V., Alling, D. W. et al. (1986) Antibody to hepatitis B core antigen as a paradoxical marker for non-A, non-B hepatitis agents in donated blood. *Annals of Internal Medicine*, **104**, 488–95.

Krajden, M., Zhao, J., Bourke, C., Scalia, V., Gill, P. & Lau, W. (1996) Detection of hepatitis C virus by PCR in second-generation enzyme immunoassay-seropositive blood donor by using matched pairs of fresh frozen plasma and pilot tube sera. *Journal of Clinical Microbiology*, **34**, 2191–5.

Krams, S. M., Fox, C. K., Beatty, P. R. et al. (1998) Human hepatocytes produce an isoform of Fas that inhibits apoptosis. *Transplantation*, **65**, 713–21.

Krawczynski, K., Beach, M. J., Bradley, D. W. et al. (1992a) Hepatitis C virus antigen in hepatocytes: immunomorphologic detection and identification. *Gastroenterology*, **103**, 622–9.

Krawczynski, K., Beach, M., Bradley, D. W., Meeks, E. & Spelbring, J. E. (1992b) Immunosuppression and pathogenic studies of acute hepatitis C virus (HCV) infection in chimpanzees. *Hepatology*, **2**, 131A.

Kroes, A. C. M., Quint, W. G. V. & Heijtink, R. A. (1991) Significance of isolated hepatitis B core antibodies detected by enzyme immunoassay in a high risk population. *Journal of Medical Virology*, **35**, 96–100.

Krugman, S. & Gocke, D. S. (1978) Acute viral hepatitis. In *Viral Hepatitis*, Vol. XV, ed. L. H. Smith, Jr, pp. 30–47. Philadelphia, PA: Saunders.

Kuchroo, V. K., Das, M. P., Brown, J. A. et al. (1995) B7-1 and B7-2 costimulatory molecules activate differentially the Th1/Th2 developmental pathways: application to autoimmune disease therapy. *Cell*, **80**, 707–18.

Kudesia, G., Ball, G. & Irving, W. L. (1995) Vertical transmission of hepatitis C. *Lancet*, **345**, 1122.

Kuhnl, P., Seidl, S., Stangel, W., Beyer, J., Sibrowski, W. & Flik, J. (1989) Antibody to hepatitis C virus in German blood donors. *Lancet*, **ii**, 324.

Kumar, A., Haque, J., Lacoste, J., Hiscott, J. & Williams, B. R. G. (1994b) Double-stranded RNA-dependent protein kinase activates transcription factor NF-κB by phosphorylating IκB. *Proceedings of the National Academy of Sciences of the USA*, **91**, 6288–92.

Kumar, U., Monjardino, J. & Thomas H. C. (1994a) Hypervariable region of hepatitis C virus envelope glycoprotein (E2/NS1) in an agammaglobulinemic patient. *Gastroenterology*, **106**, 1072–5.

Kuo, G., Choo, Q. L., Alter, H. J. et al. (1989) An assay for circulating antibodies to a major etiologic virus of human non-A, non-B hepatitis. *Science*, **244**, 362–4.

Kurosaki, M., Enomoto, N., Marumo, F. & Sato, C. (1995) Variations in the core region of hepatitis C virus genomes in patient with chronic hepatitis. *Archives of Virology*, **140**, 1087–94.

Kurosaki, M., Enomoto, N., Murakami, T. et al. (1997) Analysis of genotypes and amino acid residues 2209 to 2248 of the NS5A region of hepatitis C virus in relation to the response to interferon-β therapy. *Hepatology*, **25**, 750–3.

Kwok, S. & Higuchi, R. (1989) Avoiding false positives with PCR. *Nature*, **339**, 237–8.

Kwong, A. D. & Risano, C. (1998) Development of a hepatitis C virus RNA helicase high throughput assay. In *Antiviral Methods and Protocols*, eds. D. Kinchington & R. F. Schinazi, Ch. 9. Totowa, NJ: Humana Press.

Kwong, A. D., Kim, J. L. & Lin, C. (2000) Structure and function of hepatitis C virus NS3 helicase. *Current Topics in Microbiology and Immunology*, **242**, 171–96.

Kyono, K., Miyashiro, M. & Taguchi, I. (1998) Detection of hepatitis C virus helicase activity using the scintillation proximity assay system. *Analytical Biochemistry*, **257**, 120–6.

La Civita, L., Zignego, A. L., Monti, M., Longombardo, G., Pasero, G. & Ferri, C. (1995) Mixed cryoglobulinemia as a possible preneoplastic disorder. *Arthritis and Rheumatism*, **38**, 1859–60.

Lai, K. N., Lai, F. M., Leung, N. W. Y., Lo, S. T. & Tam, J. S. (1990a) Hepatitis with isolated serum antibody to hepatitis B core antigen. A variant of non-A, non-B hepatitis? *American Journal of Clinical Pathology*, **93**, 79–83.

Lai, M. E., Mazzoleni, A. P., Argiolu, F. et al. (1994) Hepatitis C virus in multiple episodes of acute hepatitis in polytransfused thalassaemic children. *Lancet*, **343**, 388–90.

Lai, M. M. C. & Ware C. F. (2000) Hepatitis C virus core protein: possible roles in viral pathogenesis. *Current Topics in Microbiology and Immunology*, **242**, 117–34.

Lai, M. Y., Chen, P. J., Yang, P. M., Sheu, J. C., Sung, J. L. & Chen, D. S. (1990b) Identification and characterization of intrahepatic hepatitis B virus DNA in HBsAg-seronegative patients with chronic liver disease and hepatocellular carcinoma in Taiwan. *Hepatology*, **12**, 575–81.

Lai, M. Y., Kao, J. H., Yang, P. M. et al. (1996) Long term efficacy of ribavirin plus interferon alfa in the treatment of chronic hepatitis C. *Gastroenterology*, **111**, 1307–12.

Lai, V. C. H., Zhong, W. D., Skelton, A. et al. (2000) Generation and characterization of a hepatitis C virus NS3 protease-dependent bovine viral diarrhea virus. *Journal of Virology,* **74,** 6339–47.

Lam, N. P., DeGuzman, L. J., Pitrak, D. & Layden, T. J. (1994) Clinical and histologic predictors of response to interferon-alpha in patients with chronic hepatitis C viral infection. *Digestive Disease and Sciences,* **39,** 2660–4.

Lanford, R. E., Sureau, C., Jacob, J. R., White, R. & Fuerst, T. R. (1994) Demonstration of *in vitro* infection of chimpanzee hepatocytes with hepatitis C virus using strand-specific RT/PCR. *Virology,* **202,** 606–14.

Lanzavecchia, A. (1997) Understanding the mechanisms of sustained signaling and T cell activation. *Journal of Experimental Medicine,* **185,** 1717–19.

Larkin, J., Clayton, M., Sun, B. et al. (1999) Hepatitis B virus transgenic SCID mouse model of chronic liver disease. *Nature Medicine,* **5,** 907–12.

Lau, G. K. K., Fang, J. W. S., Wu, P. C., Davis, G. L. & Lau, J. Y. N. (1994) Detection of hepatitis C virus genome in formalin-fixed paraffin-embedded liver tissue by *in situ* reverse transcription polymerase chain reaction. *Journal of Medical Virology,* **44,** 406–9.

Lau, J. Y. N., Alexander, G. J. M. & Alberti, A. (1991) Viral hepatitis. *Gut,* **32**(Suppl.), 47–62.

Lau, J. Y. N., Davis, G. L., Kniffen, J. et al. (1993) Significance of serum hepatitis C virus RNA levels in chronic hepatitis C. *Lancet,* **341,** 1501–4.

Lawal, Z., Petrik, J., Wong, V. S., Alesander, G. J. & Allain, J. P. (1997) Hepatitis C virus genomic variability in untreated and immunosuppressed patients. *Virology,* **228,** 107–11.

Lechmann, M., Ihlenfeldt, H. G., Braunschweiger, I. et al. (1996) T- and B-cell responses to different hepatitis C virus antigens in patients with chronic hepatitis C infection and in healthy anti-hepatitis C virus-positive blood donors without viremia. *Hepatology,* **24,** 790–5.

Lee, C. (1996) Transfusion-transmitted disease. *Baillière's Clinical Haematology,* **9,** 369–94.

Lee, G. H., Merlino, G. & Fausto, N. (1992) Development of liver tumors in transforming growth factor α transgenic mice. *Cancer Research,* **52,** 5162–70.

Lee, S. B. & Esteban, M. (1994) The interferon-induced double-stranded RNA activated protein kinase induces apoptosis. *Virology,* **199,** 491–6.

Lee, S. R., Wood, C. L., Lane, M. J. et al. (1995) Increased detection of hepatitis C virus infection in commercial plasma donors by a third-generation screening assay. *Transfusion,* **35,** 845–9.

Lee, S. W., Cho, J. H. & Sung, Y. C. (1998) Optimal induction of hepatitis C virus envelope-specific immunity by bicistronic plasmid DNA inoculation with the granulocyte-macrophage colony-stimulating factor gene. *Journal of Virology,* **72,** 8430–6.

Lee, T. H., Finegold, M. J., Shen, R. F., DeMayo, J. L., Woo, S. L. C. & Butel, J. S. (1990) Hepatitis B virus transactivator X protein is not tumorigenic in transgenic mice. *Journal of Virology,* **64,** 5939–47.

Lee, W. M. (1993) The silent epidemic of hepatitis C. *Gastroenterology,* **104,** 661–2.

Lefkowitch, J. H. & Apfelbaum, T. F. (1989) Non-A, non-B hepatitis: characterization of liver biopsy pathology. *Journal of Clinical Gastroenterology,* **11,** 225–32.

Lefkowitch, J. H., Schiff, E. R., Davis, G. L. et al. and the Hepatitis Interventional Therapy Group (1993) Pathological diagnosis of chronic hepatitis C: a multicenter comparative study with chronic hepatitis B. *Gastroenterology,* **104,** 595–603.

Le Guen, B., Squadrito, G., Nalpas, B., Berthelot, P., Pol, S. & Brechot, C. (1997) Hepatitis C virus genome complexity correlates with response to interferon therapy: a study in French patients with chronic hepatitis C. *Hepatology*, **25**, 1250–4.

Leinbach, S. S., Bhat, R. A., Xia, S. M. et al. (1994) Substrate specificity of the NS3 serine proteinase of hepatitis C virus as determined by mutagenesis at the NS3/NS4A junction. *Virology*, **204**, 163–9.

Leite-de-Moraes, M. C. & Dy, M. (1997) Natural killer T cells: a potent cytokine-producing cell population. *European Cytokine Network*, **8**, 229–37.

Lenzi, M., Ballardini, G., Fusconi, M. et al. (1990) Type 2 autoimmune hepatitis and hepatitis C virus infection. *Lancet*, **335**, 258–9.

Lerat, H., Berby, F., Trabaud, M. A. et al. (1996) Specific detection of hepatitis C virus minus strand RNA in hemapoietic cells. *Journal of Clinical Investigation*, **97**, 845–51.

Leroux-Roels, G., Esquivel, C. A., DeLeys, R. et al. (1996) Lymphoproliferative responses to hepatitis C virus core, E1, E2, and NS3 in patients with chronic hepatitis C infection treated with interferon alpha. *Hepatology*, **23**, 8–16.

Lesburg, C. A., Cable, M. B., Ferrari, E., Hong, Z., Mannarino, A. F. & Weber, P. C. (1999) Crystal structure of the RNA-dependent RNA polymerase from hepatitis C virus reveals a fully encircled active site. *Nature Structural Biology*, **6**, 937–43.

Li, J. S., Tong, S. P., Vitvitski, L., Lepot, D. & Trepo, C. (1991) Two French genotypes of hepatitis C virus: homology of the predominant genotype with the prototype American strain. *Gene*, **105**, 167–72.

Li, J. S., Vitvitski, L., Tong, S. P. & Trepo, C. (1994) Identification of the third major genotype of hepatitis C virus in France. *Biochemical and Biophysical Research Communications*, **199**, 1474–81.

Li, X., Jeffers, L. J., Shao, L. et al. (1995) Identification of hepatitis C virus by immunoelectron microscopy. *Journal of Viral Hepatitis*, **2**, 227–34.

Liang, T. J., Jeffers, L. J., Reddy, K. R. et al. (1993) Viral pathogenesis of hepatocellular carcinoma in the United States. *Hepatology*, **18**, 1326–33.

Liaw, Y. F., Lee, C. S., Tsai, S. L. et al. (1995) T cell mediated autologous hepatocytotoxicity in patients with chronic hepatitis C virus infection. *Hepatology*, **22**, 1368–73.

Liaw, Y. F., Tsai, S. L., Sheen, I. S. et al. (1998) Clinical and virological course of chronic hepatitis B virus infection with hepatitis C and D virus markers. *American Journal of Gastroenterology*, **93**, 354–9.

Lieber, A., Vrancken Peeters, M. J., Meuse, L., Fausto, N., Perkins, J. & Kay, M. A. (1995) Adenovirus mediated urokinase gene transfer induces liver regeneration and allows for efficient retrovirus transduction of hepatocytes *in vivo. Proceedings of the National Academy of Sciences of the USA*, **92**, 6210–14.

Lieber, A., He, C. Y., Polyak, S. J., Gretch, D. R., Barr, D. & Kay, M. A. (1996) Elimination of hepatitis C virus RNA in infected human hepatocytes by adenovirus-mediated expression of ribozymes. *Journal of Virology*, **70**, 8782–91.

Lima, W. F., Brown-Driver, V., Fox, M., Hanecak, R. & Bruice, T. W. (1997) Combinatorial screening and rational optimization for hybridization to folded hepatitis C virus RNA of oligonucleotides with biological antisense activity. *Journal of Biological Chemistry*, **272**, 626–38.

Lin, C. & Rice, C. M. (1995) The hepatitis C virus NS3 serine proteinase and NS4A cofactor: establishment of a cell-free *trans*-processing assay. *Proceedings of the National Academy of Sciences of the USA*, **92**, 7622–6.

Lin, C., Lindenbach, B. D., Pragai, B., McCourt, D. W. & Rice, C. M. (1994a) Processing of the hepatitis C virus E2-NS2 region: identification of p7 and two distinct E2-specific products with different C termini. *Journal of Virology*, **68**, 5063–73.

Lin, C., Pragai, B. M., Grakoui, A., Xu, J. & Rice, C. M. (1994b) Hepatitis C virus NS3 serine proteinase: *trans*-cleavage requirements and processing kinetics. *Journal of Virology*, **68**, 8147–57.

Lin, C., Thomson, J. A. & Rice, C. M. (1995) A central region in the hepatitis C virus NS4A protein allows formation of an active NS3-NS4A serine proteinase complex *in vivo* and *in vitro*. *Journal of Virology*, **69**, 4373–80.

Lin, C., Wu, J. W., Hsiao, K. & Su, M. S. S. (1997) The hepatitis C virus NS4A protein: interactions with NS4B and NS5A proteins. *Journal of Virology*, **71**, 6465–71.

Lin-Chu, M., Tsai, S. J., Watanabe, J. & Nishioka, K. (1990) The prevalence of anti-HCV among Chinese voluntary blood donors in Taiwan. *Transfusion*, **30**, 471–3.

Linnen, J., Wages, J. Jr, Zhang-Keck, Z. Y. et al. (1996) Molecular cloning and disease association of hepatitis G virus: a transfusion-transmissible agent. *Science*, **271**, 505–8.

Liou, T. C., Chang, T. T., Young, K. C., Lin, X. Z., Lin, C. Y. & Wu, H. L. (1992) Detection of HCV RNA in saliva, urine, seminal fluid, and ascites. *Journal of Medical Virology*, **37**, 197–202.

Liu, Q., Tackney, C., Bhat, R. A., Prince, A. M. & Zhang, P. (1997) Regulated processing of hepatitis C virus core protein is linked to subcellular localization. *Journal of Virology*, **71**, 657–62.

Livak, K. J., Flood, S. J. A., Marmaro, J., Giusti, W. & Deetz, K. (1995) Oligonucleotides with fluorescent dyes at opposite ends provide a quenched probe system useful for detecting PCR product and nucleic acid hybridization. *PCR Methods Applications*, **4**, 357–62.

Lo, S. Y., Selby, M., Tong, M. & Ou, J. H. (1994) Comparative studies of the core gene products of two-different hepatitis C virus isolates: two alternative forms determined by a single amino acid substitution. *Virology*, **199**, 124–31.

Lo, S. Y., Masiarz, F., Hwang, S. B., Lai, M. M. C. & Ou, J. H. (1995) Differential subcellular localization of hepatitis C virus core gene products. *Virology*, **213**, 455–61.

Lo, S. Y., Selby, M. J. & Ou, J. H. (1996) Interaction between hepatitis C virus core protein and E1 envelope protein. *Journal of Virology*, **70**, 5177–82.

Lohmann, V., Korner, F., Herian, U. & Bartenschlager, R. (1997) Biochemical properties of hepatitis C virus NS5B RNA-dependent RNA polymerase and identification of amino acid sequence motifs essential for enzymatic activity. *Journal of Virology*, **71**, 9416–28.

Lohmann, V., Roos, A., Korner, F., Koch, J. O. & Bartenschlager, R. (1998) Biochemical and kinetic analysis of NS5B RNA-dependent RNA polymerase of the hepatitis C virus. *Virology*, **249**, 108–18.

Lohmann, V., Korner, F., Koch, J.-O., Herian, U., Theilmann, L. & Bartenschlager, R. (1999)

Replication of subgenomic hepatitis C virus RNA in a hepatoma cell line. *Science*, **285**, 110–13.

Lohr, H. F., Goergen, B., Meyer zum Buschenfelde, K. H. & Gerken, G. (1995) HCV replication in mononuclear cells stimulates anti-HCV secreting B cells and reflects nonresponsiveness to interferon-alpha. *Journal of Medical Virology*, **46**, 314–20.

Lohse, A. W., Gerken, G., Mohr, H. et al. (1995) Relation between autoimmune liver disease and viral hepatitis: Clinical and serological characteristics in 859 patients. *Zeitschrift für Gastroenterologie*, **33**, 527–33.

Lopez-Labrador, F. X., Ampurdanes, S., Forns, X. et al. (1997) Hepatitis C virus (HCV) genotypes in Spanish patients with HCV infection: relationship between HCV genotype 1b, cirrhosis and hepatocellular carcinoma. *Journal of Hepatology*, **27**, 959–65.

Loriot, M. A., Bronowicki, J. P., Lagorce, D. et al. (1999) Permissiveness of human biliary epithelial cells to infection by hepatitis C virus. *Hepatology*, **29**, 1587–95.

Love, A., Smaradottir, A., Thorsteinsson, S. B., Stanzeit, B. & Weidell, A. (1995) Hepatitis C virus genotypes among blood donors and their recipients in Iceland determined by polymerase chain reaction. *Vox Sanguinus*, **69**, 18–22.

Love, R. A., Parge, H. E., Wickersham, J. A. et al. (1996) The crystal structure of hepatitis C virus NS3 proteinase reveals a trypsin-like fold and a structural zinc binding site. *Cell*, **87**, 331–42.

Lu, H. H. & Wimmer, E. (1996) Poliovirus chimeras replicating under the translational control of genetic elements of hepatitis C virus reveal unusual properties of the internal ribosomal entry site of hepatitis C virus. *Proceedings of the National Academy of Sciences of the USA*, **93**, 1412–17.

Lu, M., Funsch, B., Wiese, M. & Roggendorf, M. (1995) Analysis of hepatitis C virus quasispecies populations by temperature gradient gel electrophoresis. *Journal of General Virology*, **76**, 881–7.

Lu, W., Lo, S. Y., Chen, M., Wu, K. J., Fung, Y. K. T. & Ou, J. H. (1999) Activation of p53 tumor suppressor by hepatitis C virus core protein. *Virology*, **264**, 134–41.

Lubin, I., Faktotowich, Y., Lapidot, T. et al. (1991) Engraftment and development of human T and B cells in mice after bone marrow transplantation. *Science*, **252**, 427–31.

Lunel, F. & Musset, L. (1998) Hepatitis C virus infection and cryoglobulinemia. *Journal of Hepatology*, **29**, 848–55.

Lunel, F., Cresta, P., Vitour, D. et al. (1999) Comparative evaluation of hepatitis C virus RNA quantitation by branched DNA, NASBA, and monitor asays. *Hepatology*, **29**, 528–35.

Luo, G., Hamatake, R. K., Mathis, D. M. et al. (2000) *De novo* initiation of RNA synthesis by the RNA-dependent RNA polymerase (NS5B) of hepatitis C virus. *Journal of Virology*, **74**, 851–63.

Luppi, M., Ferrari, M. G., Bonaccorsio, G. et al. (1996) Hepatitis C virus infection in subsets of neoplastic lymphoproliferations not associated with cryoglobulinemia. *Leukemia*, **10**, 351–5.

MacCallum, F. O. (1947) Homologous serum jaundice. *Lancet*, **ii**, 691–2.

Maggi, F., Fornai, C., Vatteroni, M. L. et al. (1997) Differences in hepatitis C virus quasispecies composition between liver, peripheral blood mononuclear cells and plasma. *Journal of General Virology*, **78**, 1521–5.

Maisonneuve, P., Laurian, Y., Guerois, C. et al. (1991) Antibody to hepatitis C (anti C 100-3) in French hemophiliacs. *Nouvelle Revue Française d'Hematologie*, **33**, 263–6.

Maisonneuve, P., Courouce, A. M., Ferrer le Coeur, F. et al. (1992) Anti-HCV and recipients: situation in hemophiliacs in 1991. *Revue Française de Transfusion et d'Hemobiologie*, **35**, 193–8.

Major, M. E. & Feinstone, S. M. (1997) The molecular virology of hepatitis C. *Hepatology*, **25**, 1527–38.

Major, M. E. & Feinstone, S. M. (2000) Characterization of hepatitis C virus infectious clones in chimpanzees: long-term studies. *Current Topics in Microbiology and Immunology*, **242**, 279–98.

Major, M. E., Mihalik, K., Fernandez, J. et al. (1999) Long-term follow-up of chimpanzees inoculated with the first infectious clone for hepatitis C virus. *Journal of Virology*, **73**, 3317–25.

Makris, M., Preston, F. E., Rosendaal, F. R., Underwood, J. C., Rice, K. M. & Triger, D. R. (1996) The natural history of chronic hepatitis C in haemophiliacs. *British Journal of Haematology*, **94**, 746–52.

Malik, A. H. & Lee, W. M. (2000) Chronic hepatitis B virus infection: treatment strategies for the next millennium. *Annals of Internal Medicine*, **132**, 723–31.

Manabe, N., Chevallier, M., Chossegros, P. et al. (1993) Interferon-α2b therapy reduces liver fibrosis in chronic non-A, non-B hepatitis: a quantitative histological evaluation. *Hepatology*, **18**, 1344–9.

Mangia, A., Gentile, R., Casavilla, I. et al. (1999) HLA class II favors clearance of HCV infection and progression of the chronic liver damage. *Journal of Hepatology*, **30**, 984–9.

Mannucci, P. M., Schimpf, K., Brettler, D. B. et al. (1990) Low risk for hepatitis C in haemophiliacs given a high-purity, pasteurized factor VIII-concentrate. *Annals of Internal Medicine*, **113**, 27–32.

Mannucci, P. M., Schimpf, K., Abe, T. et al. (1992) Low risk of viral infection after administration of vapor-heated factor VIII concentrate. *Transfusion*, **32**, 134–8.

Mansell, C. J. & Locarnini, S. A. (1995) Epidemiology of hepatitis C in the east. *Seminars in Liver Disease*, **15**, 15–32.

Manzin, A., Candela, M., Solforosi, L., Gabrielli, A. & Clementi, M. (1999) Dynamics of hepatitis C viremia after plasma exchange. *Journal of Hepatology*, **31**, 389–93.

Marcellin, P., Boyer, N., Giostra, E. et al. (1991) Recombinant human α-interferon in patients with chronic non-A, non-B hepatitis. A multicenter, randomized, controlled trial from France. *Hepatology*, **13**, 393–7.

Marshall, R. L., Laffler, T. G., Cerney, M. B., Sustachek, J. C., Kratochvil, J. D. & Morgan, R. L. (1994) Detection of HCV RNA by the asymmetric gap ligase chain reaction. *PCR Methods and Applications*, **4**, 80–4.

Martell, M., Esteban, J. I., Quer, J. et al. (1992) Hepatitis C virus (HCV) circulates as a population of differently but closely related genomes: quasispecies nature of HCV genome distribution. *Journal of Virology*, **66**, 3225–9.

Martell, M., Gomez, J., Esteban, J. I. et al. (1999) High-throughput real-time reverse transcription–PCR quantitation of hepatitis C virus RNA. *Journal of Clinical Microbiology*, **37**, 327–32.

Martinot-Peignoux, M., Marcellin, P., Pouteau, M. et al. (1995) Pretreatment serum hepatitis C virus RNA levels and hepatitis C virus genotype are the main and independent prognostic factors of sustained response to interferon alfa therapy in chronic hepatitis C. *Hepatology*, 22, 1050–6.

Marusawa, H., Hijikata, M., Chiba, T. & Shimotohno, K. (1999) Hepatitis C virus core protein inhibits Fas- and tumor necrosis factor alpha-mediated apoptosis via NF-κB activation. *Journal of Virology*, 73, 4713–20.

Matsubara, T., Sumazaki, R. & Takita, H. (1995) Mother-to-infant transmission of hepatitis C virus: a prospective study. *European Journal of Pediatrics*, 154, 973–8.

Matsuda, J., Suzuki, M., Nozaki, C. et al. (1998) Transgenic mouse expressing a full-length hepatitis C virus cDNA. *Japanese Journal of Cancer Research*, 89, 150–8.

Matsumoto, M., Hwang, S. B., Jeng, K. S., Zhu, N. & Lai, M. M. C. (1996) Homotypic interaction and multimerization of hepatitis C virus core protein. *Virology*, 218, 43–51.

Matsumoto, M., Hsieh, T. Y., Zhu, N. et al. (1997) Hepatitis C virus core protein interacts with the cytoplasmic tail of lymphotoxin-β receptor. *Journal of Virology*, 71, 1301–9.

Matsuura, A., Kinebuchi, M., Chen, H. Z. et al. (2000) NKT cells in the rat: organ-specific distribution of NK T cells expressing distinct V alpha 14 chains. *Journal of Immunology*, 164, 3140–8.

Mattsson, L., Sonnerborg, A. & Weiland, O. (1993) Outcome of acute symptomatic non-A, non-B hepatitis: a 13 year followup study of hepatitis C virus markers. *Liver*, 13, 274–8.

Mattson, S., Weiland, O. & Glaumann, H. (1990) Application of a numerical scoring system for assessment of histological outcome in patients with chronic posttransfusion non-A, non-B, hepatitis with or without antibodies to hepatitis C. *Liver*, 10, 257–63.

Maugh, T. H. (1980) Where is the hepatitis C virus? *Science*, 210, 999–1000.

Maurer, N., Mori, A., Palmer, L. et al. (1999) Lipid-based systems for the intracellular delivery of genetic drugs. *Molecular Membrane Biology*, 16, 129–40.

Mauser-Bunschoten, E. P., Bresters, D., van Drimmelen, A. A. et al. (1995) Hepatitis C infection and viremia in Dutch hemophilia patients. *Journal of Medical Virology*, 45, 241–6.

Mazzella, G., Accogli, E., Sottili, S. et al. (1996) Alpha interferon treatment may prevent hepatocellular carcinoma in HCV related liver cirrhosis. *Journal of Hepatology*, 24, 141–7.

McCormick, S. E., Goodman, Z. D., Maydonovitch, C. L. & Sjogren, M. H. (1996) Evaluation of liver histology, ALT elevation, and HCV RNA titer in patients with chronic hepatitis C. *American Journal of Gastroenterology*, 91, 1516–22.

McFarlane, I. G., Tolley, P., Major, G., McFarlane, B. M. & Williams, R. (1983) Development of an enzyme-linked immunosorbent assay (ELISA) for antibodies against the liver specific membrane lipoprotein (LSP). *Journal of Immunological Methods*, 64, 215–25.

McFarlane, I. G., Smith, H. M., Johnson, P. J., Bray, G. P., Vergani, D. & Williams, R. (1990) Hepatitis C virus antibodies in chronic active hepatitis. Pathogenetic factor or false positive results? *Lancet*, 335, 754–7.

McHutchison, J. G. & Poynard, T. (1999) Combination therapy with interferon plus ribavirin for the initial treatment of chronic hepatitis C. *Seminars in Liver Disease*, 19, 57–65.

McKechnie, V. M., Mills, P. R. & McCruden, E. A. (2000) The NS5A gene of hepatitis C virus in patients treated with interferon alpha. *Journal of Medical Virology*, 60, 367–78.

McKiernan, S. & Kelleher, D. (2000) Immunogenetics of hepatitis C virus. *Journal of Viral Hepatitis*, **7**(Suppl. 1), 13–14.

McOmish, F., Yap, P. L., Dow, B. C. et al. (1994) Geographical distribution of hepatitis C virus genotypes in blood donors–An international collaborative survey. *Journal of Clinical Microbiology*, **32**, 884–92.

McQuillan, G. M., Alter, M. J., Moyer, L. A., Lambert, S. B. & Margolis, H. S. (1997) A population based serologic study of hepatitis C virus infection in the United States. In *Viral Hepatitis and Liver Disease*, eds. M. Rizzetto, R. H. Purcell, J. L. Gerin & G. Verme, pp. 267–70. Turin, Italy: Edizioni Minerva Medica.

Mecchia, M., Casato, M., Tufi, R. et al. (1996) Nonrheumatoid IgM in human hepatitis C virus supergroups. *Proceedings of the National Academy of Sciences of the USA*, **87**, 2057–61.

Meisel, H., Reip, A., Faltus, B. et al. (1995) Transmission of hepatitis C virus to children and husbands by women infected with contaminated anti-D immunoglobulin. *Lancet*, **345**, 1209–11.

Mendel, I., Muraine, M., Riachi, G. et al. (1997) Detection and genotyping of the hepatitis C RNA in tear fluid from patients with chronic hepatitis C. *Journal of Medical Virology*, **51**, 231–3.

Meurs, E. F., Galabru, J., Barber, G. N., Katze, M. G. & Hovanessian, A. G. (1993) Tumor suppressor function of the interferon-induced double stranded RNA activated protein kinase. *Proceedings of the National Academy of Sciences of the USA*, **90**, 232–6.

Meyers, J. D., Dienstag, J. L., Purcel, R. H., Thomas, L. D. & Holmes, K. K. (1977) Parenterally transmitted non-A, non-B hepatitis: an epidemic reassessed. *Annals of Internal Medicine*, **87**, 57–9.

Mezey, E., Potter, J. J., Slusser, R. J. & Abdi, W. (1977) Changes in hepatic collagen metabolism in rats produced by chronic ethanol feeding. *Laboratory Investigation*, **36**, 206–14.

Michalak, J. P., Wychowski, C., Choukhi, A. et al. (1997) Characterization of truncated forms of the hepatitis C virus glycoproteins. *Journal of General Virology*, **78**, 2299–306.

Miller, R. H. & Purcell, R. H. (1990) Hepatitis C virus shares amino acid sequence similarity with pestiviruses and flaviviruses as well as members of two plant virus supergroups. *Proceedings of the National Academy of Sciences of the USA*, **87**, 2057–61.

Mink, M. A., Benichou, S., Madaule, P., Tiollais, P., Prince, A. M. & Inchauspe, G. (1994) Characterization and mapping of a B-cell immunogenic domain in hepatitis C virus E2 glycoprotein using a yeast peptide library. *Virology*, **200**, 246–55.

Minuk, G. Y. (1999) The influence of host factors on the natural history of chronic hepatitis C viral infections. *Journal of Viral Hepatitis*, **6**, 271–6.

Minutello, M. A., Pileri, P., Unutmaz, D. et al. (1993) Compartmentalization of T lymphocytes to the site of disease: intrahepatic CD4$^+$ T cells specific for the protein NS4 of hepatitis C virus in patients with chronic hepatitis C. *Journal of Experimental Medicine*, **178**, 17–25.

Mishida, N., Fukuda, Y., Kokuryu, H. et al. (1993) Role and mutational heterogeneity of the *p53* gene in hepatocellular carcinoma. *Cancer Research*, **53**, 368–72.

Misiani, R., Bellavita, P., Fenili, D. et al. (1994) Interferon alfa-2a therapy in cryoglobulinemia associated with hepatitis C virus. *New England Journal of Medicine*, **330**, 751–6.

Missale, G., Bertoni, R., Lamonaca, V. et al. (1996) Different clinical behaviors of acute hepatitis

C virus infection are associated with different vigor of the anti-viral cell-mediated immune response. *Journal of Clinical Investigation,* **98,** 706–14.

Mita, E. & Hayashi, N. (1997) Apoptosis in human diseases: role of Fas system in liver cell injury by viral hepatitis. *Rinsho Byor (Japanese Journal of Clinical Pathology),* **45,** 477–82.

Mita, E., Hayashi, N., Kanazawa, Y. et al. (1994) Hepatitis C virus genotype and RNA titer in the progression of type C chronic liver disease. *Journal of Hepatology,* **21,** 468–73.

Miyamoto, H., Okamoto, H., Sato, K., Tanaka, T. & Mishiro, S. (1992) Extraordinarily low density of hepatitis C virus estimated by sucrose density gradient centrifugation and the polymerase chain reaction. *Journal of General Virology,* **73,** 715–18.

Mizokami, M., Gojobori, T. & Lau, J. Y. N. (1994) Molecular evolutionary virology: its application to hepatitis C virus. *Gastroenterology,* **107,** 1181–2.

Mizuno, M., Yamada, G., Tanaka, T., Shimotohno, K., Takatani, M. & Tsuji, T. (1995) Virion-like structures in HeLa G cells transfected with the full-length sequence of the hepatitis C virus genome. *Gastroenterology,* **109,** 1933–40.

Mizushima, H., Hijikata, H., Asabe, S. I., Hirota, M., Kimura, K. & Shimotohno, K. (1994) Two hepatitis C virus glycoprotein E2 products with different C termini. *Journal of Virology,* **68,** 6215–22.

Mizutani, T., Kato, N., Hirota, M., Sugiyama, K., Murakami, A. & Shimotohno, K. (1995) Inhibition of hepatitis C virus replication by antisense oligonucleotide in culture cells. *Biochemical and Biophysical Research Communications,* **212,** 906–11.

Mizutani, T., Kato, N., Ikeda, M., Sugiyama, K. & Shimotohno, K. (1996a) Long term human T cell culture system supporting hepatitis C virus replication. *Biochemical and Biophysical Research Communications,* **227,** 822–6.

Mizutani, T., Kato, N., Saito, S., Ikeda, M., Sugiyama, K. & Shimitohno, K. (1996b) Characterization of hepatitis C virus replication in cloned cells obtained from a human T cell leukemia virus type 1 infected cell line, MT-2. *Journal of Virology,* **70,** 7219–23.

Mohr, L., Shankara, S., Yoon, S. K. et al. (2000) Gene therapy of hepatocellular carcinoma *in vitro* and *in vivo* in nude mice by adenoviral transfer of the *Escherichia coli* purine nucleoside phosphorylase gene. *Hepatology,* **31,** 606–14.

Monath, T. P. (1990) Flaviviruses. In *Virology,* eds. B. N. Fields & D. M. Knipe, pp. 763–70. New York: Raven Press.

Monazahian, M., Bohme, I., Bonk, S. et al. (1999) Low-density lipoprotein receptor as a candidate receptor for hepatitis C virus. *Journal of Medical Virology,* **57,** 223–9.

Mondelli, M., Alberti, A., Tremolada, F., Williams, R., Eddleston, A. L. W. F. & Realdi, G. (1986) *In vitro* cell-mediated cytotoxicity for autologous liver cells in chronic non-A, non-B hepatitis. *Clinical Experimental Immunology,* **63,** 147–55.

Mondelli, M. U., Cerino, A., Boender, P. et al. (1994) Significance of the immune system to a major, conformational B-cell epitope on the hepatitis C virus NS3 region defined by a human monoclonal antibody. *Journal of Virology,* **68,** 4829–36.

Montesano, R., Hainaut, P. & Wild, C. P. (1997) Hepatocellular carcinoma: from gene to public health. *Journal of the National Cancer Institute,* **89,** 1844–51.

Monteverde, A., Ballare, M. & Pileri, S. (1997) Hepatic lymphoid aggregates in chronic hepatitis C and mixed cryoglobulinemia. *Springer Seminars in Immunopathology,* **19,** 99–110.

Moradpour, D., Englert, C., Wakita, T. & Wands, J. R. (1996) Characterization of cell lines allowing tightly regulated expression of hepatitis C virus core protein. *Virology,* **222**, 51–63.

Moradpour, D., Kary, P., Rice, C.M. & Blum, H.E. (1998) Continuous human cell lines inducibly expressing hepatitis C virus structural and nonstructural proteins. *Hepatology,* **28**, 192–201.

Moretta, L., Ciccone, E., Mingari, M.C., Biassoni, R. & Moretta, A. (1994) Human natural killer cells: origin, clonality, specificity, receptors. *Advances in Immunology,* **55**, 341–58.

Morgenstern, K.A., Landro, J.A., Hsiao, K., Lin, C., Yong, G. & Su, M.S.S. (1997) Polynucleo-tide modulation of the protease nucleoside triphosphatase and helicase activities of a hepatitis C virus NS3-NS4A complex isolated from transfected COS cells. *Journal of Virology,* **71**, 3767–75.

Mori, S., Kato, N., Yagyu, A. et al. (1992) A new type of hepatitis C virus in patients in Thailand. *Biochemical and Biophysical Research Communications,* **183**, 334–42.

Moriya, K., Yotsuyanagi, H., Shintani, Y. et al. (1997) Hepatitis C virus core protein induces hepatic steatosis in transgenic mice. *Journal of General Virology,* **78**, 1527–31.

Moriya, K., Fujie, H., Shintani, Y. et al. (1998) The core protein of hepatitis C virus induces hepatocellular carcinoma in transgenic mice. *Nature Medicine,* **4**, 1065–7.

Moser, C., Stettler, P., Tratschin, J.D. & Hofmann, M.A. (1999) Cytopathogenic and non-cytopathogenic RNA replicons of classical swine fever virus. *Journal of Virology,* **73**, 7787–94.

Mosley, J.W. (1992) Transmission of hepatitis C by pasteurised factor VIII. *Lancet,* **340**, 1160–1.

Mosley, J.W., Redeker, A.G., Feinstone, S.M. & Purcell, R.H. (1977) Multiple hepatitis viruses in multiple attacks of acute viral hepatitis. *New England Journal of Medicine,* **296**, 75–8.

Mosmann, T.R., Cherwinski, H., Bond, M.W., Giedlin, M.A. & Coffman, R.L. (1986) Two types of murine helper T cell clones. I. Definition according to profiles of lymphokine activities and secreted proteins. *Journal of Immunology,* **136**, 2348–57.

Mossier, J.F., Scoaze, J.Y., Marcellin, P., Degott, C., Benahmou, J.P. & Feldmann, G. (1994) Expression of cytokine-dependent immune adhesion molecules by hepatocytes. *Gastroen-terology,* **107**, 1457–68.

Muchmore, E., Popper, H., Peterson, D.A., Miller, M.F. & Lieberman, H.M. (1988) Non-A, non-B hepatitis related hepatocellular carcinoma in a chimpanzee. *Journal of Medical Primatology,* **17**, 235–46.

Muerhoff, A.S., Leary, T.P., Simons, J.N. et al. (1995) Genomic organization of GB viruses A and B: two new members of the Flaviviridae associated with GB agent hepatitis. *Journal of Virology,* **69**, 5621–30.

Muller, H.M., Pfaff, E., Goeser, T., Kallinowski, B., Solbach, C. & Theilmann, L. (1993) Peripheral blood leukocytes serve as a possible extrahepatic site for hepatitis C virus replica-tion. *Journal of General Virology,* **74**, 669–76.

Munro, J., Briggs, J.D. & McCruden, E.A.B. (1996) Detection of a cluster of hepatitis C infections in a renal transplant unit by analysis of sequence variation of the NS5A gene. *Journal of Infectious Diseases,* **174**, 177–80.

Murakami, Y., Hayashi, K., Hirohashi, S. & Sekiya, T. (1991) Aberations of the tumor sup-pressor p53 and retinoblastoma genes in human hepatocellular carcinomas. *Cancer Research,* **51**, 5520–5.

Murphy, D., Willems, B. & Delage, G. (1994) Use of the 5' noncoding region for genotyping hepatitis C virus. *Journal of Infectious Diseases,* **169**, 473–5.

Murray, J. S., Madri, J., Tite, J., Carding, S. R. & Bottomly, K. (1989) MHC control of CD4[+] T cell subset activation. *Journal of Experimental Medicine*, **170**, 2135–40.

Murray, J. S., Pfeiffer, C., Madri, J. & Bottomly, K. (1992) Major histocompatibility (MHC) control of CD4 T cell subset activation. II. A single peptide induces either humoral or cell mediated responses in mice of distinct MHC genotype. *European Journal of Immunology*, **22**, 559–65.

Nagai, H., Pineau, P., Tiollais, P., Buendia, M. A. & Dejean, A. (1997) Comprehensive allelotyping of human hepatocellular carcinoma. *Oncogene*, **14**, 2927–33.

Nagao, Y., Sata, M., Tanikawa, K., Itoh, K. & Kameyama, T. (1995) Lichen planus and hepatitis C virus in the northern Kyushu region of Japan. *European Journal of Clinical Investigation*, **25**, 910–14.

Nagao, Y., Sata, M., Ide, T. et al. (1996) Development and exacerbation of oral lichen planus during and after interferon therapy for hepatitis C. *European Journal of Clinical Investigation*, **26**, 1171–4.

Naito, M., Hayashi, N., Hagiwara, H. et al. (1994) Serum hepatitis C virus RNA quantity and histological features of hepatitis C virus carriers with persistently normal ALT levels. *Hepatology*, **19**, 871–5.

Naito, M., Hayashi, N., Moribe, T. et al. (1995) Hepatitis C viral quasispecies in hepatitis C virus carriers with normal liver enzymes and patients with type C chronic liver disease. *Hepatology*, **22**, 407–12.

Nakagawa, H., Shimomura, H., Hasui, T., Tsuji, H. & Tsuji, T. (1994) Quantitative detection of hepatitis C virus genome in liver tissue and circulation by competitive reverse transcription-polymerase chain reaction. *Digestive Diseases and Sciences*, **39**, 225–33.

Nakajima, N., Kijikata, M., Yoshikura, H. & Shimizu, Y. K. (1996) Characterization of long term cultures of hepatitis C virus. *Journal of Virology*, **70**, 3325–9.

Nakamoto, Y., Guidotti, L. G., Pasquetto, V., Schreiber, R. D. & Chisari, F. V. (1997) Differential target cell sensitivity to CTL-activated death pathways in hepatitis B virus transgenic mice. *Journal of Immunology*, **158**, 5692–7.

Nakano, I., Maertens, G., Major, M. E. et al. (1997) Immunization with plasmid DNA encoding hepatitis C virus envelope E2 antigenic domains induces antibodies whose immune reactivity is linked to the injection mode. *Journal of Virology*, **71**, 7101–9.

Nakao, T., Enomoto, N., Takada, N., Takada, A. & Date, T. (1991) Typing of hepatitis C virus genomes by restriction fragment length polymorphism. *Journal of General Virology*, **72**, 2105–12.

Naldini, L., Blomer, U., Gallay, P., Ory, D., Mulligan, R., Gage, F. H., Verma, I. M. & Trono, D. (1996) *In vivo* gene delivery and stable transduction of nondividing cells by a lentiviral vector. *Science*, **272**, 263–7.

Naoumov, N. V., Chokshi, S., Metivier, E., Maertens, G., Johnson, P. J. & Williams, R. (1997) Hepatitis C virus infection in the development of hepatocellular carcinoma in cirrhosis. *Journal of Hepatology*, **27**, 331–6.

Nardone, G., Romano, M., Calabro, A. et al. (1996) Activation of fetal promoters of insulinlike growth factor II gene in hepatitis C virus-related chronic hepatitis, cirrhosis, and hepatocellular carcinoma. *Hepatology*, **23**, 1304–12.

Nasoff, M. S., Zebedee, S. L., Inchauspe, G. & Prince, A. M. (1991) Identification of an immunodominant epitope within the capsid protein of hepatitis C virus. *Proceedings of the National Academy of Sciences of the USA*, **88**, 5462–6.

Navas, S., Bosch, O., Castillo, I., Marriott, E. & Carreno, V. (1995) Porphyria cutanea tarda and hepatitis C and B viruses infection: a retrospective study. *Hepatology*, **21**, 279–84.

Negro, F. (1998) Detection of hepatitis C virus RNA in liver tissue: an overview. *Italian Journal of Gastroenterology and Hepatology*, **30**, 205–10.

Negro, F., Pacchioni, D., Shimizu, Y. et al. (1992) Detection of intrahepatic replication of hepatitis C virus RNA by *in situ* hybridization and comparison with histopathology. *Proceedings of the National Academy of Sciences of the USA*, **89**, 2247–51.

Negro, F., Giostra, E., Krawczynski, K. et al. (1998) Detection of intrahepatic hepatitis C virus replication by strand-specific semi-quantitative RT-PCR: preliminary application to the liver transplantation model. *Journal of Hepatology*, **29**, 1–11.

Nelson, D. R., Marousis, C. G., Davis, G. L. et al. (1997) The role of hepatitis C virus specific cytotoxic T lymphocytes in chronic hepatitis C. *Journal of Immunology*, **158**, 1473–81.

Nelson, D. R., Marousis, C. G., Ohno, T., Davis, G. L. & Lau, J. Y. N. (1998) Intrahepatic hepatitis C virus specific cytotoxic T lymphocyte activity and response to interferon alfa therapy in chronic hepatitis C. *Hepatology*, **28**, 225–30.

Neumann, A. U., Lam, N. P., Dahari, H. et al. (1998) Hepatitis C viral dynamics in vivo and the antiviral efficacy of interferon-α therapy. *Science*, **282**, 103–7.

Niederau, C., Lange, S., Heintges, T. et al. (1998) Prognosis of chronic hepatitis C: results of a large prospective cohort study. *Hepatology*, **28**, 1687–95.

NIH (1997) National Institutes of Health Consensus Development Conference Panel statement: management of hepatitis C. *Hepatology*, **26**(Suppl. 1), 2–10.

Nishida, N., Fukuda, Y., Kokuryu, H. et al. (1992) Accumulation of allelic loss on arms of chromosomes 13q, 16q and 17p in advanced stages of human hepatocellular carcinoma. *International Journal of Cancer*, **51**, 862–8.

Nishida, N., Fukuda, Y., Komeda, T. et al. (1994) Amplification and overexpression of the cyclin D1 gene in aggressive human hepatocellular carcinoma. *Cancer Research*, **54**, 3107–10.

Nishiguchi, S., Kuroki, T., Ueda, T. et al. (1992) Detection of hepatitis C virus antibody in the absence of viral RNA in patients with autoimmune hepatitis. *Annuals of Internal Medicine*, **116**, 21–5.

Nishiguchi, S., Kuroki, T., Nakatani, S. et al. (1995) Randomized trial of effects of interferon-α on incidence of hepatocellular carcinoma in chronic active hepatitis C with cirrhosis. *Lancet*, **346**, 1051–5.

Nishizawa, T., Okamoto, H., Konishi, K., Yoshizawa, H., Miyakawa, Y. & Mayumi, M. (1997) A novel DNA virus (TTV) associated with elevated transaminase levels in posttransfusion hepatitis of unknown etiology. *Biochemical and Biophysical Research Communications*, **241**, 92–7.

Niu, J., Kumar, U., Monjardino, J., Goldin, R., Rosin, D. & Thomas, H. C. (1995) Hepatitis C virus replication in hepatocellular carcinoma. *Journal of Clinical Pathology*, **48**, 880–2.

Niu, M. T., Alter, M. J., Kristensen, C. & Margolis, H. S. (1992) Outbreak of hemodialysis-associated non-A, non-B hepatitis and correlation with antibody to hepatitis C virus. *American Journal of Kidney Diseases*, **4**, 345–52.

Niu, M. T., Coleman, P. J. & Alter, M. J. (1993) Multicenter study of hepatitis C virus infection in chronic hemodialysis patients and hemodialysis center staff members. *American Journal of Kidney Diseases*, **22**, 568–73.

Nolandt, O., Kern, V., Muller, H. et al. (1997) Analysis of hepatitis C virus core protein interaction domains. *Journal of General Virology*, **78**, 1331–40.

Norkrans, G., Frosner, G., Hermodsson, S. & Iwarson, S. (1980) Multiple hepatitis attacks in drug addicts. *Journal of the American Medical Association*, **243**, 1056–8.

Nose, H., Imazeki, F., Ohto, M. & Omata, M. (1993) *p53* gene mutations and 17p allelic deletions in hepatocellular carcinoma from Japan. *Cancer*, **72**, 355–60.

Nouri-Aria, K. T., Sallie, R., Mizokami, M., Portmann, B. C. & Williams, R. (1995) Intrahepatic expression of hepatitis C virus antigens in chronic liver disease. *Journal of Pathology*, **175**, 77–83.

Nousbaum, J. B., Stanislas, P., Nalpas, B., Landais, P., Berthelot, P. & Brechot, C. (1995) Hepatitis C virus type 1b (II) infection in France and Italy. *Annuals of Internal Medicine*, **122**, 161–8.

Novak, J. E. & Kirkegaard, K. (1991) Improved method for detecting negative strands used to demonstrate specificity of plus strand encapsidation and the ratio of positive to negative strands in infected cells. *Journal of Virology*, **65**, 3384–7.

Ogasawara, J., Watanabe-Fukunaga, R., Adachi, M. et al. (1993) Lethal effects of the anti-Fas antibody in mice. *Nature*, **364**, 806–9.

Ogata, N., Alter, H. J., Miller, R. H. & Purcell, R. H. (1991) Nucleotide sequence and mutation rate of the H strain of hepatitis C virus. *Proceedings of the National Academy of Sciences of the USA*, **88**, 3392–6.

Ohashi, K., Marion, P. L., Nakai, H. et al. (2000) Sustained survival of human hepatocytes in mice: a model for *in vivo* infection with human hepatitis B and hepatitis delta viruses. *Nature Medicine*, **6**, 327–31.

Ohishi, M., Sakisaka, S., Harada, M., et al. (1999) Detection of hepatitis C virus and hepatitis C virus replication in hepatocellular carcinoma by *in situ* hybridization. *Scandinavian Journal of Gastroenterology*, **34**, 432–8.

Ohnishi, K., Nomura, F. & Nakano, M. (1991) Interferon therapy for acute posttransfusion non-A, non-B hepatitis: response with respect to anti-hepatitis C virus antibody status. *American Journal of Gastroenterology*, **86**, 1041–9.

Ohta, K., Ueda, T., Nagai, S. et al. (1993) Pathogenesis of idiopathic pulmonary fibrosis: is hepatitis C virus involved? *Nihon Kyobu Shikkan Gakkai Zasshi (Japanese Journal of Thoracic Diseases)*, **31S**, 32–5.

Ohto, H., Terazawa, S., Sasaki, N. The Vertical Transmission of Hepatitis C Virus Collaborative Study Group (1994) Transmission of hepatitis C virus from mother to infants. *New England Journal of Medicine*, **30**, 744–50.

Okamoto, H., Okada, S., Sugiyama, Y. et al. (1990) The 5′-terminal sequence of the hepatitis C virus genome. *Japanese Journal of Experimental Medicine*, **60**, 167–77.

Okamoto, H., Kojima, M., Okada, S. et al. (1992a) Genetic drift of hepatitis C virus during an 8.2 year infection in a chimpanzee: variability and stability. *Virology*, **190**, 894–9.

Okamoto, H., Kurai, K., Okada, S. et al. (1992b) Full-length sequence of a hepatitis C virus genome having poor homology to reported isolates: comparative study of four distinct genotypes. *Virology*, **188**, 331–41.

Okamoto, H., Sugiyama, Y., Okada, S. et al. (1992c) Typing hepatitis C virus by polymerase chain reaction with type-specific primers: application to clinical surveys and tracing infectious sources. *Journal of General Virology*, **73**, 673–9.

Okamoto, H., Kojima, M., Sakamoto, M. et al. (1994) The entire nucleotide sequence and classification of a hepatitis C virus isolate of a novel genotype from an Indonesian patient with chronic liver disease. *Journal of General Virology*, **75**, 629–35.

Okamoto, H., Kobata, S., Tokita, H. et al. (1996) A second-generation method of genotyping hepatitis C virus by the polymerase chain reaction with sense and antisense primers deduced from the core gene. *Journal of Virological Methods*, **57**, 31–45.

Okazaki, M., Hino, K., Fujii, K., Kobayashi, N. & Okita, K. (1996) Hepatic Fas antigen expression before and after interferon therapy in patients with chronic hepatitis C. *Digestive Diseases and Sciences*, **41**, 2453–8.

Okuda, K., Hayashi, H., Kobayashi, S. & Irie, Y. (1995) Mode of hepatitis C infection not associated with blood transfusion among chronic hemodialysis patients. *Journal of Hepatology*, **23**, 28–31.

Oldach, D. (1999) 'Real-time' polymerase chain reaction. *Gastroenterology*, **116**, 763–4.

Omata, M., Iwama, S., Sumida, M., Ito, Y. & Okuda, K. (1981) Clinicopathological study of acute non-A, non-B post transfusion hepatitis: histological features of liver biopsies in acute phase. *Liver*, **1**, 201–8.

Onji, M., Kikuchi, T., Michitaka, K., Saito, I., Miyamura, T. & Ohta, Y. (1991) Detection of hepatitis C virus antibody in patients with autoimmune hepatitis and other chronic liver diseases. *Gastroenterologia Japonica*, **26**, 182–6.

Onodera, H., Ukai, K., Suzuki, M. & Minami, Y. (1997) Incidence of hepatocellular carcinoma after interferon therapy in patients with chronic hepatitis C. *Tohoku Journal of Experimental Medicine*, **18**, 275–83.

Oshima, M., Tsuchiya, M., Yagasaki, M. et al. (1991) cDNA clones of Japanese hepatitis C virus genomes derived from a single patient show sequence heterogeneity. *Journal of General Virology*, **72**, 2805–9.

Oshita, M., Hayashi, N., Kasahara, A. et al. (1994) Increased serum hepatitis C virus RNA levels among alcoholic patients with chronic hepatitis C. *Hepatology*, **20**, 1115–20.

Ostapowicz, G., Watson, K. J., Locarnini, S. A. & Desmond, P. V. (1998) Role of alcohol in the progression of liver disease caused by hepatitis C virus infection. *Hepatology*, **27**, 1730–5.

Overton, H., Mcmillan, D., Gillespie, F. & Mills, J. (1995) Recombinant baculovirus expressed NS3 proteinase of hepatitis C virus shows activity in cell based and *in vitro* assays. *Journal of General Virology*, **76**, 3009–19.

Owen-Schaub, L. B., Zhang, W., Cusack, J. C. et al. (1995) Wild-type human p53 and a temperature-sensitive mutant induce Fas/APO-1 expression. *Molecular and Cellular Biology*, **15**, 3032–40.

Pancholi, P., Liu, Q., Tricoche, N., Zhang, P., Perkus, M. E. & Prince, A. M. (2000) DNA prime-canarypox boost with polycistronic hepatitis C virus (HCV) genes generates potent immune responses to HCV structural and nonstructural proteins. *Journal of Infectious Diseases*, **182**, 18–27.

Paolini, C., DeFrancesco, R. & Gallinari, P. (2000a) Enzymatic properties of hepatitis C virus NS3-associated helicase. *Journal of General Virology*, **81**, 1335–45.

Paolini, C., Lahm, A., DeFrancesco, R. & Gallinari, P. (2000b) Mutational analysis of hepatitis C virus NS3-associated helicase. *Journal of General Virology*, **81**, 1649–58.

Papa, S., Rinaldi, M., Mangia, A. et al. (1998) Development of a multigenic plasmid vector for HCV DNA immunization. *Research in Virology*, **149**, 315–9.

Par, A. (1990) Antibodies to hepatitis C virus in Hungary. *Lancet*, **336**, 123.

Pasquinelli, C., Shoenberger, J., Chung, J. et al. (1997) Hepatitis C virus core and E2 protein expression in transgenic mice. *Hepatology*, **25**, 719–27.

Patel, T. & Gores, G. J. (1995) Apoptosis and hepatobiliary disease. *Hepatology*, **21**, 1725–41.

Paterlini, P., Driss, F., Nalpas, B. et al. (1993) Persistence of hepatitis B and hepatitis C viral genomes in primary liver cancers from HBsAg-negative patients: a study of a low-endemic area. *Hepatology*, **17**, 20–9.

Paterlini, P., Poussin, K., Kew, M., Franco, D. & Brechot, C. (1995) Selective accumulation of the X transcript of hepatitis B virus in patients negative for hepatitis B surface antigen with hepatocellular carcinoma. *Hepatology*, **21**, 313–21.

Patijn, G. A., Liever, A., Schowalter, D. B., Schwall, R. & Kay, M. A. (1998) Hepatocyte growth factor induces hepatocyte proliferation *in vivo* and allows for efficient retroviral-mediated gene transfer in mice. *Hepatology*, **28**, 707–16.

Patterson, J. L. & Fernandez-Larson, R. (1990) Molecular action of ribavirin. *Reviews in Infectious Diseases*, **12**, 1132–46.

Pawlotsky, J. M. & Germanidis, G. (1999) The non-structural 5A protein of hepatitis C. *Journal of Viral Hepatitis*, **6**, 343–56.

Pawlotsky, J. M., Germanidis, G., Newuann, A. U., Pellerin, M., Frainais, P. O. & Dhumeaux, D. (1998) Interferon resistance of hepatitis C virus genotype 1b: relationship to nonstructural 5A gene quasispecies mutations. *Journal of Virology*, **72**, 2795–805.

Pawlotsky, J. M., Germanidis, G., Frainais, P. O. et al. (1999) Evolution of the hepatitis C virus second envelope protein hypervariable region in chronically infected patients receiving alpha interferon therapy. *Journal of Virology*, **73**, 6490–9.

Pearson, C. I., van Ewijik, W. & McDevitt, H. O. (1997) Induction of apoptosis and T helper 2 (Th2) responses correlates with peptide affinity for the major histocompatibility complex in self-reactive T cell receptor transgenic mice. *Journal of Experimental Medicine*, **185**, 583–99.

Peng, S. Y., Lai, P. L. & Hsu, H. C. (1993) Amplification of the c-*myc* gene in human hepatocellular carcinoma: biologic significance. *Journal of the Formosan Medical Association*, **92**, 866–70.

Pereira, A. (1999) Cost-effectiveness of transfusing virus-inactivated plasma instead of standard plasma. *Transfusion*, **39**, 479–87.

Pereira, B. J. G., Milford, E. L., Kirkman, R. L. et al. (1992) Prevalence of hepatitis C virus RNA in organ donors positive for hepatitis C antibody and in the recipients of their organs. *New England Journal of Medicine*, **327**, 910–15.

Pestova, T. V., Shatsky, I. N., Fletcher, S. P., Jackson, R. J., Hellen, C. (1998) A prokaryotic-like mode of cytoplasmatic eukaryotic ribosome binding to the initiation codon during internal translation of hepatitis C virus and classical swine fever virus RNAs. *Genes and Development,* **12,** 67–83.

Petrosillo, N., Puro, V. & Ippolito, G. (1994) Prevalence of hepatitis C antibodies in health-care workers. *Lancet,* **344,** 339–40.

Pfeiffer, C., Stein, J., Southwood, S., Ketelaar, H., Sette, A. & Bottomly, K. (1995) Altered peptide ligands can control CD4 T lymphocyte differentiation *in vivo. Journal of Experimental Medicine,* **181,** 1569–74.

Piazza, M., Borgia, G. & Picciotto, L. (1995) Detection of hepatitis C virus-RNA by polymerase chain reaction in dental surgeries. *Journal of Medical Virology,* **45,** 40–2.

Picciotto, A., Campo, N., Brizzolara, R. et al. (1997) HCV-RNA levels play an important role independently of genotype in predicting response to interferon therapy. *European Journal of Gastroenterology and Hepatology,* **9,** 67–9.

Pieroni, L., Santolini, E., Fipaldini, C., Pacini, L., Migliaccio, G. & La Monica, N. (1997) *In vitro* study of the NS2-3 proteinase of hepatitis C virus. *Journal of Virology,* **71,** 6373–80.

Pileri, P., Uematsu, Y., Campagnoli, S. et al. (1998) Binding of hepatitis C virus to CD81. *Science,* **282,** 938–41.

Pizzi, E., Tramontano, A., Tomei, L. et al. (1994) Molecular model of the specificity pocket of the hepatitis C virus protease: implications for substrate recognition. *Proceedings of the National Academy of Sciences of the USA,* **91,** 888–92.

Poch, O., Sauvaget, I., Delarue, M. & Tordo, N. (1989) Identification of four conserved motifs among the RNA dependent polymerase encoding elements. *EMBO Journal,* **8,** 3867–74.

Polyak, S. J., Faulkner, G., Carithers, R. L. Jr, Corey, L. & Gretch, D. R. (1997) Assessment of hepatitis C virus quasispecies heterogeneity by gel shift analysis: correlation with response to interferon therapy. *Journal of Infectious Diseases,* **175,** 1101–7.

Ponzetto, A., Fiume, L., Forzani, B. et al. (1991) Adenine arabinoside monophosphate and acyclovir monophosphate coupled to lactosaminated albumin reduce woodchuck hepatitis virus viremia at doses lower than the unconjugated drugs. *Hepatology,* **14,** 16–24.

Poralla, T., Hutteroth, T. H., zum Buschenfelde, K. H. M. (1984) Cellular cytotoxicity against autologous hepatocytes in acute and chronic non-A, non-B hepatitis. *Gut,* **25,** 114–20.

Poulsen, H. & Christoffersen, P. (1969) Abnormal bile duct epithelium in liver biopsies with histological signs of viral hepatitis. *Acta Pathologica Microbiologie in Scandinavica,* **76,** 383–90.

Poynard, T., Leroy, V., Cohard, M. et al. (1996) Meta-analysis of interferon randomized trials in the treatment of viral hepatitis C: effects of dose and duration. *Hepatology,* **24,** 778–89.

Poynard, T., Bedosa, P. & Opolon, P. (1997) Natural history of liver fibrosis progression in patients with chronic hepatitis C. *Lancet,* **349,** 825–32.

Pozzato, G., Kaneko, S., Moretti, M. et al. (1994) Different genotypes of hepatitis C virus are associated with different severity of chronic liver disease. *Journal of Medical Virology,* **43,** 291–6.

Preugschat, F., Averett, D. R., Clarke, B. E. & Porter, D. J. T. (1996) A steady-state and pre-steady-state kinetic analysis of the NTPase activity associated with the hepatitis C virus NS3 helicase domain. *Journal of Biological Chemistry,* **271**, 24449–57.

Preugschat, F., Danger, D. P., Carter, L. H., Davis, R. G. & Porter, D. J. T. (2000) Kinetic analysis of the effect of mutagenesis of W501 and V432 of the hepatitis C virus NS3 helicase domain on ATPase and strand-separating activity. *Biochemistry,* **39**, 5174–83.

Prieto, M., Olaso, V., Verdu, C. et al. (1995) Does the healthy hepatitis C carrier state really exist? An analysis using polymerase chain reaction. *Hepatology,* **22**, 413–7.

Prince, A. M. (1983) Non-A, non-B hepatitis viruses. *Annual Review of Microbiology,* **37**, 217–32.

Prince, A. M., Brotman, B., Grady, G. F. et al. (1974) Long-incubation post-transfusion hepatitis without serological evidence of exposure to hepatitis B virus. *Lancet,* **ii**, 241–6.

Prince, A. M., Huima-Byron, T., Williams, B. A. A., Bardina, L. & Brotman, B. (1984) Isolation of a virus from chimpanzee liver cell cultures inoculated with sera containing the agent of non-A, non-B hepatitis. *Lancet,* **ii**, 1071–5.

Prince, A. M., Brotman, B., Huima-Bryon, T., Pascual, D., Jaffery, M. & Inchauspe, G. (1992) Immunity in hepatitis C infection. *Journal of Infectious Diseases,* **165**, 438–43.

Prince, A. M., Huima-Bryon, T., Parker, T. S. & Levine, D. M. (1996) Visualization of hepatitis C virions and putative defective interfering particles isolated from low density lipoproteins. *Journal of Viral Hepatitis,* **3**, 11–17.

Prince, A. M., Pascual, D., Meruelo, D. et al. (2000) Strategies for evaluation of enveloped virus inactivation in red cell concentrates using hypericin. *Photochemistry and Photobiology,* **71**, 188–95.

Puoti, M., Zonaro, A., Ravaggi, A., Marin, M. O., Castelnuovo, F. & Cariani, E. (1992) Hepatitis C virus RNA and antibody response in the clinical course of acute hepatitis C virus infection. *Hepatology,* **16**, 877–81.

Purcell, R. H. (1994) Hepatitis viruses: changing patterns of human disease. *Proceedings of the National Academy of Sciences of the USA,* **91**, 2401–6.

Qin, L. X., Tang, Z. Y., Sham, J. S. et al. (1999) The association of chromosome 8p deletion and tumor metastasis in human hepatocellular carcinoma. *Cancer Research,* **59**, 5662–5.

Qin, X. Q., Tao, N., Dergay, A. et al. (1998) Interferon-β gene therapy inhibits tumor formation and causes regression of established tumors in immune deficient mice. *Proceedings of the National Academy of Sciences of the USA,* **95**, 14411–16.

Quan, C. M., Krajden, M., Zhao, J. & Chan, A. W. (1993) High performance liquid chromatography to assess the effect of serum storage conditions on the detection of hepatitis C virus by polymerase chain reaction. *Journal of Virological Methods,* **43**, 299–308.

Quinti, I., Hassan, N. F., El Salman, D. et al. (1995) Hepatitis C virus specific B cell activation: IgG and IgM detection in acute and chronic hepatitis C. *Journal of Hepatology,* **23**, 640–7.

Rabinowitz, J. E. & Samulski, R. J. (1998) Adeno-associated virus expression system for gene transfer. *Current Opinion in Biotechnology,* **9**, 470–5.

Ramsay, A. J., Ruby, J. & Ramshaw, I. A. (1993) A case for cytokines as effector molecules in the resolution of virus infection. *Immunology Today,* **14**, 155–7.

Rashid, A., Wang, J. S., Qian, G. S., Lu, B. X., Hamilton, S. R. & Groopman, J. D. (1999) Genetic alterations in hepatocellular carcinomas: association between loss of chromosome 4q and p53 gene mutations. *British Journal of Cancer,* **80**, 59–66.

Ray, R. B., Lagging, L. M., Meyer, K., Steele, R. & Ray, R. (1995) Transcriptional regulation of cellular and viral promoters by the hepatitis C virus core protein. *Virus Research,* **37**, 209–20.

Ray, R. B., Meyer, K. & Ray, R. (1996a) Suppression of apoptotic cell death by hepatitis C virus core preotein. *Virology,* **226**, 176–82.

Ray, R. B., Lagging, L. M., Meyer, K. & Ray, R. (1996b) Hepatitis C virus core protein cooperates with *ras* and transforms primary rat embryo fibroblasts to tumorigenic phenotype. *Journal of Virology,* **70**, 4438–43.

Ray, R. B., Steele, R., Meyer, K. & Ray, R. (1997) Transcriptional repression of p53 promoter by hepatitis C core protein. *Journal of Biological Chemistry,* **272**, 10983–6.

Ray, R. B., Stelle, R., Meyer, K. & Ray, R. (1998a) Hepatitis C virus core protein represses $p21^{WAF1/CIP1/SDI1}$ promoter activity. *Gene,* **208**, 331–6.

Ray, R. B., Meyer, K., Steele, R., Shrivastava, A., Aggarwal, B. B. & Ray, R. (1998b) Inhibition of tumor necrosis factor (TNF-alpha)-mediated apoptosis by hepatitis C virus core protein. *Journal of Biological Chemistry,* **273**, 2256–9.

Ray, S. C., Wang, Y. M., Laeyendecker, O., Ticehurst, J. R., Villano, S. A. & Thomas, D. L. (1999) Acute hepatitis C virus structural gene sequences as predictors of persistent viremia: hyper-variable region 1 as a decoy. *Journal of Virology,* **73**, 2938–46.

Reed, K. E., Grakoui, A. R. & Rice, C. M. (1995) Hepatitis C virus encoded NS2-3: cleavage site mutagenesis and requirements for bimolecular cleavage. *Journal of Virology,* **69**, 4127–36.

Reed, K. E., Xu, J. & Rice, C. M. (1997) Phosphorylation of the hepatitis C virus NS5A protein *in vitro* and *in vivo*: properties of the NS5A-associated kinase. *Journal of Virology,* **71**, 7187–97.

Reed, K. E., Gorbalenya, A. E. & Rice, C. M. (1998) The NS5A/NS5 proteins from three genera of the family Flaviviridae are phosphorylated by associated serine/threonine kinases. *Journal of Virology,* **72**, 6199–206.

Reesink, H. W. & van der Poel, C. L. (1989) Blood transfusion and hepatitis: Still a threat? *Blut,* **58**, 1–6.

Rehermann, B. & Chisari, F. V. (2000) Cell mediated immune responses to the hepatitis C virus. *Current Topics in Microbiology and Immunology,* **242**, 299–325.

Rehermann, B., Chang, K. M., McHutchinson, J. G., Kokka, R., Houghton, M. & Chisari, F. V. (1996a) Quantitative analysis of the peripheral blood cytotoxic T lymphocyte response in patients with chronic hepatitis C virus infection. *Journal of Clinical Investigation,* **98**, 1432–40.

Rehermann, B., Chang, K. M., McHutchinson, J. G., Kokka, R., Houghton, M. & Chisari, F. V. (1996b) Differential cytotoxic T lymphocyte responsiveness to the hepatitis B and C viruses in chronically infected patients. *Journal of Virology,* **70**, 7092–102.

Reichard, O., Andersson, J., Schvarcz, R. & Weiland, O. (1991) Ribavirin treatment for chronic hepatitis C. *Lancet,* **337**, 1058–61.

Reichard, O., Yun, Z. B., Sonnerborg, A. & Weiland, O. (1993) Hepatitis C viral RNA titers in serum prior to, during, and after oral treatment with ribavirin for chronic hepatitis C. *Journal of Medical Virology,* **41**, 99–102.

Reichard, O., Norkrans, G., Fryden, A., Braconier, J. H., Sonnerborg, A. & Weiland, O. (1998) Alfa-interferon and ribavirin versus alfa-interferon alone as therapy for chronic hepatitis C: a randomized, double-blind, placebo-controlled study. *Lancet,* **351,** 83–7.

Reid, A. E., Koziel, M. J., Aiza, I. et al. (1999) Hepatitis C virus genotypes and viremia and hepatocellular carcinoma. *American Journal of Gastrenterology,* **94,** 1619–26.

Resti, M., Azzari, C., Lega, L. et al. (1995) Mother-to-infant transmission of hepatitis C virus. *Acta Paediatrica,* **84,** 251–5.

Reynolds, J. E., Kaminski, A., Kettinen, H. J. et al. (1995) Unique features of internal initiation of hepatitis C virus RNA translation. *EMBO Journal,* **14,** 6010–20.

Reynolds, J. E., Kaminski, A., Carroll, A. R., Clarke, B. E., Rowlands, D. J. & Jackson, R. J. (1996) Internal initiation of translation of hepatitis C virus RNA: the ribosome entry site is at the authentic initiation codon. *RNA,* **2,** 867–78.

Rice, C. M. & Walker, C. M. (1995) Hepatitis C virus specific T lymphocyte responses. *Current Opinion in Immunology,* **7,** 532–8.

Rice, P. S., Smith, D. B., Simmonds, P. & Holmes, E. (1993) Heterosexual transmission of hepatitis C virus. *Lancet,* **342,** 1052–3.

Richards, O. C. & Ehrenfeld, E. (1998) Effects of poliovirus 3AB protein on 3D polymerase-catalyzed reaction. *Journal of Biological Chemistry,* **273,** 12832–40.

Richman, D. D. (2000) The impact of drug resistance on the effectiveness of chemotherapy for chronic hepatitis B. *Hepatology,* **32,** 866–7.

Rijnbrand, R. C. A. & Lemon, S. M. (2000) Internal ribosome entry site mediated translation in hepatitis C virus replication. *Current Topics in Microbiology and Immunology,* **242,** 85–116.

Rijnbrand, R., Bredenbeck, P., van der Straaten, T. et al. (1995) Almost the entire 5' non-translated region of hepatitis C virus is required for cap-independent translation. *FEBS,* **365,** 115–9.

Rijnbrand, R., Abbink, T. E. M., Haasnoot, P. C. J., Spaan, W. J. M. & Bredenbeek, P. J. (1996) The influence of AUG codons in the hepatitis C virus 5' nontranslated region on translation and mapping of the translation initiation window. *Virology,* **226,** 47–56.

Roberts, I. M. & Harrison, B. D. (1970) Inclusion bodies and tubular structures in *Chenopodium amaranticolor* plants infected with strawberry latent ringspot virus. *Journal of General Virology,* **7,** 47–54.

Roberts, J. M., Searle, J. W. & Cooksley, W. G. E. (1993) Histological patterns of prolonged hepatitis C virus infection. *Gastroenterologica Japanica,* **28,** 901–5.

Rockstroh, J. K., Spengler, U., Sudhop, T. et al. (1996) Immunosuppression may lead to progression of hepatitis C virus-associated liver disease in haemophiliacs coinfected with HIV. *American Journal of Gastroenterology,* **91,** 2563–8.

Rodriguez-Inigo, E., Bartolome, J., de Lucas, S. et al. (1999) Histological damage in chronic hepatitis C is not related to the extent of infection in the liver. *American Journal of Pathology,* **154,** 1877–81.

Roehl, H. H., Parsley, T. B., Ho, T. V. & Semler, B. L. (1997) Processing of a cellular polypeptide by 3CD proteinase is required for poliovirus ribonucleoprotein complex formation. *Journal of Virology,* **71,** 578–85.

Roizman, B. & Palese, P. (1996) Multiplication of viruses: an overview. In *Virology,* eds. B. N. Fields, D. M. Knipe & P. M. Howley. Philadelphia, PA: Lippinchott-Raven.

Romeo, R., Colombo, M., Rumi, M. et al. (1996a) Lack of association between type of hepatitis C virus, serum load and severity of liver disease. *Journal of Viral Hepatitis,* 3, 183–90.

Romeo, R., Tommasini, M. A., Rumi, M. G. et al. (1996b) Genotypes in the progression of hepatitis C related cirrhosis and development of hepatocellular carcinoma. *Hepatology,* 24, 153A.

Rosa, D., Campagnoli, S., Moretto, C. et al. (1996) A quantitative test to estimate neutralizing antibodies to the hepatitis C virus: cytofluorometric assessment of envelope glycoprotein 2 binding to target cells. *Proceedings of the National Academy of Sciences of the USA,* 93, 1759–63.

Rosen, H. R., Hinrichs, D. J., Gretch, D. R. et al. (1999) Association of multispecific CD4+ response to hepatitis C and severity of recurrence after liver transplantation. *Gastroenterology,* 117, 926–32.

Rosman, A. S., Paronetto, F., Galvin, K., Williams, R. J. & Lieber, C. S. (1993) Hepatitis C virus antibody in alcoholic patients: association with the presence of portal and/or lobular hepatitis. *Archives of Internal Medicine,* 153, 965–9.

Rousell, R. H., Budinger, M. D., Pirofsky, B. & Schiff, R. I. (1991) Prospective study on the hepatitis safety of intravenous immunoglobulin, pH 4.25. *Vox Sanguinis,* 60, 65–8.

Ruggieri, A., Harada, T., Matsuura, Y. & Miyamura, T. (1997) Sensitization to Fas-mediated apoptosis by hepatitis C virus core protein. *Virology,* 229, 68–76.

Ruiz, J., Qian, C., Drozdzik, M. & Prieto, J. (1999) Gene therapy of viral hepatitis and hepatocellular carcinoma. *Journal of Viral Hepatitis,* 6, 17–34.

Rumi, M., Del Ninno, E., Parravicini, M. L. et al. (1996) A prospective, randomized trial comparing lymphoblastoid to recombinant interferon alpha 2a as therapy for chronic hepatitis C. *Hepatology,* 24, 1366–70.

Sabatino, G., Ramenghi, L. A., diMarzio, M. & Pizzigallo, E. (1996) Vertical transmission of hepatitis C virus: an epidemiological study on 2980 pregnant women in Italy. *European Journal of Epidemiology,* 12, 443–7.

Saito, I., Miyamura, T., Ohbayahsi, A. et al. (1990) Hepatitis C virus infection is associated with the development of hepatocellular carcinoma. *Proceedings of the National Academy of Sciences of the USA,* 87, 6547–9.

Saito, T., Sherman, G. J., Kurokohchi, K. et al. (1997) Plasmid DNA-based immunization for hepatitis C virus structural proteins: immune responses in mice. *Gastroenterology,* 112, 1321–30.

Sakamoto, M., Hirohashi, S., Tsuda, H. et al. (1988) Increasing incidence of hepatocellular carcinoma possibly associated with non-A, non-B hepatitis in Japan, disclosed by hepatitis B virus DNA analysis of surgically resected cases. *Cancer Research,* 48, 7294–7.

Sakamoto, N., Enomoto, N., Kurosaki, M., Marumo, F. & Sato, C. (1994) Detection and quantification of hepatitis C virus RNA replication in the liver. *Journal of Hepatology,* 20, 593–7.

Sakamoto, N., Wu, C. H. & Wu, G. Y. (1996) Intracellular cleavage of hepatitis C virus RNA and inhibition of viral protein translation by hammerhead ribozymes. *Journal of Clinical Investigation,* 98, 2720–8.

Sakamuro, D., Furukawa, T. & Takegami T. (1995) Hepatitis C virus nonstructural protein NS3 transforms NIH3T3 cells. *Journal of Virology*, **69**, 3893–6.

Salazar-Mather, T. P., Orange, J. S. & Biron, C. A. (1998) Early murine cytomegalovirus (MCMV) infection induces liver natural killer (NK) cell inflammation and protection through macrophage inflammatory protein 1α (MIP-1α)-dependent pathways. *Journal of Experimental Medicine*, **187**, 1–14.

Saldanha, J. & Minor, P. H. (1996a) Collaborative study to assess the suitability of an HCV-RNA reference sample for detection of an HCV-RNA in plasma pools by PCR. *Vox Sanguinis*, **70**, 148–51.

Saldanha, J. & Minor, P. H. (1996b) Incidence of hepatitis C virus RNA in anti-HCV negative plasma pools and blood products. *Vox Sanguinis*, **70**, 232–4.

Saldanha, J., Lelie, N. & Heath, A. (1999) WHO Collaborative Study Group: establishment of the first international standard for nucleic acid amplification technology (NAT) assays for HCV RNA. *Vox Sanguinis*, **76**, 149–58.

Sandres, K., Dubois, M., Passquier, C. et al. (2000) Genetic heterogeneity of hypervariable region 1 of the hepatitis C virus (HCV) genome and sensitivity of HCV to alpha interferon therapy. *Journal of Virology*, **74**, 661–8.

Sangar, D. V. & Carroll, A. R. (1998) A tale of two strands: reverse-transcriptase polymerase chain reaction detection of hepatitis C virus replication. *Hepatology*, **28**, 1173–6.

Sansonno, D., Cornacchiulo, V., Iacobelli, A. R., De Stefano, R., Lospalluti, M. & Dammacco, F. (1995) Localization of hepatitis virus antigens in liver and skin tissues of chronic hepatitis C virus infected patients with mixed cryoglobulinemia. *Hepatology*, **21**, 305–12.

Sansonno, D., Cornacchiulo, V., Racanelli, V. & Dammacco, F. (1997) *In situ* simultaneous detection of hepatitis C virus RNA and hepatitis C virus-related antigens in hepatocelluar carcinoma. *Cancer*, **80**, 22–33.

Santolini, E., Migliaccio G. & La Monica, N. (1994) Biosynthesis and biochemical properties of the hepatitis C virus core protein. *Journal of Virology*, **68**, 3631–41.

Santolini, E., Pacini, L., Fipaldini, C., Migliaccio, G. & La Monica, N. (1995) The NS2 protein of hepatitis C virus is a transmembrane polypeptide. *Journal of Virology*, **69**, 7461–71.

Santoni-Rugiu, E., Nagy, P., Jensen, M. R., Factor, V. M. & Thorgeirsson, S. S. (1996) Evolution of neoplastic development in the liver of transgenic mice coexpressing c-*myc* and transforming growth factor α. *American Journal of Pathology*, **149**, 407–28.

Santoni-Rugiu, E., Jensen, M. R., Factor, V. M. & Thorgiersson, S. S. (1999) Acceleration of c-*myc*-induced hepatocarcinogenesis by co-expression of transforming growth factor (TGF)-alpha in transgenic mice is associated with TGF-beta1 signaling disruption. *American Journal of Pathology*, **154**, 1693–700.

Sarobe, P., Pendleton, C. D., Akatsuka, T. et al. (1998) Enhanced *in vitro* potency and *in vivo* immunogenicity of a CTL epitope from hepatitis C virus core protein following amino acid replacement at secondary HLA-A2.1 binding positions. *Journal of Clinical Investigation*, **102**, 1239–48.

Sarrazin, C., Kornetzky, I., Ruster, B. et al. (2000a) Mutations within the E2 and NS5A protein in patients infected with hepatitis C virus type 3a and correlation with treatment response. *Hepatology*, **31**, 1360–70.

Sarrazin, C., Teuber, G., Kokka, R., Rabenau, H. & Zeuzem, S. (2000b) Detection of residual hepatitis C virus RNA by transcription-mediated amplification in patients with complete virologic response according to polymerase chain reaction-based assays. *Hepatology*, **32**, 818–23.

Sartori, M., La Terra, G., Aglietta, M., Manzin, A., Navino, C. & Verzetti, G. (1993) Transmission of hepatitis C via blood splash into conjunctiva. *Scandinavian Journal of Infectious Diseases*, **25**, 270–1.

Satoh, S., Tanji, Y., Hijikata, M., Kimura, K. & Shimotohno, K. (1995) The N-terminal region of hepatitis C virus nonstructural protein 3 (NS3) is essential for stable complex formation with NS4A. *Journal of Virology*, **69**, 4255–60.

Sawada, M., Takada, A., Takase, S. & Takada, N. (1993) Effects of alcohol on the replication of hepatitis C virus. *Alcohol* (Suppl. 1B), 85–90.

Sawanpanyalert, P., Boonmar, S., Maeda, T., Matsuura, Y. & Miyamura, T. (1996) Risk factors for hepatitis C virus infection among blood donors in an HIV-epidemic area in Thailand. *Journal of Epidemiology and Community Health*, **50**, 174–7.

Schalm, S. W., Weiland, O., Hansen, B. E. et al. (1999) Interferon–ribavirin for chronic hepatitis C with and without cirrhosis: analysis of individual patients data of six controlled studies. *Gastroenterology*, **117**, 408–13.

Schinazi, R. F., Ilan, E., Black, P. L., Yao, X. & Dagan, S. (1999) Cell-based and animal models for hepatitis B and C viruses. *Antiviral Chemistry and Chemotherapy*, **10**, 99–114.

Schirmacher, P., Held, W. A., Yang, D., Chisari, F. V., Rustum, Y. & Rogler, C. E. (1992) Reactivation of insulin-like growth factor II during hepatocarcinogenesis in transgenic mice suggests a role in malignant growth. *Cancer Research*, **52**, 2549–56.

Schluger, L. K., Sheiner, P. A., Thung, S. N. et al. (1996) Severe recurrent cholestatic hepatitis C following orthotopic liver transplantation. *Hepatology*, **23**, 971–6.

Schmid, M., Pirovino, M., Altorfer, J., Gudat, F. & Bianchi, L. (1982) Acute hepatitis non-A, non-B: are there any specific light microscopic features? *Liver*, **2**, 61–7.

Schmidt, M., Frey, B., Kaluza, K. & Sobek, H. (1996) Application of heat-labile uracil-DNA glycosylase in improved carryover prevention techninque. *Biochemica*, **2**, 13–15.

Schmit, C. M., McKillop, L. H., Cahill, P. A. & Sitzmann, J. V. (1997) Increased MAPK expression and activity in primary human hepatocellular carcinoma. *Biochemical and Biophysical Research Communications*, **236**, 54–8.

Schreiber, G. B., Busch, M. P., Kleinman, S. H. & Korelitz, J. (1996a) The risk of transfusion-transmitted viral infections. *New England Journal of Medicine*, **334**, 661–5.

Schreiber, G. B., Busch, M. P., Kleinman, S. H. for the Retrovirus Epidemiology Donor Study (1996b) The risk of transfusion-transmitted viral infections. *New England Journal of Medicine*, **334**, 1685–90.

Schupper, H., Hayashi, P., Scheffel, J. et al. (1993) Peripheral blood mononuclear cell responses to recombinant hepatitis C virus antigens in patients with chronic hepatitis C. *Hepatology*, **18**, 1055–60.

Schvarcz, R., Nystrom, B., Oksanen, A. & Sonnerborg, A. (1995) Prevention of nosocomial transmission of hepatitis C virus. *Lancet*, **346**, 190.

Schwarcz, R., von Sydow, M. & Weiland, O. (1990) Autoimmune chronic active hepatitis: changing reactivity for antibodies to hepatitis C virus after immunosuppressive therapy. *Scandinavian Journal of Gastroenterology*, **25**, 1175–80.

Seeff, L. B. (1991) Hepatitis C from a needlestick injury. *Annuals of Internal Medicine*, **115**, 411.

Seeff, L. B. (1992) Acute viral hepatitis. In *Liver and Biliary Diseases*, ed. N. Kaplowitz, pp.252–278, Philadelphia, PA: Williams & Wilkins.

Seeff, L. B. (1995) Natural history of viral hepatitis, type C. *Seminars in Gastrointestinal Diseases*, **6**, 20–7.

Seeff, L. B. (1997) Natural history of hepatitis C. *Hepatology*, **26**(Suppl. 1), 21–8.

Seeff, L. B. (1998) The natural history of hepatitis C. A quandary. *Hepatology*, **28**, 1710–12.

Seeff, L. B., Wright, E. C., Zimmerman, H. J. & McCollum, R. W. (1975) Cooperative studies group. VA cooperative study of post-transfusion hepatitis and responsible risk factors. *American Journal of Medical Sciences*, **270**, 355–62.

Seeff, L. B., Buskell-Bales, Z., Wright, E. C. et al. (1992) Long-term mortality after transfusion-associated non-A, non-B hepatitis. *New England Journal of Medicine*, **327**, 1906–11.

Seipp, S., Mueller, H. M., Pfaff, E., Stremmel, W., Theilmann, L. & Goeser, T. (1997) Establishment of persistent hepatitis C virus infection and replication *in vitro*. *Journal of General Virology*, **78**, 2467–76.

Seishima, M., Takemura, M., Saito, K., Ando, K. & Noma, A. (1997) Increased serum soluble Fas (sFas) concentrations in HCV-positive patients with liver cirrhosis. *Journal of Hepatology*, **27**, 424–5.

Sellner, L. N., Coelen, R. J. & Mackenzie, J. S. (1992) Reverse transcriptase inhibits Taq polymerase activity. *Nucleic Acids Research*, **20**, 1487–90.

Serfaty, L., Chazouilleres, O., Poujol-Robert, A. et al. (1997) Risk factors for cirrhosis in patients with chronic hepatitis C virus infection: results of a case-control study. *Hepatology*, **26**, 776–9.

Seto, B., Goleman, W. G., Iwarson, S. & Gerety, R. J. (1984) Detection of reverse transcriptase activity in association with the non-A, non-B hepatitis agent(s). *Lancet*, **ii**, 941–3.

Shan, M., Liu, K. & Fang, H. (1999) DNA vaccination of the induction of immune responses by codelivery of IL-12 expression vector with hepatitis C structural antigens. *Chung Hua Kan Tsang Ping Tsa Chih*, **7**, 236–9.

Sharara, A. I. (1997) Chronic hepatitis C. *Southern Medical Journal*, **90**, 872–7.

Sheu, J. C., Lin, Y. W., Chou, H. C. et al. (1999) Loss of heterozygosity and microsatellite instability in hepatocellular carcinoma in Taiwan. *British Journal of Cancer*, **80**, 468–76.

Shields, P. L., Morland, C. M., Salmon, M., Clin, S., Hubacher, S. G. & Adams, D. H. (1999) Chemokine and chemokine receptor interactions provide a mechanism for selective T cell recruitment to specific liver compartments within hepatitis C infected liver. *Journal of Immunology*, **163**, 6236–43.

Shih, C. M., Lo, S. J., Miyamura, T., Chen, S. Y. & Lee, Y. H. W. (1993) Suppression of hepatitis B virus expression and replication by hepatitis C virus core protein in HuH-7 cells. *Journal of Virology*, **67**, 5823–32.

Shih, C. M., Chen, C. M., Chen, S. Y. & Lee, Y. H. W. (1995) Modulation of the *trans*-suppression activity of hepatitis C virus core protein by phosphorylation. *Journal of Virology*, **69**, 1160–71.

Shimada, A., Shiota, G., Miyata, H. et al. (1998) Aberrant expression of double-stranded RNA-dependent protein kinase in hepatocytes of chronic hepatitis and differentiated hepatocellular carcinoma. *Cancer Research*, **58**, 4434–8.

Shimizu, Y. K. & Yoshikura, H. (1994) Multicycle infection of hepatitis C virus in cell culture and inhibition by alpha and beta interferons. *Journal of Virology,* **68,** 8406–8.

Shimizu, Y. K., Feinstone, S. M., Purcell, R. H., Alter, H. J. & London, W. T. (1979) Non-A, non-B hepatitis: ultrastructural evidence for two agents in experimentally infected chimpanzees. *Science,* **205,** 197–200.

Shimizu, Y. K., Oomura, M., Abe, K. et al. (1985) Production of antibody associated with non-A, non-B hepatitis in a chimpanzee lymphoblastoid cell line established by in vitro transformation with Epstein–Barr virus. *Proceedings of the National Academy of Sciences of the USA,* **82,** 2138–42.

Shimuzu, Y. K., Purcell, R. H., Gerin, J. L., Feinstone, S. M., Ono, Y. & Shikata, T. (1986) Further studies by immunofluorescence of the monoclonal antibodies associated with experimental non-A, non-B hepatitis in chimpanzees and their relation to D hepatitis. *Hepatology,* **6,** 1329–33.

Shimizu, Y. K., Iwamoto, A., Hijikata, M., Purcell, R. H. & Yoshikura, H. (1992) Evidence for *in vitro* replication of hepatitis C virus genome in a human T-cell line. *Proceedings of the National Academy of Sciences of the USA,* **89,** 5477–81.

Shimizu, Y. K., Purcell, R. H. & Yoshikura, H. (1993) Correlation between the infectivity of hepatitis C virus *in vivo* and its infectivity *in vitro*. *Proceedings of the National Academy of Sciences of the USA,* **90,** 6037–41.

Shimizu, Y. K., Hijikata, M., Iwamoto, A., Alter, H. J., Purcell, R. H. & Yoshikura, H. (1994) Neutralizing antibodies against hepatitis C virus and the emergence of neutralization escape mutant viruses. *Journal of Virology,* **68,** 1494–1500.

Shimizu, Y., Yamaji, K., Masuho, Y. et al. (1996) Identification of the sequence of NS4A required for enhanced cleavage of the NS5A/5B site by hepatitis C virus NS3 proteinase. *Journal of Virology,* **70,** 127–32.

Shimoike, T., Mimori, S., Tani, H., Matsuura, Y. & Miyamura, T. (1999) Interaction of hepatitis C virus core protein with viral sense RNA and suppression of its translation. *Journal of Virology,* **73,** 9718–25.

Shindo, M., Di Bisceglie, A. M. & Silver, J. (1991) Quantitation of hepatitis C virus RNA in serum using the polymerase chain reaction and a colorimetric enzymatic detection system. *Hepatology,* **14,** 64A.

Shindo, M., Di Bisceglie, A. M., Biswas, R., Mihalik, K. & Feinstone, S. M. (1992) Hepatitis C virus replication during acute infection in the chimpanzee. *Journal of Infectious Diseases,* **166,** 424–7.

Shindo, M., Di Bisceglie, A. M., Akatsuka, T. et al. (1994) The physical state of the negative strand of hepatitis C virus RNA in the serum of patients with chronic hepatitis C. *Proceedings of the National Academy of Sciences of the USA,* **91,** 8719–23.

Shindo, M., Arai, K., Sokawa, Y. & Okuno, T. (1995) The virological and histological states of anti-hepatitis C virus positive subjects with normal liver biochemical values. *Hepatology,* **22,** 418–25.

Shindo, M., Hanada, K., Koya, S., Arai, K., Sokawa, Y. & Okuno, T. (1996) The clinical significance of changes in genetic heterogeneity of the hypervariable region 1 in chronic hepatitis C with interferon therapy. *Hepatology,* **24,** 1018–23.

Shinkai, Y., Rathbun, G., Lam, K. P. et al. (1992) Rag-2 deficient mice lack mature lymphocytes owing to an inability to initiate V (D) rearrangment. *Cell*, **68**, 855–67.

Shirachi, R., Shiraishi, H., Tateda, A., Kikuchi, K. & Ishida, N. (1978). Hepatitis 'C' antigen in non-A, non-B post-transfusion hepatitis. *Lancet*, **ii**, 853–6.

Shoji, I., Suzuki, T., Chieda, S. et al. (1995) Proteolytic activity of NS3 serine proteinase of hepatitis C virus efficiently expressed in *Escherichia coli*. *Hepatology*, **22**, 1648–55.

Shresta, S., Pham, C. T., Thomas, D. A., Graubert, T. A. & Ley, T. J. (1998) How do cytotoxic lymphocytes kill their targets? *Current Opinion in Immunology*, **10**, 581–7.

Shrivastava, A., Manna, S. K., Ray, R. & Aggarwal, B. B. (1998) Ectopic expression of hepatitis C virus core protein differentially regulates nuclear transcription factors. *Journal of Virology*, **72**, 9722–8.

Shukla, D. D., Hoyne, P. A. & Ward, C. W. (1995) Evaluation of complete genome sequences and sequences of individual gene products for the classification of hepatitis C viruses. *Archives of Virology*, **140**, 1747–61.

Sidhu, G. S., Stahl, R. E., El-Sadr, W. & Zolla-Payner, S. (1983) Ultrastructural markers of AIDS. *Lancet*, **i**, 990–91.

Silini, E., Bono, F., Cividini, A. et al. (1995) Differential distribution of hepatitis C virus genotypes in patients with and without liver function abnormalities. *Hepatology*, **21**, 285–90.

Sillekens, P. T. (1996) Qualitative and quantitative NASBA for detection of human immunodeficiency virus type 1 and hepatitis C virus infection. *Transplantation Proceedings*, **28**, 2941–4.

Simmonds, P. (1998) Variability of the hepatitis C virus genome. *Current Studies in Hematology and Blood Transfusion*, **62**, 38–63.

Simmonds, P., Holmes, E. C., Cha, T. A. et al. (1993) Classification of hepatitis C virus into six major genotypes and a series of subtypes by phylogenetic analysis of the NS-5 region. *Journal of General Virology*, **74**, 2391–9.

Simmonds, P., Mellor, J., Nuchprayoon, C., Tanpraseri, S. & Smith, D. R. (1997) Molecular epidemiology and classification of variants of hepatitis C virus found in South East Asia. In *Viral hepatitis and liver disease*, eds. M. Rizzetto, R. H. Purcell, J. L. Gerin & G. Verme, pp. 187–94. Torino, Italy: Edizioni Minerva Medica.

Simo, R., Hernandez, C., Genesca, J., Jardi, R. & Mesa, J. (1996) High prevalence of hepatitis C virus infection in diabetic patients. *Diabetes Care*, **19**, 998–1000.

Simons, J. N., Leary, T. P., Dawson, G. J. et al. (1995a) Isolation of novel virus-like sequences associated with human hepatitis. *Nature Medicine*, **1**, 564–9.

Simons, J. N., Pilotmatias, T. J., Leary, T. P. et al. (1995b) Identification of two flavirvirus-like genomes in the GB hepatitis agent. *Proceedings of the National Academy of Sciences of the USA*, **92**, 3401–5.

Sizova, D. V., Kolupaeva, V. G., Pestova, T. V., Shatsky, I. N. & Hellen, C. (1998) Specific interaction of eukaryotic translation initiation factor 3 with the 5' nontranslated regions of hepatitis C virus and classical swine fever virus RNAs. *Journal of Virology*, **72**, 4775–82.

Slagle, B. L., Lee, T. H., Medina, D., Finegold, M. J. & Butel, J. S. (1996) Increased sensitivity to the hepatocarcinogen diethylnitrosamine in transgenic mice carrying the hepatitis B virus X gene. *Molecular Carcinogenesis*, **15**, 261–9.

Smyth, R., Keenan, E., Dorman, A. & O'Connor, J. (1995) Hepatitis C infection among injecting drug users attending the National Drug Treatment Centre. *Israel Journal of Medical Sciences*, **164**, 267–8.

Song, M. K., Lee, S. W., Suh, Y. S., Le, K. J. & Sung, Y. C. (2000) Enhancement of immuno-globulin G2a and cytotoxic T lymphocyte responses by a booster immunization with recombinant hepatitis C virus E2 protein in E2 DNA primed mice. *Journal of Virology*, **74**, 2920–5.

Song, O. K., Cho, O. H., Hahm, B. & Jang, S. K. (1996) Development of an *in vivo* assay system suitable for screening inhibitors of hepatitis C viral protease. *Molecules and Cells*, **6**, 183–9.

Soto, B., Sanchez-Quijano, A., Rodrigo, L. et al. (1997) Human immunodeficiency virus infection modifies the natural history of chronic parenterally acquired hepatitis C with an unusually rapid progression to cirrhosis. *Journal of Hepatology*, **26**, 1–5.

Spangberg, K. & Schwartz, S. (1999) Poly(C)-binding protein interacts with the hepatitis C virus 5' untranslated region. *Journal of General Virology*, **80**, 1371–6.

Spertini, O. & Frei, P. C. (1982) Demonstration of a single antigen–antibody system in 28 patients with non-A, non-B viral hepatitis. *Lancet*, **ii**, 899–903.

Sporn, M. B. & Roberts, A. B. (1989) Transforming growth factor β. Multiple actions and potential clinical applications. *Journal of the American Medical Association*, **262**, 938–41.

Squadrito, G., Leone, F., Sartori, M. et al. (1997) Mutations in the nonstructural 5A region of hepatitis C virus and response of chronic hepatitis C to interferon alpha. *Gastroenterology*, **113**, 567–72.

Steinkuhler, C., Urbani, A., Tomei, L. et al. (1996) Activity of purified hepatitis C virus proteinase NS3 on peptide substrates. *Journal of Virology*, **70**, 6694–700.

Steinkuhler, C., Biasiol, G., Brunetti, M. et al. (1998) Product inhibition of the hepatitis C virus NS3 protease. *Biochemistry*, **37**, 8899–905.

Stempniak, M., Hostomska, Z., Nodes, B. R. & Hostomsky, Z. (1997) The NS3 proteinase domain of hepatitis C virus is a zinc-containing enzyme. *Journal of Virology*, **71**, 2881–6.

Stevens, C. E., Aach, R. D., Hollinger, F. B. et al. (1984) Hepatitis B virus antibody in blood donors and the occurrence of non-A, non-B hepatitis in transfusion recipients: an analysis of the Transfusion-transmitted Viruses Study. *Annals of Internal Medicine*, **101**, 733–8.

Strassburg, C. P., Obermayer-Straub, P. & Manns, M. P. (1996) Autoimmunity in hepatitis C and D virus infection. *Journal of Viral Hepatitis*, **3**, 49–59.

Su, H., Chang, J. C., Xu, S. M. & Kan, Y. W. (1996) AFP-positive hepatocellular carcinoma cells by adeno-associated virus transfer of the herpes simplex virus thymidine kinase. *Human Gene Therapy*, **7**, 463–70.

Suda, T., Okazaki, T., Naito, Y. et al. (1995) Expression of the Fas ligand in cells of T cell lineage. *Journal of Immunology*, **154**, 3806–13.

Sudo, K., Inoue, H., Shimizu, Y. et al. (1996) Establishment of an *in vitro* assay system for screening hepatitis C virus protease inhibitors using high performance liquid chromatography. *Antiviral Research*, **32**, 9–18.

Sudo, K., Matsumoto, Y., Matsushima, M. et al. (1997) Novel hepatitis C virus protease inhibitors: thiazolidine derivatives. *Biochemical and Biophysical Research Communications*, **238**, 643–7.

Sugg, U., Schenzle, D. & Hess, G. (1988) Antibodies to hepatitis B core antigen in blood donors screened for alanine aminotransferase level and hepatitis non-A, non-B in recipients. *Transfusion,* **28**, 386–8.

Sugiyama, K., Kato, N., Ikeda, M. et al. (1997) *Japanese Journal of Cancer Research,* **88**, 925–7.

Sulaiman, H. A., Noer, H. M., Endardjo, S. & Hoyaranda, E. (1991) The prevalence of antibody to hepatitis C virus (anti-HCV) in patients with acute and chronic liver diseases in Jakarta, Indonesia. *Gastroenterology Japan,* **26**, 179–83.

Sun, B., Pan, J., Gerber, M. & Feitelson, M. A. (1999) Evidence for consistent HCV replication in HepG2 cells. *Antiviral Therapy,* 4(Suppl. 4), A94.

Sun, D. X., Zhang, F. G., Geng, Y. Q. & Xi, D. S. (1996) Hepatitis C transmission by cosmetic tattooing in women. *Lancet,* **347**, 541.

Suzich, J. A., Tamura, J. K., Palmer-Hill, F. et al. (1993) Hepatitis C virus NS3 polynucleotide-stimulated nucleoside triphosphatase and comparison with the related pestivirus and flavivirus enzymes. *Journal of Virology,* **67**, 6152–8.

Suzuki, R., Matsuura, Y., Suzuki, T. et al. (1995a) Nuclear localization of the truncated hepatitis C virus core protein with its hydrophobic C terminus deleted. *Journal of General Virology,* **76**, 53–61.

Suzuki, T., Sato, M., Chieda, S. et al. (1995b) *In vivo* and *in vitro trans*-cleavage activity of hepatitis C virus serine proteinase expressed by recombinant baculoviruses. *Journal of General Virology,* **76**, 3021–9.

Sypek, J. P., Chung, C. L., Mayor, S. E. H. et al. (1993) Resolution of cutaneous leishmaniasis: interleukin 12 initiates a protective T helper type 1 immune response. *Journal of Experimental Medicine,* **177**, 1797–802.

Tabor, E., Gerety, R. J., Drucker, J. A. et al. (1978) Transmission of non-A, non-B hepatitis from man to chimpanzee. *Lancet,* **i**, 463–6.

Tabor, E., April, M., Seeff, L. B. & Gerety, R. J. (1979) Acute non-A, non-B hepatitis. Prolonged presence of the infectious agent in blood. *Gastroenterology,* **76**, 680–4.

Tabor, E., Seeff, L. B. & Gerety, R. J. (1980) Chronic non-A, non-B hepatitis carrier state. *New England Journal of Medicine,* **303**, 139–43.

Tai, C. L., Chi, W. K., Chen, D. S. & Hwang, L. H. (1996) The helicase activity associated with hepatitis C virus nonstructural protein 3 (NS3). *Journal of Virology,* **70**, 8477–84.

Takada, N., Takase, S., Takada, A. & Date, T. (1993) Differences in the hepatitis C virus genotypes in different countries. *Journal of Hepatology,* **17**, 277–83.

Takahara, T., Hayashi, N., Miyamoto, Y. et al. (1995) Expression of the hepatitis C virus genome in rat liver after cationic liposome-mediated *in vivo* gene transfer. *Hepatology,* **21**, 746–51.

Takahashi, M., Yamada, G., Miyamoto, R., Doi, T., Endo, H. & Tsuji, T. (1993) Natural history of chronic hepatitis C. *American Journal of Gastroenterology,* **88**, 240–3.

Takaki, A., Wiese, M., Maertens, G. et al. (2000) Cellular immune responses persist and humoral responses decrease two decades after recovery from a single-source outbreak of hepatitis C. *Nature Medicine,* **6**, 578–82.

Takamizawa, A., Mori, C., Fuke, I. et al. (1991) Structure and organization of the hepatitis C virus genome isolated from human carriers. *Journal of Virology,* **65**, 1105–13.

Takeda, S., Shibata, M., Morishima, T. et al. (1992) Hepatitis C virus infection in hepatocellular carcinoma. *Cancer,* **70,** 2255–9.

Takehara, T., Hayashi, N., Mita, E. et al. (1993) Detection of the minus strand of hepatitis C virus RNA by reverse transcription and polymerase chain reaction: implications for hepatitis C virus replication in infected tissue. *Hepatology,* **15,** 387–90.

Takeuchi, T., Katsume, A., Tanaka, T. et al. (1999) Real-time detection system for quantification of hepatitis C virus genome. *Gastroenterology,* **116,** 636–42.

Takikawa, S., Ishii, K., Aizaki, H. et al. (2000) Cell fusion activity of hepatitis C virus envelope proteins. Journal of Virology, **74,** 5066–74.

Taliani, M., Bianchi, E., Narjes, F. et al. (1996) A continuous assay of hepatitis C virus protease based on resonance energy transfer depsipeptide substrates. *Analytical Biochemistry,* **240,** 60–7.

Tamori, A., Nishiguchi, S., Kubo, S. et al. (1999) Possible contribution to hepatocarcinogenesis of X transcript of hepatitis B virus in Japanese patients with hepatitis C virus. *Hepatology,* **29,** 1429–34.

Tan, S. L., Nakao, H., He, Y. P. et al. (1999) NS5A, a nonstructural protein of hepatitis C virus, binds growth factor receptor-bound protein 2 adaptor protein in a Src homology 3 domain/ ligand-dependent manner and perturbs mitogenic signaling. *Proceedings of the National Academy of Sciences of the USA,* **96,** 5533–8.

Tanaka, K., Sata, M., Uchimura, Y., Suzuki, H. & Tankkawa, K. (1998) Long-term evaluation of interferon therapy in hepatitis C virus-associated cirrhosis: does IFN prevent development of hepatocellular carcinoma? *Oncology Reports,* **5,** 205–8.

Tanaka, S., Takenaka, K., Matsumata, T., Mori, R. & Sugimachi, K. (1996) Hepatitis C virus replication is associated with expression of transforming growth factor-α and insulin-like growth factor-II in cirrhotic livers. *Digestive Diseases and Sciences,* **41,** 208–15.

Tanaka, T., Kato, N., Cho, M. J. & Shimotohno, K. (1995) A novel sequence found at the 3' terminus of hepatitis C virus genome. *Biochemical and Biophysical Research Communications,* **215,** 744–9.

Tanaka, Y., Enomoto, N., Kojima, S. et al. (1993) Detection of hepatitis C virus RNA in the liver by *in situ* hybridization. *Liver,* **13,** 203–8.

Tang, L., Tanaka, Y., Enomoto, N., Marumo, F. & Sato, C. (1995) Detection of hepatitis C virus RNA in hepatocellular carcinoma by *in situ* hybridization. *Cancer,* **76,** 2211–16.

Taniguchi, S., Okamoto, H. & Sakamoto, M. (1993) A structurally flexible and antigenically variable N-terminal domain of the hepatitis C virus E2/NS1 protein: implication for an escape from antibody. *Virology,* **195,** 297–301.

Tanimoto, A., Ide, Y., Arima, N., Sasaguri, Y. & Padmanabhan, R. (1997) The amino terminal deletion mutants of hepatitis C virus nonstructural proteins NS5A function as transcriptional activators in yeast. *Biochemical and Biophysical Research Communications,* **236,** 360–4.

Tanji, Y., Hijikata, M., Hirowatari, Y. & Shimotohno, K. (1994a) Identification of the domain required for *trans*-cleavage activity of hepatitis C viral serine proteinase. *Gene,* **145,** 215–19.

Tanji, Y., Hijikata, M., Hirowatari, Y. & Shimotohno, K. (1994b) Hepatitis C virus polyprotein processing kinetics and mutagenic analysis of serine proteinase-dependent cleavage. *Journal of Virology,* **68,** 8418–24.

Tanji, Y., Hijikata, M., Satoh, S., Kaneko, T. & Shimotohno, K. (1995a) Hepatitis C virus encoded nonstructural protein NS4A has versatile functions in viral protein processing. *Journal of Virology*, **69**, 1575–81.

Tanji, Y., Kaneko, T., Satoh, S. & Shimotohno, K. (1995b) Phosphorylation of hepatitis C virus-encoded nonstructural protein NS5A. *Journal of Virology*, **69**, 3980–6.

Tao, Q., Wei, L., Chang, J., Wang, H. & Sun, Y. (1998) Relationship between interferon therapy and variability in nonstructural gene 5B of hepatitis C virus. *Journal of Gastroenterology*, **33**, 684–93.

Tarao, K., Rino, Y., Ohkawa, S. et al. (1999) Association between high serum alanine aminotransferase levels and more rapid development and higher rate of incidence of hepatocellular carcinoma in patients with hepatitis C virus-associated cirrhosis. *Cancer*, **86**, 589–95.

Taylor, D. R., Shi, S. T., Romano, P. R., Barber, G. N. & Lai, M. M. (1999) Inhibition of the interferon-inducible protein kinase by HCV E2 protein. *Science*, **285**, 107–10.

Telfer, P., Sabin, C., Devereux, H., Scott, F., Dusheiko, G. & Lee, C. (1994) The progression of HCV associated liver disease in a cohort of haemophilic patients. *British Journal of Haematology*, **87**, 555–61.

Thiel, V., Siddell, S. G. & Herold, J. (1998) Replication and transcription of HCV 299E replicons. *Advances in Experimental Medicine and Biology*, **440**, 109–13.

Thomas, D. L., Zenilman, J. M., Alter, H. J., Shih, J. W., Galai, N., Galai, N. & Quinn, T. C. (1995) Sexual transmission of hepatitis C virus among patients attending sexually transmitted disease clinics in Baltimore–an analysis of 309 sex partnerships. *Journal of Infectious Diseases*, **171**, 768–75.

Thomas, D. L., Shih, J. W., Alter, H. J. et al. (1996) Effect of human immunodeficiency virus on hepatitis C virus infection among injection drug users. *Journal of Infectious Diseases*, **174**, 690–5.

Thomson, B. J., Doran, M., Lever, A. M. L. & Webster, A. D. B. (1987) Alpha-interferon therapy for non-A, non-B hepatitis transmitted by gammaglobulin replacement therapy. *Lancet*, **i**, 539–41.

Thomssen, R., Bonk, S., Propfe, C., Heermann, K. H., Kochel, H. G. & Uy, A. (1992) Association of hepatitis C virus in human sera with β-lipoprotein. *Medical Microbiology and Immunology*, **181**, 293–300.

Thomssen, R., Bonk, S. & Thiel, A. (1993) Density heterogeneities of hepatitis C virus in human sera due to the binding of beta-lipoproteins and immunoglobulins. *Medical Microbiology and Immunology*, **182**, 329–34.

Tibbs, C., Donaldson, P., Underhill, J., Thomson, L., Manabe, K. & Williams, R. (1996) Evidence that the HLA DQA1*03 allele confers protection from chronic HCV infection in northern European caucasoids. *Hepatology*, **24**, 1342–5.

Tine, F., Magrin, S., Craxi, A. & Pagliaro, L. (1991) Interferon for non-A, non-B chronic hepatitis: a meta-analysis of randomized clinical trials. *Journal of Hepatology*, **13**, 192–9.

Tokita, H., Okamoto, H., Tsuda, F. et al. (1994) Hepatitis C virus variants from Vietnam are classifiable into the seventh, eighth, and ninth major gene groups. *Proceedings of the National Academy of Sciences of the USA*, **91**, 11022–6.

Tokita, H., Okamoto, H., Luengrojanakul, P. et al. (1995) Hepatitis C virus variants from

Thailand classifable into five novel genotypes in the sixth (6b), seventh (7c, 7d) and ninth (9b, 9c) major genetic groups. *Journal of General Virology*, **76**, 2329–35.

Tokita, H., Okamoto, H., Iiuka, H. et al. (1996) Hepatitis C virus variants from Jakarta, Indonesia classifable into novel genotypes in the second (2e and 2f), tenth (10a) and eleventh (11a) genetic groups. *Journal of General Virology*, **77**, 293–301.

Tomei, L., Failla, C., Vitale, R. L., Bianchi, E. & DeFrancesco, R. (1996) A central hydrophobic domain of the hepatitis C virus NS4A protein is necessary and sufficient for the activation of the NS3 proteinase. *Journal of General Virology*, **77**, 1065–70.

Tomonaga, T. & Levens, D. (1995) Heterogeneous nuclear ribonucleoprotein K is a DNA-binding transactivator. *Journal of Biological Chemistry*, **270**, 4875–81.

Tong, M. J., El-Farra, N. S., Reikes, A. R. & Co, R. L. (1995) Clinical outcomes after transfusion-associated hepatitis C. *New England Journal of Medicine*, **332**, 1463–6.

Toyoda, H., Fukuda, Y., Koyama, Y., Takamatsu, J., Saito, H. & Hayakawa, T. (1997) Effect of immunosuppression on composition of quasispecies population of hepatitis C virus in patients with chronic hepatitis C coinfected with human immunodeficiency virus. *Journal of Hepatology*, **26**, 975–82.

Toyoda, H., Kumada, T., Nakano, S. et al. (2000) The effect of retreatment with interferon-alpha on the incidence of hepatocellular carcinoma in patients with chronic hepatitis C. *Cancer*, **88**, 58–65.

Toyonaga, T., Hino, O., Sugai, S. et al. (1994) Chronic active hepatitis in transgenic mice expressing interferon-gamma in the liver. *Proceedings of the National Academy of Sciences of the USA*, **91**, 614–8.

Tremolada, F., Casarin, C., Tagger, A. et al. (1991) Antibody to hepatitis C virus in post transfusion hepatitis. *Annals of Internal Medicine*, **114**, 277–81.

Tremolada, F., Casarin, C., Alberti, A. et al. (1992) Long-term follow-up of non-A, non-B (type C) posttransfusion hepatitis. *Journal of Hepatology*, **16**, 273–81.

Trepo, C., Vitvitski, L., Degros, F. et al. (1983) Correlations between non-A, non-B (NANB) and hepatitis B (HB) markers: further evidence suggestive of cross reactivity between two distinct agents. In *Second International Symposium on Viral Hepatitis*, ed. F. Deinhardt. pp. 137–40, New York: Marcel Dekker.

Trowbridge, R. & Gowans, E. J. (1998) Identification of novel sequences at the 5′ terminus of the hepatitis C virus genome. *Journal of Viral Hepatitis*, **5**, 95–8.

Tsai, S. L., Liaw, Y. F., Chen, M. H., Huang, C. Y. & Kuo, G. C. (1997) Detection of type 2-like T-helper cells in hepatitis C infections: implication for chronicity. *Hepatology*, **25**, 449–58.

Tsai, S. L., Chen, Y. M., Chen, M. H. et al. (1998) Hepatitis C virus variants circumventing cytotoxic T lymphocyte activity as a mechanism of chronicity. *Gastroenterology*, **115**, 954–65.

Tsiquaye, K., N. & Zuckerman, A. J. (1979) New human hepatitis virus. *Lancet*, **i**, 1135–6.

Tsuchihara, K., Tanaka, T., Hijikata, M. et al. (1997) Specific interaction of polypyrimidine tract-binding protein with the extreme 3′-terminal structure of the hepatitis C virus genome, the 3′X. *Journal of Virology*, **71**, 6720–6.

Tsuchihara, K., Hijikata, M., Fukuda, K., Kuroki, T., Yamamoto, N. & Shimotohno, K. (1999) Hepatitis C virus core protein regulates cell growth and signal transduction pathway transmitting growth stimuli. *Virology*, **258**, 100–7.

Tsukiyama-Kohara, K., Iizuka, N., Kohara, M. & Nomoto, A. (1992) Internal ribosome entry site within hepatitis C virus RNA. *Journal of Virology*, **66**, 1476–83.

Tsutsui, H., Matsui, K., Okamura, H. & Nakanishi, K. (2000) Pathophysiological roles of interleukin-18 in inflammatory liver diseases. *Immunological Reviews*, **174**,192–209.

Uchida, T., Shikata, T., Tanaka, E. & Kiyosawa, K. (1994) Immunoperoxidase staining of hepatitis C virus in formalin-fixed, paraffin-embedded needle liver biopsies. *Virchows Archives*, **424**, 465–9.

Ueda, H., Ullrich, S. J., Ngo, L., Feitelson, M. A. & Jay G. (1995) Functional inactivation but not structural mutation of p53 causes liver cancer. *Nature Genetics*, **9**, 41–7.

Urashima, T., Saigo, K., Kobayashi, S. et al. (1997) Identification of hepatitis B virus integration in hepatitis C virus-infected hepatocellular carcinoma. *Journal of Hepatology*, **26**, 771–8.

Urbani, A., Bazzo, R., Nardi, M. C. et al. (1998) The metal binding site of the hepatitis C virus NS3 proteinase. A spectroscopic study. *Journal of Biological Chemistry*, **273**, 18760–9.

Usuda, S., Yoshizawa, K., Yabu, K. & Kiyosawa, K. (1993) Immunological responses against an autologous human hepatocellular carcinoma cell line. *Journal of Gastroenterology and Hepatology*, **8**, 517–23.

Uyttendaele, S., Claeys, H., Mertens, W., Verhaert, H. & Vermylen, C. (1994) Evaluation of third-generation and confirmatory assays for HCV antibodies. *Vox Sanguinis*, **66**, 122–9.

Valitutti, S., Muller, S., Dessing, M. & Lanzavecchis, A. (1996) Different responses are elicited in cytotoxic T lymphocytes by different levels of T cell receptor occupancy. *Journal of Experimental Medicine*, **183**, 1917–21.

Valli, M. B., Bertolini, L., Lucovacci, S., Ponzetto, A. & Carloni, G. (1995) Detection of a 5' UTR variation in the HCV genome after long term *in vitro* infection. *Research in Virology*, **146**, 285–8.

Valli, M. B., Carloni, G. & Manzin, A. (1997) Hepatitis C virus infection of a Vero cell clone displaying efficient virus cell binding. *Research in Virology*, **148**, 181–6.

van der Poel, C. L. (1999) Hepatitis C virus and blood transfusion: past and present risks. *Journal of Hepatology*, **31**(Suppl. 1), 101–6.

van der Poel, C. L., Reesink, H. W., Lelie, P. N. et al. (1989) Anti-hepatitis C antibodies and non-A, non-B posttransfusion hepatitis in The Netherlands. *Lancet*, **ii**, 297–8.

van der Poel, C. L., Reesink, H. W., Schaasberg, W. et al. (1990a) Infectivity of blood seropositive for hepatitis C virus antibodies. *Lancet*, **335**, 558–60.

van der Poel, C. L., Reesink, H. W., Schaasberg, W. et al. (1990b) Infectivity of blood seropositive for hepatitis C virus antibodies. *Lancet*, **335**, 558–60.

van der Poel, C. L., Cuypers, H. T., Reesink, H. W. et al. (1991a) Confirmation of hepatitis C virus infection by new four-antigen recombinant immunoblot assay. *Lancet*, **337**, 317–9.

van der Poel, C. L., Reesink, H. W., Mauser-Bunschoten, E. P. et al. (1991b) Prevalence of anti-HCV antibodies confirmed by recombinant immunoblot in different population subsets in The Netherlands. *Vox Sanguinis*, **61**, 30–6.

van der Poel, C. L., Bresters, D., Reesink, H. W. et al. (1992) Early antihepatitis C virus response with second generation C200/C22 ELISA. *Vox Sanguinis*, **62**, 208–12.

van der Poel, C. L., Cuypers, H. T. & Reesink, H. W. (1994) Hepatitis C virus six years on. *Lancet*, **344**, 1475–9.

Vargas, V., Castella, L. & Esteban, J. I. (1990) High frequency of antibodies to the hepatitis C virus among patients with hepatocellular carcinoma. *Annuals of Internal Medicine*, **112**, 232–3.

Varnavski, A. N. & Khromykh, A. A. (1999) Noncytopathic flavivirus replicon RNA based system for expression and delivery of heterologous genes. *Virology*, **255**, 366–75.

Vernelen, K., Claeys, H., Verhaert, H., Volckaerts, A. & Vermylen, C. (1994) Significance of NS3 and NS5 antigens in screening for HCV antibody. *Lancet*, **343**, 853.

Villa, E., Ferreti, I., DePalma, M. et al. (1991) HCV RNA in serum asymptomatic blood donors involved in post-transfusion hepatitis. *Journal of Hepatology*, **13**, 256–9.

Villamil, F. G., Hu, K.-Q., Yu, C.-H. et al. (1995) Detection of hepatitis C virus with RNA polymerase chain reaction in fulminant hepatic failure. *Hepatology*, **22**, 1379–86.

Vitvitski, L., Trepo, C. & Hantz, O. (1980) Use of the cross-reactivity between hepatitis B and non-A, non-B viruses for the identification and detection of non-A, non-B 'e' antigen. *Journal of Virological Methods*, **1**, 149–56.

von Boehmer, H. (1997) Lymphotoxins: from cytotoxicity to lymphoid organogenesis. *Proceedings of the National Academy of Sciences of the USA*, **94**, 8926–7.

Vrielink, H., van der Poel, C. L., Reesink, H. W., Zaaijer, H. L. & Lelie, P. N. (1995) Transmission of hepatitis C virus by anti-HCV negative blood transfusion: a case report. *Vox Sanguinis*, **68**, 55–6.

Wakita, T., Taya, C., Katsume, A. et al. (1998) Efficient conditional transgene expression in hepatitis C virus cDNA transgenic mice mediated by the Cre/loxP system. *Journal of Biological Chemistry*, **273**, 9001–6.

Walker, C. M. (1997) Comparative features of hepatitis C virus infection in humans and chimpanzees. *Springer Seminars in Immunopathology*, **19**, 85–98.

Wands, J. R., Bruns, R. R., Carlson, R. I., Ware, A., Menitove, J. E. & Isslebacher, K. J. (1982) Monoclonal IgM radioimmunoassay for hepatitis B surface antigen: high binding activity in serum that is unreactive with conventional antibodies. *Proceedings of the National Academy of Sciences of the USA*, **79**, 1277–81.

Wands, J. R., Fujita, Y. K., Isslebacher, K. J. et al. (1986) Identification and transmission of hepatitis B virus-related variants. *Proceedings of the National Academy of Sciences of the USA*, **83**, 6608–12.

Wang, C., Sarnow, P. & Siddiqui, A. (1993) Translation of human hepatitis C virus RNA in cultured cells is mediated by an internal ribosome binding mechanism. *Journal of Virology*, **67**, 3338–44.

Wang, C., Sarnow, P. & Siddiqui, A. (1994) A conserved helical element is essential for internal initiation of translation of hepatitis C virus RNA. *Journal of Virology*, **68**, 7301–7.

Wang, C., Le, S. Y., Ali, N. & Siddiqui, A. (1995) An RNA pseudoknot is an essential structural element of the internal ribosome entry site located with the hepatitis C virus 5' noncoding region. *RNA*, **1**, 526–37.

Wang, J. T., Wang, T. H., Shen, J. C., Lin, S. M., Lin, J. T. & Chen, D. S. (1992) Effects of anticoagulants and storage of blood samples on efficacy of the polymerase chain reaction assay for hepatitis C virus. *Journal of Clinical Microbiology*, **30**, 750–3.

Wang, W. Y., Preville, P., Morin, N., Mounir, S., Cai, W. Z. & Siddiqui, M. A. (2000) Hepatitis C viral IRES inhibition by phenazine and phenazine-like molecules. *Bioorganic and Medicinal Chemistry Letters*, **10**, 1151–4.

Watanabe, T., Katagiri, J., Kojima, H. et al. (1987) Studies on transmission of human non-A, non-B hepatitis to marmosets. *Journal of Medical Virology*, **22**, 143–56.

Watanabe, J., Minegishi, K., Mitsumori, T. et al. (1990) Prevalence of anti-HCV antibody in blood donors in the Tokyo area. *Vox Sanguinis*, **59**, 86–8.

Weiland, O., Zhang, Y. Y. & Widell, A. (1993) Serum HCV RNA levels in patients with chronic hepatitis C given a second course of interferon alpha-2b treatment after relapse following initial treatment. *Scandinavian Journal of Infectious Diseases*, **25**, 25–30.

Weiner, A. J., Kuo, G., Bradley, D. W. et al. (1990) Detection of hepatitis C viral sequences in non-A, non-B hepatitis. *Lancet*, **335**, 1–3.

Weiner, A. J., Brauer, M. J., Rosenblatt, J. et al. (1991) Variable and hypervariable domains are found in the regions of HCV corresponding to the flavivirus envelope and NS1 proteins and the pestivirus envelope glycoproteins. *Virology*, **180**, 842–8.

Weiner, A. J., Geysen, H. M., Christopherson, C. et al. (1992) Evidence for immune selection of hepatitis C virus (HCV) putative envelope glycoprotein variants: potential role in chronic HCV infections. *Proceedings of the National Academy of Sciences of the USA*, **89**, 3468–72.

Weiner, A. J., Erickson, A. L., Kansopon, J. et al. (1995) Persistent hepatitis C virus infection in a chimpanzee is associated with emergence of a cytotoxic T lymphocyte escape variant. *Proceedings of the National Academy of Sciences of the USA*, **92**, 2755–9.

Wejstal, R., Hermodsson, S. & Norkrans, G. (1991) Long term follow up of chronic hepatitis non-A, non-B with especial reference to hepatitis C. *Liver*, **11**, 143–8.

Welch, P. J., Yei, S. & Barber, J. R. (1998) Ribozyme gene therapy for hepatitis C virus infection. *Clinical and Diagnostic Virology*, **10**, 163–71.

Welch, P. J., Tritz, R., Yei, S., Leavitt, M., Yu, M. & Barber, J. (1996) A potential therapeutic application of hairpin ribozymes: *in vitro* and *in vivo* studies of gene therapy for hepatitis C virus infection. *Gene Therapy*, **3**, 994–1001.

Wentworth, P. A., Sette, A., Celis, E. et al. (1996) Identification of A2-restricted hepatitis C virus-specific cytotoxic T lymphocyte epitopes from conserved regions of the viral genome. *International Immunology*, **8**, 651–9.

Wheeler, M. D., Kono, H., Rusyn, I. et al. (2000) Chronic ethanol increases adeno-associated viral transgenic expression in rat liver via oxidant and NFκ-B dependent mechanisms. *Hepatology*, **32**, 1050–9.

Widell, A., Shev, S., Mansson, S. et al. (1994) Genotyping of hepatitis C virus isolates by a modified polymerase chain reaction assay using type specific primers: epidemiological applications. *Journal of Medical Virology*, **44**, 272–9.

Wild, C. P. & Hall, A. J. (2000) Primary prevention of hepatocellular carcinoma in developing countries. *Mutation Research*, **462**, 381–93.

Wiley, T. E., McCarthy, M., Breidt, L., McCarthy, M. & Layden, T. J. (1998) Impact of alcohol in the histological and clinical progression of hepatitis C infection. *Hepatology*, **28**, 805–9.

Wilson, J. J., Polyak, S. J., Day, T. D. & Gretch, D. R. (1995) Characterization of simple and complex hepatitis C virus quasispecies by heteroduplex gel shift analysis: correlation with nucleotide sequencing. *Journal of General Virology*, **76**, 1763–71.

Wimmer, E., Hellen, C. U. & Cao, X. (1993) Genetics of poliovirus. *Annual Reviews of Genetics*, **27**, 353–426.

Wolk, B., Sansonno, D., Krausslich, H. G. et al. (2000) Subcellular localization, stability, and *trans*-cleavage competence of the hepatitis C virus NS3-NS4A complex expressed in tetracycline-regulated cell lines. *Journal of Virology*, **74**, 2293–304.

Wong, D. C., Purcell, R. H., Sreenivasan, M. A., Prasad, S. R. & Pavri, K. M. (1980) Epidemic and endemic hepatitis in India: evidence for a non-A, non-B hepatitis virus aetiology. *Lancet*, **ii**, 876–9.

Wong, D. K., Dudley, D. D., Afdhal, N. H. et al. (1998) Liver derived CTL in hepatitis C virus infection: breadth and specificity of responses in a cohort of persons with chronic infection. *Journal of Immunology*, **160**, 1479–88.

Wong, S., Mehta, A. E., Faiman, C., Berard, L., Ibbott, T. & Minuk, G. Y. (1996) Absence of serologic evidence for hepatitis C virus infection in patients with Hashimoto's thyroiditis. *Hepatogastroenterology*, **43**, 420–1.

Wooster, R., Bignell, G., Lancaster, J. et al. (1995) Identification of the breast cancer susceptibility gene BRCA2. *Nature*, **378**, 789–92.

Wreghitt, T. G., Gray, J. J., Allain, J. P. et al. (1994) Transmission of hepatitis C virus antibody by organ transplantation in the United Kingdom. *Journal of Hepatology*, **20**, 768–72.

Wu, C. H. & Wu, G. Y. (1998) Targeted inhibition of hepatitis C virus directed gene expression in human hepatoma cell lines. *Gastroenterology*, **114**, 1304–12.

Wu, G. Y. & Wu, C. H. (1992) Specific inhibition of hepatitis B viral gene expression *in vitro* by targeted antisense oligonucleotides. *Journal of Biological Chemistry*, **267**, 12436–9.

Wu, J., Liu, P., Zhu, J. L., Maddukuri, S. & Zern, M. A. (1998) Increased liver uptake of liposomes and improved targeting efficacy by labeling with asialofetuin in rodents. *Hepatology*, **27**, 772–8.

Wu, R. R., Mizokami, M., Lau, J. Y. et al. (1995) Seroprevalence of hepatitis C virus infection and its genotype in Lanzhou, western China. *Journal of Medical Virology*, **45**, 174–8.

Wyke, R. J., Tsiquaye, K. N., Thornton, A. et al. (1979) Transmission of non-A, non-B hepatitis to chimpanzees by factor IX concentrates after fatal complications in patients with chronic liver disease. *Lancet*, **i**, 520–4.

Xiao, W., Berta, S. C., Lu, M. M., Moscioni, A. D., Tazelaar, J. & Wilson, J. M. (1998) Adeno-associated virus as a vector for liver directed gene therapy. *Journal of Virology*, **72**, 10222–6.

Xie, Z. C., Riezu-Boj, J. I., Lasarte, J. J. et al. (1998) Transmission of hepatitis C virus infection to tree shrews. *Virology*, **244**, 513–20.

Xu, L. Z., Larzul, D., Delaporte, E., Brechot, C. & Kremsdorf, D. (1994) Hepatitis C virus genotype 4 is highly prevalent in central Africa (Gabon). *Journal of General Virology*, **75**, 2393–8.

Yamada, G., Takatani, M., Kishi, F. et al. (1995) Efficacy of interferon alfa therapy in chronic hepatitis C patients depends primarily on hepatitis C virus RNA level. *Hepatology*, **22**, 1351–4.

Yamada, K., Mori, A., Seki, M. et al. (1998) Critical point mutations for hepatitis C virus NS3 proteinase. *Virology*, **246**, 104–12.

Yamada, M., Kakumu, S., Yoshioka, K. et al. (1994a) Hepatitis C virus genotypes are not responsible for development of serious liver disease. *Digestive Diseases and Sciences*, **39**, 234–9.

Yamada, N., Tanihara, K., Mizokami, M. et al. (1994b) Full-length sequence of the genome of hepatitis C virus type 3a: comparative study with different genotypes. *Journal of General Virology*, **75**, 3279–84.

Yamakawa, Y., Seta, M., Suzuki, H., Neguchi, S. & Tanikawa, K. (1996) Higher elimination rate of hepatitis C virus among women. *Journal of Viral Hepatitis*, **3**, 317–21.

Yamamoto, C., Enomoto, N., Kurosaki, M. et al. (1997) Nucleotide sequence variations in the internal ribosome entry site of hepatitis C virus-1b: no association with efficacy of interferon therapy or serum HCV RNA levels. *Hepatology*, **26**, 1616–20.

Yamamoto, M., Hayashi, N., Miyamoto, Y. et al. (1995) *In vivo* transfection of hepatitis C virus complementary DNA into rodent liver by asialoglycoprotein receptor mediated gene delivery. *Hepatology*, **22**, 847–55.

Yamashita, T., Kaneko, S., Yukiriro, S. et al. (1998) RNA dependent RNA polymerase activity of the soluble recombinant hepatitis C virus NS5B protein truncated at the C-terminal region. *Journal of Biological Chemistry*, **273**, 15479–86.

Yan, Y., Li, Y., Munshi, S. et al. (1998) Complex of NS3 proteinase and NS4A peptide of BK strain hepatitis C virus: a 2.2A resolution structure in a hexagonal crystal form. *Protein Science*, **7**, 837–47.

Yanagi, M., St. Clair, M., Emerson, S. U., Purcell, R. H. & Bukh, J. (1999) *In vivo* analysis of the 3' untranslated region of the hepatitis C virus after *in vitro* mutagenesis of an infectious cDNA clone. *Proceedings of the National Academy of Sciences of the USA*, **96**, 2291–5.

Yang, P. M., Su., I. J., Lai, M. Y. et al. (1988) Immunohistochemical studies on intrahepatic lymphocyte infiltrates in chronic type B hepatitis with special emphasis on the activation status of lymphocytes. *American Journal of Gastroenterology*, **83**, 948–53.

Yang, Y., Nunes, F., Berencsi, K., Furth, E. E., Gonczol, E. & Wilson, J. M. (1994) Cellular immunity to viral antigens limits E1-deleted adenoviruses for gene therapy. *Proceedings of the National Academy of Sciences of the USA*, **91**, 4407–11.

Yano, M., Yaatsuhasi, H., Inoue, O., Inoduchi, K. & Koga, M. I. (1993) Epidemiology and long term prognosis of hepatitis C virus infection in Japan. *Gut*, **34**(Suppl.), 13–16.

Yao, N. & Weber, P. C. (1998) Helicase, a target for novel inhibitors of hepatitis C virus. *Antiviral Therapy*, **3**(Suppl. 3), 93–97.

Yao, T., Degli Esposti, S., Huang, L., Arnon, R., Spangenberger, A. & Zern, M. A. (1994) Inhibition of carbon tetrachloride induced liver injury by liposomes containing vitamin E. *American Journal of Physiology*, **30**, G476–84.

Yen, J. H., Chang, S. C., Hu, C. R. et al. (1995) Cellular proteins specifically bind to the 5' noncoding region of hepatitis C virus RNA. *Virology*, **208**, 723–32.

Ying, H., Zaks, T. Z., Wang, R. F. et al. (1999) Cancer therapy using a self-replicating RNA vaccine. *Nature Medicine*, **5**, 823–7.

Yoo, B. J., Selby, M., Choe, J. et al. (1995) Transfection of a differentiated human hepatoma cell line Huh7 with *in vitro* transcribed hepatitis C virus HCV RNA and establishment of a long term culture persistently infected with HCV. *Journal of Virology*, **69**, 32–8.

Yoshikura, H., Hijikata, M., Nakajima, N. & Shimizu, Y. K. (1996) Replication of hepatitis C virus. *Journal of Viral Hepatitis*, **3**, 3–10.

Yoshioka, K., Kakumu, S., Wakita, T. et al. (1992) Detection of hepatitis C virus by polymerase chain reaction and response to interferon-alpha therapy: relationship to genotypes of hepatitis C virus. *Hepatology*, **16**, 293–9.

Yoshizawa, H., Akahane, Y., Itoh, Y. et al. (1980) Virus-like particles in a plasma fraction (fibrinogen) and in the circulation of apparently healthy blood donors capable of inducing non-A, non-B hepatitis in humans and chimpanzees. *Gastroenterology*, **79**, 512–20.

Yoshizawa, H., Itoh, Y., Iwakiri, S. et al. (1981) Demonstration of two different types of non-A, non-B hepatitis by reinjection and cross-challenge studies in chimpanzees. *Gastroenterology*, **81**, 107–13.

You, L. R., Chen, C. M., Yeh, T. S. et al. (1999) Hepatitis C virus core protein interacts with cellular putative RNA helicase. *Journal of Virology*, **73**, 2842–53.

Young, D. C., Tuschall, D. M. & Flanegan, J. B. (1985) Poliovirus RNA-dependent RNA polymerase and host cell protein synthesize product RNA twice the size of poliovirion RNA *in vitro*. *Journal of Virology*, **54**, 256–64.

Young, H. A. & Hardy, K. J. (1995) Role of interferon-gamma in immune cell regulation. *Journal of Leukocyte Biology*, **58**, 373–81.

Young, K. K. Y., Resnick, R. M. & Myers, T. W. (1993) Detection of hepatitis C virus RNA by a combined reverse transcription-polymerase chain reaction assay. *Journal of Clinical Microbiology*, **31**, 882–6.

Yu, S. H., Nagayama, K., Enomoto, N., Izumi, N., Marumo, F. & Sato, C. (2000) Intrahepatic mRNA expression of interferon-inducible antiviral genes in liver diseases: dsRNA-dependent protein kinase overexpression and RNase L inhibitor suppression in chronic hepatitis C. *Hepatology*, **32**, 1089–95.

Yu, M. C., Tong, M. J., Coursaget, P., Ross, R. K., Govindarajan, S. & Henderson, B. E. (1990) Prevalence of hepatitis B and C viral markers in black and white patients with hepatocellular carcinoma in the United States. *Journal of the National Cancer Institute*, **82**, 1038–41.

Yuan, F., Baxter, L. T. & Jain, R. K. (1991) Pharmacokinetic analysis of two-step approach using bifunctional and enzyme-conjugated antibodies. *Cancer Research*, **51**, 3119–30.

Yuan, Z. H., Kumar, U., Thomas, H. C., Wen, Y. M. & Monjardino, J. (1997) Expression, purification, and partial characterization of HCV RNA polymerase. *Biochemical and Biophysical Research Communications*, **232**, 231–5.

Yuki, N., Hayashi, N., Moribe, T. et al. (1997) Relation of disease activity during chronic hepatitis C infection to complexity of hypervariable region 1 quasispecies. *Hepatology*, **25**, 439–44.

Zaaijer, H. L., Cuypers, H. T. M., Reesink, H. W. et al. (1993) Reliability of polymerase chain reaction for detection of hepatitis C virus. *Lancet*, **341**, 722–4.

Zanetti, A. R., Tanzi, E., Paccagnini, S. & the Lombardy Study Group on Vertical HCV Transmission (1995) Mother to infant transmission of hepatitis C virus. *Lancet*, **345**, 289–91.

Zein, N. N., Poterucha, J. J., Gross, J. B. Jr et al. (1996) Increased risk of hepatocellular carcinoma in patients infected with hepatitis C genotype 1b. *American Journal of Gastroenterology*, **91**, 2560–2.

Zern, M. A. & Kresina, T. F. (1997) Hepatic drug delivery and gene therapy. *Hepatology*, **25**, 484–91.

Zeuzem, S. (2000) Hepatitis C virus: kinetics and quasispecies evolution during anti-viral therapy. *Forum*, **10**, 32–42.

Zeuzem, S., Franke, A., Lee, J. H., Herrmann, G., Ruster, B. & Roth, W. K. (1996) Phylogenetic analysis of hepatitis C virus isolates and their correlation to viremia, liver function tests, and histology. *Hepatology,* **24**, 1003–9.

Zeuzem, S., Feinman, S. V., Rasenack, J. et al. (2000) Peginterferon alfa-2a in patients with chronic hepatitis C. *New England Journal of Medicine,* **343,**1666–72.

Zhang, H., Hanecak, R., Brown-Driver, V. et al. (1999) Antisense oligonucleotide inhibition of hepatitis C virus (HCV) gene expression in livers of mice infected with an HCV-vaccinia virus. *Antimicrobial Agents and Chemotherapy,* **43**, 347–53.

Zhong, W. D., Ferrari, E., Lesburg, C. A. et al. (2000) Template/primer requirements and single nucleotide incorporation by hepatitis C virus nonstructural protein 5B polymerase. *Journal of Virology,* **74**, 9134–43.

Zhu, M., London, W. T., Duan, L.-X. & Feitelson, M. A. (1993). The value of hepatitis B X antigen as a prognostic marker in the development of hepatocellular carcinoma. *International Journal of Cancer,* **55**, 571–6.

Zhu, N., Khoshnan, A., Schneider, R. et al. (1998) Hepatitis C virus core protein binds to the cytoplasmic domain of tumor necrosis factor (TNF) receptor 1 and enhances TNF-induced apoptosis. *Journal of Virology,* **72**, 3691–7.

Zibert, A., Schreier, E. & Roggendorf, M. (1995) Antibodies in human sera specific to hypervariable region 1 of hepatitis C virus can block viral attachment. *Virology,* **208**, 653–61.

Zignego, A. L. & Brechot, C. (1999) Extrahepatic manifestations of HCV infection: facts and controversies. *Journal of Hepatology,* **31**, 369–76.

Zignego, A. L., Ferri, C., Giannini, C. et al. (1997a) Analysis of HCV infection in mixed cryoglobulinemia and B cell non-Hodgkin's lymphoma: evidence for a pathogenetic role. *Archives of Virology,* **142**, 545–55.

Zignego, A. L., Gianneli, F., Marrocchi, M. E., Giannini, C., Gentilini, P. & Ferri, C. (1997b) Frequency of *bcl-2* rearrangement in patients with mixed cryoglobulinemia and HCV positive liver diseases. *Clinical and Experimental Rheumatology,* **15**, 711–12.

Zinkernagel, R. M., Moskophidis, D., Kundig, T., Oehen, S., Pircher, H. P. & Hengartner, H. (1993) Effector T cell induction and T cell memory versus peripheral deletion of T cells. *Immunological Reviews,* **131**, 198–223.

Zuck, T. F., Sherwood, W. C. & Bove, J. R. (1987) A review of recent events related to surrogate testing of blood to prevent non-A, non-B posttransfusion hepatitis. *Transfusion,* **27**, 203–6.

Zuckerman, J., Clewley, G., Griffiths, P. & Cockcroft, A. (1994) Prevalence of hepatitis C antibodies in clinical health-care workers. *Lancet,* **343**, 1618–20.

Zylberberg, H. & Pol, S. (1996) Reciprocal interactions between human immunodeficiency virus and hepatitis C virus infections. *Clinical Infectious Diseases,* **23**, 1117–25.

Index

Printed in the United States
by Baker & Taylor Publisher Services